Allocating Scarce Medical Resources

The Clinical Medical Ethics Series
H. Tristram Engelhardt, Jr. and Kevin Wm. Wildes, S.J., Series Editors

Allocating Scarce Medical Resources

Roman Catholic Perspectives

H. TRISTRAM ENGELHARDT, JR.
AND MARK J. CHERRY, EDITORS

GEORGETOWN UNIVERSITY PRESS / WASHINGTON, D.C.

Georgetown University Press, Washington, D.C.
© 2002 by Georgetown University Press. All rights reserved.
Printed in the United States of America

10 9 8 7 6 5 4 3 2 1   2002

This volume is printed on acid-free offset book paper.

Library of Congress Cataloging-in-Publication Data

Allocating scarce medical resources : Roman Catholic perspectives / H. Tristram
Engelhardt, Jr. and Mark J. Cherry, editors.
     p. cm. — (Clinical medical ethics series)
   Includes bibliographical references and index.
   ISBN 0-87840-882-7 (pbk. : alk. paper)
     1. Medical ethics. 2. Christian ethics—Catholic authors. I. Engelhardt, H. Tristram
(Hugo Tristram), 1941– II. Cherry, Mark J. III. Clinical medical ethics (Washington, D.C.)

R725.55 .A43 2002
174′.2—dc21   2001040800

Contents

PART IV / MORAL THEOLOGICAL PERSPECTIVES

PART V / MORAL AND PUBLIC POLICY CHALLENGES

PART VI / FROM A DIFFERENT POINT OF VIEW: JEWISH, ORTHODOX, AND PROTESTANT PERSPECTIVES

PART VII / CRITICAL COMMENTARY

Preface

The essays that make up this book grew out of papers that were written and rewritten during and after a series of meetings involving a small working group of theologians, philosophers, and physicians. The first meeting was held in Schaan, the Principality of Liechtenstein, August 30–September 1, 1997. The second and third meetings were held in Houston, February 7–10 and October 24–27, 1998. The fourth and final meeting was convened in the precincts of Dublin, May 13–16, 1999. Out of the conversations sustained at these meetings, the major papers were rewritten, recast, and refocused four times. The book, in short, grew out of a dialogue sustained during a period of some three years. So, too, the Consensus Statement grew out of a discussion of this group of scholars. Long after the last meeting in 1999, it was the subject of interchanges by e-mail, fax, and post. The result is this volume and its reflections on Roman Catholic moral theological insights into the proper allocation of medical resources, using critical care as a heuristic example.

A number of individuals must be thanked who did not in the end contribute essays, but who were discussion partners as well as members of an Editorial Advisory Board that aided in reviewing and focusing the essays. These people include Francesc Abel, S.J.; Emanuel Agius; Angeles tan Alora; Antonio Autiero; Gerhold K. Becker; Baruch A. Brody; Nicholas Capaldi; Ned Cassem, S.J.; Dimitri Cozby; George Eber; Ruiping Fan; Curtis Freeman; Harvey Gordon; Diego Gracia; Stanley Hauerwas; Henk ten Have; Ana Smith Iltis; B. Andrew Lustig; Therese Lysaught; Jose Mainetti; Gerald McKenny; Lisa Rasmussen; Al Rosenfeld; Giovanni Russo; Mark Siegler; Allyne Smith; David Solomon; Charles Sprung; William Stempsey, S.J.; Carole Bailey Stoneking; Laurence P. Ulrich; and Laurie Zoloth.

H. Tristram Engelhardt, Jr.

Acknowledgment

The editors would like to express our thanks to *Christian Bioethics* for permission to reprint the "Consensus Statement" of the Working Group on Roman Catholic Approaches to Determining Appropriate Critical Care in this volume.

PART I

Moral Responsibility and High Technology: An Introduction

Infinite Expectations and Finite Resources: A Roman Catholic Perspective on Setting Limits to Critical Care, or, Can Roman Catholic Moral Theology Offer More than Secular Morality Provides?

H. Tristram Engelhardt, Jr.

HUMAN FINITUDE AND ITS MEDICAL DISCONTENTS

This is as much a volume on moral theology as one on bioethics, at least if one understands theology as a discursive reflection on the moral requirements of God. It addresses moral issues involved in limiting access to medical treatment, using critical care as a heuristic point of focus in order to determine the nature of the moral guidance that Roman Catholic moral theology can bring to this cluster of issues. Throughout the industrial and the developing worlds, new and costly diagnostic and therapeutic interventions have spurred a rise in health care costs, both in absolute terms and as a percentage of gross domestic product. Critical care dramatically illustrates the drama of these cost pressures: The use of intensive care generates some 15–20 percent of health care hospital costs in the United States. It also contributes significantly to costs in all industrial countries. Critical care places special burdens on health care budgets and the energies of health care units. And critical care is an especially attractive area for study, because it is one of the few areas where there are good clinical predictive measures regarding the likelihood of survival or death. As a result, one can with increasing accuracy predict the likelihood of saving lives and at what cost. Still, one can rarely be sure there is no chance of success, only that the likelihood is very remote and at great cost. Critical care forces one to face how to gamble with life and death in the face of finitude. Though there is an emerging literature focusing on the appropriate use of critical care resources, the secular bioethical literature remains underdeveloped.[1]

There have been some attempts to frame a Christian—indeed, a Roman Catholic—perspective on these issues, but they have only provided beginnings (Wildes 1995). This work uses the example of critical care to frame a moral understanding of the appropriate limits on access to medical treatment, drawing on moral insights from within Roman

Catholicism. Because critical care involves choices in the face of finitude, it invites existential questions regarding the meaning of life, the nature of a good death, and the appropriate use of limited resources. For those who know that the prize of human life is immortality, the question arises of how much must be invested in marginally postponing death or of achieving a very small chance for long-term survival, when the real goal is eternal life.

After a rather modest level of investment, the availability of high-technology health care does not on average contribute dramatically to life expectancy. After a low level of health care expenditure, among countries the differences in life expectancy at birth are minor in comparison with the differences in life expectancy due to being male or female, rich or poor, high status or low status (Iglehart 1990; Marmot et al. 1991; Anderson et al. 2000). Nevertheless, high-technology health care garners attention not commanded by other social services, which may in fact have a greater impact on the likelihood of living a long life. Critical care provides an epiphany of the moral choices regarding life and death that are generated by high-technology medicine. The question arises as to at what point the use of such resources may distract from the struggle toward salvation.

From the time of at least Plato's *Republic*, medicine has engaged attention because of the possibility it offers of postponing death and preserving health (Hamilton and Cairns 1961, 404–11). Even for Plato, medicine was associated with an arrogation of powers that threatened to undermine virtue. Plato's reflections on Herodicus and on health care generally touch many of our contemporary concerns and raise the issue of determining the proper limits to health care investments. If health care in Plato's time posed the question of setting limits, this is even more the case in the face of contemporary high-technology health care interventions, such as those that frame the environment of critical care. Contemporary high-technology medicine commands an attention and evokes a set of expectations that have a momentum of their own, the sum of which can be characterized as a technological imperative. There is a moral assumption that technology that can decrease the chance of dying must be used. For many persons, the very availability of high-technology interventions that can postpone death demands their use. Unlike Plato, for many any opportunity to offer any possibility of postponing death appears obligatory. If life is at stake, how can one fail to rescue another from death? If this is the only life one will ever have, how much is it worth? In the face of ultimate annihilation, what could be appropriate other than a full dedication to postponing death? Such assumptions tempt us to expend huge sums in the pursuit of small chances of incrementally postponing death. The result is often to construe critical care physicians as standing in a godlike position, from which they must make decisions whether to extend life or to accept death.

Plato and the pagan Greeks recognized that medicine can be the source of a temptation to hubris (Amundsen 1978). For Christians, the temptation is even clearer. The hope progressively to set aside one's finitude so as marginally to postpone death can be regarded as recapitulating the temptation of Eden: to gain divine power without God. For the Christian after the Fall who recognizes that the only way to Resurrection is through the Cross, the temptation is especially troubling. How should one regard the use of critical care when it only slightly delays death? How should one balance the concern for this life with a recognition that attempting to save life at all costs will likely distract from the struggle toward salvation? Can the recognition of humanity's ultimate destiny aid in discerning how properly to make decisions not just for particular patients but regarding policy bearing on the availability of critical care units generally? How many critical care beds should one staff? And if there are not enough critical care beds available for all who could benefit from them, on what principle should one decide who should have access, as well as who may or should be denied access?

Because some may always wish to postpone death somewhat further, and because resources for such postponement are always limited, intensive care units and critical care medicine bring into focus many of the problems encountered generally in developing allocatory health care policy. The decisions have an added force because one can often gauge outcomes better than in other areas of medicine. Patients in a critical care unit tend to have numerous physiological values measured and are followed carefully in a confined environment, so one can determine under what circumstances which patients are likely to have what likelihood of survival (Knaus et al. 1991). One can also measure the costs involved in securing survival. The result is that one has in hand significant information about the likelihood of success as well as the costs involved in gaining success. Against this background, one is faced with the questions that constitute the drama of bioethical decision making and health care policy:

- How much money should be invested to save life and at what likelihood of success?
- How should one's answers change, given different likely qualities of life?
- Should one use critical care for patients who would survive but only in a persistent vegetative state?
- How should one consider survival, with likely significant compromise in the ability to engage actively in the activities of daily life?
- How should one's answers change, given different likely lengths of survival?
- What costs should one take into consideration, in addition to financial costs?

All these questions and more must then be recast in the light of what insight, if any, Christianity can bring to the issue of determining how allocatory health care policy should be shaped:

- Are there insights regarding critical care that can be garnered from a religious perspective, particularly a Christian perspective?
- Is there a single Christian perspective?
- Is there a special knowledge that Christians can contribute to these policy matters?
- Is it possible that a Christian approach would at times conflict with secular understandings of the appropriate use of health care resources?
- Is there necessarily a compatibility between Christian and secular approaches, and if not, how would one come to terms with any tensions or conflicts?
- Should Christian insights be offered to society as a whole? Or provided only to or within Christian institutions?
- What is the special contribution to be made in all of this by Roman Catholic moral theology?

Any attempt by Christians to think through the appropriate limits to the use of critical care leads to more foundational issues concerning the relationship between secular and Christian bioethics:

- Can a Christian bioethics be a particular ethics and still remain an ethics worthy of the name?
- Can the moral life be fully understood only within the Christian faith?
- If a Christian bioethics claims special moral insights, is it sectarian?

The conflict between the aspiration to a particular moral message—indeed, a specifically Christian moral message—and the universality of moral rationality lies at the heart of the debates that shaped the essays in this volume. Indeed, this tension is at the core of the identity crisis of much of contemporary Western Christianity.

THE BIOETHICS OF ALLOCATION: A PLURALITY OF MORAL VISIONS

Numerous difficulties have plagued the project of devising a moral account for the allocation of health care resources. In great measure, the challenge has turned on the problem of facing inequalities and limits when they bear not just on health and disability, but on life itself. Much public policy has been developed in terms of a disingenuous commitment to providing all citizens equally with all the care from which they could benefit. Such an approach to health care policymaking is at best deceptive and at worst involves a corruptive false consciousness, which makes forthright health care policymaking impossible. It is not possible to provide all with (1) the best of care, (2) equal care, (3) physician and patient choice, while (4) still containing costs. One must compromise on one or more points. If resources are not unlimited, then one must limit choice and provide a basic package but not the best of care. And if one is not to impose intrusive governmental constraints, one must accept numerous forms of inequalities. One is then pressed to confront such questions as:

- How does one define adequate health care in general, and adequate critical care in particular?
- May one legitimately restrict the freedom to purchase better basic care? That is, how does one come to terms with fundamental conflicts between freedom and equality?
- In particular, if one determines that there is a basic amount of care that should be provided to all—given a particular likelihood of success in achieving a particular quality and length of life—may those who wish and have the resources purchase care that would otherwise not be provided? May they pay more so as to assume costly but less promising gambles?

Roman Catholicism has addressed this rich complex of concerns for more than 400 years under such rubrics as ordinary versus extraordinary care, proportionate versus disproportionate care, in order to draw a line between obligatory and nonobligatory care.[2] It is worth noting that this tradition has not traditionally focused on achieving equal care, but rather that basic amount of care one should provide within a particular context. One has been obliged to treat in proportion to the social status of the individual who was ill. This tradition has also taken into account considerations such as financial, psychological, and social costs; the likelihood of success; the length of life likely to be achieved; and even the likely quality of life (e.g., one was obliged to accept treatment only "si sit spes salutis").

Recent debates regarding the notion of futile care have touched on some of the issues that have traditionally been addressed under the rubrics of ordinary versus extraordinary care (Engelhardt and Khushf 1995). It is telling that in the literature those who engage the term "futile care" are not merely concerned with those treatments that offer no prospect of success, but more especially with those that do not produce a result worthy of the effort, or that do not have a sufficient likelihood of producing an acceptable outcome. The focus of futility reflections is on treatments that bring more harm than benefit. In short, "futile care" is often used to identify disproportionate medical interventions, frequently capturing the notion that the cost of the investment may not be worth the likely gain. The difficulties involved in defining exactly what is at stake in defining "futility" (Brody and Halevy 1995) lie perhaps in the term invoking a cluster of moral concerns that share no essential element but only a family of resemblances. This heterogeneity of background considerations has led some to create procedural approaches to the determinations of futility rather than content-full guidelines (Halevy and Brody 1996). It is important to emphasize that determinations of futility are not factual determinations but performative judgments meant to establish that certain medical interventions are not obligatory, and may even be morally forbidden.

There has also been a reluctance to address forthrightly the issue of the costs (financial and other) involved in providing care. Yet financial costs inevitably play a role in determining when one is obliged to provide a treatment. For example, if critical care for a class of patients was fully successful, restoring patients to full health one out of every hundred thousand applications and cost only $1, it would likely be provided. It would save lives at the cost of $100,000 per life saved. With the same possibility of success, if the treatment cost $100,000 and if this class of patients was numerous, it would likely not be offered. One would be saving lives at the cost of $10 billion per life saved. The challenge lies in developing more precise guidelines to determine how—given a particular likelihood of success in achieving a particular length of life with a particular quality—financial costs should play a role in determining when one is no longer obliged to provide treatment. So far, the guidelines that have been elaborated have primarily addressed issues such as likely length of life and quality of life, in the sense of considering the appropriateness of critical care for persistent vegetative state and permanently obtunded patients (Society of Critical Care Ethics Committee 1994).

In addition to concerns regarding a distinction between proportionate versus disproportionate uses of resources, there have been various attempts to engage notions of justice in the allocation of resources. Such attempts have always in the end proved profoundly controversial. The controversies are at least in part a function of foundational secular moral disagreements about (1) which needs generate rights, (2) what entitlements to private property set limits on claims of social justice, and (3) when private resources establish claims to purchase better care, including better basic care, beyond any basic package provided for all.

The issue of when needs generate rights to critical care in part recapitulates the issues raised in distinguishing ordinary from extraordinary, proportionate from disproportionate care, that is, obligatory from nonobligatory care. As one moves to claims involving extraordinary or disproportionate care, putative needs no longer generate rights to or claims to health care interventions. The difficulty lies in establishing a canonical interpretive framework that can determine when which needs generate what rights for whom to what level of critical care.

Beyond the issue of claims to care, there also are disputes regarding whether care should be provided equally, as well as what sorts of equality are morally relevant. On the one hand, a concern with equality in its own right might focus on "leveling down" through what might be termed an "egalitarianism of envy." Consider, for example, three possible worlds, one in which everyone equally receives beneficial critical care interventions, a second in which one person from private resources purchases more beneficial critical care interventions than others have available, and a third in which one person receives markedly less beneficial critical care interventions because of a lack of resources. If one regards the second case as morally troubling, one is focused not on the suffering of someone who has less care, but on the inequality of someone receiving more critical care, and therefore a better chance to survive. Someone's better fortune is regarded as unfair. On the other hand, one can be concerned about "leveling up" and therefore focus on the individual who receives less beneficial critical care. Here, one is not concerned with someone having more of a chance to survive than others, but with someone having less of a chance. If one is interested in achieving the cheapest way to provide more beneficial care to such individuals, one has affirmed what can be characterized as an egalitarianism of altruism.

Which understanding of equality should play a role or be dominant in fashioning critical care allocatory policy? Why should one be morally concerned if some can purchase better care than others? Should one only be morally concerned if some cannot have any or only limited and inadequate access to basic care? Depending on how one answers such questions, one will either acquiesce in establishing a basic understanding of adequate care and allow those who can to buy better basic—as well as luxury—critical care services, or one will impose an equal standard on all as normative.

How one comes to terms with these issues will have dramatic implications for many developing countries. Consider China, which compasses communities with radically different levels of health care. Excellent critical care is now provided in many hospitals in large cities. Yet resources are insufficient for unimpeded access to critical care for all in urban areas, much less in rural areas. Should China continue to focus governmental resources on a good but spartan basic health care system, which indeed appears to deliver good health care, while encouraging a health care industry to develop for both relatively affluent Chinese as well as foreigners? Such a policy tacitly recognizes that equally distributing resources would make little difference in the care of the less affluent, but it would discourage the development of a local health care industry of excellence, while encouraging a drain of gifted physicians to other countries. In countries with internally significant differences in resource availability across classes, as well as between urban and rural areas, such choices are unavoidable. In the face of such differences and considerations, how ought one to understand claims regarding rights to, and duties to provide, critical care?

To determine which account of the generation of rights to critical care from critical care needs is normative, and which account of equality should guide policy, one must also determine which account of justice should guide the allocation of resources. This will have bearing on claims of self-determination, as well as the ownership of private resources. To resolve such controversies, one will need to turn to foundational issues. Yet moral foundational accounts appear to be dependent on particular antecedent moral intuitions, senses, notions of casuistry, or ways of balancing moral claims. That is, in order to resolve moral controversies by sound rational argument, those who do not already de facto share a content-full moral vision will need to accept common moral premises, rules of moral evidence, and rules of moral inference.

The nature of these criteria is exactly what is at issue. Because there has not been an agreement on which account of justice or which understanding of fairness should be normative, moral disputes in these as well as many other areas have remained unresolved. The depth of the disagreements is reflected in contemporary political, moral, and public policy controversies regarding the proper shaping of health care policy and the use of resources for health care. The character of these debates indicates that there is a failure to agree regarding what considerations are authoritatively normative, as well as with respect to who is in authority to bring closure to these debates (Engelhardt 1996; Wildes 2000).

The apparently interminable character of controversies in secular moral theory and the framing of moral policy regarding the appropriate allocation of resources to health care—as well as with respect to the appropriate limits to be drawn between obligatory and nonobligatory treatment—might lead one to hope that those within the various Christian moral traditions, or those within a particular Christian religion, might at least possess a sufficient commonality of understanding regarding what is morally normative, so as to be able to resolve moral controversies in this area and then provide guidance for at least the members of their own religion. After all, if Christians in general or Roman Catholics in particular possess common understandings of what views of social justice should guide health care allocatory policy, or at least possess a common view of who is in authority to resolve such controversies, then morally authoritative conclusions could be secured at least for them.

A CHRISTIAN VISION: CAN IT OFFER GUIDANCE UNAVAILABLE FROM SECULAR MORALITY AND ITS BIOETHICS?

The discussions that led to this volume explored the extent to which Christianity, in particular Roman Catholicism, can offer an understanding of the proper allocation of medical resources. There is much to suggest that the Christian approach to the allocation of resources should have a character different from that guided by general secular moral theory. After all, the Christian view of life and death is deeply at odds with the secular. Though a nonbeliever might affirm the goodness of a peaceful unforeseen death, Christians have traditionally prayed for an anticipated death (e.g., "a subitanea improvisa morte, libera nos, Domine"), recognizing that the most significant threat from serious illness is not death but dying without repentance, unreconciled with God. Presumably, any Christian account of the use of expensive and burdensome resources for the extension of life must recognize that the Christian life should be one of repentance and humility, not one of strident claims for the recruitment of resources for the extension of this life. After all, Christians should acknowledge the cardinal truth that this life is not the only life. Moreover, to focus inordinate concerns on this life and its preservation is likely to lead to treating this life as an object of idolatrous interest. In addition, Christians who understand that the Cross is the way to resurrection and eternal life will undoubtedly have a more complex or at least different understanding of suffering than those who are not Christians.

It is to this cluster of concerns, the articulation of a Christian, in particular a Roman Catholic, understanding of the appropriate limits of the use of medical resources, that the discussions that led to these essays directed their energies. After all, one might suppose that Christians might have something particular to offer to these considerations. Since the early church, Christians have reflected on the proper use of medicine. The Fathers recognize that medicine, though a prima facie good, can also distract from the pursuit of salvation. Saint Basil the Great (329–79) gives this warning in his reflections on the use of medicine.

> And, when we were commanded to return to the earth whence we had been taken and were united with the pain-ridden flesh doomed to destruction because of sin and, for the same reason, also subject to disease, the medical art was given to us to relieve the sick, in some degree at least.
>
> Now, the herbs which are the specifics for each malady do not grow out of the earth spontaneously; it is evidently the will of the Creator that they should be brought forth out of the soil to serve our need. Therefore, the obtaining of that natural virtue which is in the roots and flowers, leaves, fruits, and juices, or in such metals or products of the sea as are found especially suitable for bodily health, is to be viewed in the same way as the procuring of food and drink. Whatever requires an undue amount of thought or trouble or involves a large expenditure of effort and causes our whole life to revolve, as it were, around solicitude for the flesh must be avoided by Christians. Consequently, we must take great care to employ this medical art, if it should be necessary, not as making it wholly accountable for our state of health or illness, but as redounding to the glory of God and as a parallel to the care given the soul. In the event that medicine should fail to help, we should not place all hope for the relief of our distress in this art, but we should rest assured that He will not allow us to be tried above that which we are able to bear. (Basil 1962, 331–32)

Saint Basil then offers a warning that undue solicitude for the flesh may lead us to preserving this life at the loss of eternal life with Christ. One can quite easily become lost in the passion to postpone death.

In particular, we should not engage in health care so that our entire life revolves around our treatment. "Whatever requires an undue amount of thought or trouble or involves a large expenditure of effort and causes our whole life to revolve, as it were, around solicitude for the flesh must be avoided by Christians" (Basil 1962, 331). In this warning, Saint Basil gives greater depth to and reveals the true significance of Plato's concern in the *Republic*, Book Three, regarding the damage to virtue of the excessive use of health care.

As we reflect on drawing limits between obligatory and nonobligatory treatment, we must consider how concerns to avoid undue solicitude for the flesh should be combined with concerns appropriately to use costly resources. The Christian moral focus plausibly must be as much on avoiding sinful temptations to employ medicine to save life at all costs, thereby distorting the moral life, as on being good stewards of resources. If critical care is used improperly, patients, families, physicians, and nurses may become overly involved in the preservation of this mundane existence to the detriment of their salvation. One must consider the circumstances under which critical care may be employed without endangering the life of prayer and repentance that must characterize the Christian life under all circumstances, even in critical care units. One must also consider how involvement in care that becomes a desperate, all-consuming, and idolatrous pursuit of this life will harm families, physicians, nurses, and other caregivers.

If such reflection proves fruitful, we will articulate a set of concerns not easily appreciated in secular terms, because the cardinal considerations are transcendent. We will be led to framing a set of moral concerns about when one should not employ critical care because of the dangers it represents in certain circumstances to the spiritual life of patients, physicians, nurses, and families. Were much to be said in this area, then the Christian understanding of the proper limits on the use of critical care would be quite different from moral accounts articulated in more secular terms. This notion of moral and spiritual danger is captured by Pope Pius XII in his observation that

> normally one is held to use only ordinary means—according to the circumstances of persons, places, times, and culture—that is to say, means that do not involve any grave burden [*aucune charge extraordinaire*] for oneself or another. A more strict obligation would be too burdensome [*trop lourde*] for most men and would render the attainment of the higher, more important good too difficult. (Pope Pius XII 1957, 1031)

If certain attempts to use high-technology health care involve a distortion of the moral life and the idolatry of mere physical survival, then one will have grounds for regarding some extraordinary or disproportionate care as morally dangerous. As the literature develops, it will be interesting to gauge whether and to what extent there is the possibility of articulating such understandings within the framework of Roman Catholic moral and theological reflections. If such limitations could be established for critical care, they could then perhaps be generalized to other areas of health care intervention.

Faced with the challenge of setting limits, one might either favor the tactic of establishing concrete, content-full rules, or establishing procedures through which lines could be created. The first would be favored insofar as one shares common content-full moral premises, rules of evidence, and rules of inference. In that case, one may be able to lay out substantive guidelines to resolve controversies regarding appropriate limits to the use of critical care. Such, one would presume, should be possible for Christians. Conversely, even if one despairs of agreement regarding content-full views that respect the proper allocation of critical care, as well as the moral propriety of using critical care in particular areas, one may still be able to establish procedures to resolve controversies or appeals to authority that can be acknowledged as having the standing to guide the drawing of lines between obligatory and nonobligatory treatment. For Roman Catholicism regarding the latter, one might think of the role of the pope in shaping the magisterium. The choice in particular areas between an appeal to normative content or to moral authority will depend on the background morality one brings to the fashioning of health care policy.

The challenge of the discussions that produced this volume was to determine the extent to which Christian moral reflection can provide content-full moral guidelines or must instead rely on procedures and appeals to authority for resolutions of controversies. The employment of casuistry or the direction of a spiritual father presupposes a background moral and metaphysical context, even if it does not engage a rigid application of a set of moral guidelines or canons. Yet, in some cases, the use of a spiritual father can break free of appeals to discursively established moral content and instead be regarded as a means by which the Christian life is brought to bear not in terms of its letter but in terms of the Spirit.

It was here that the discussions that produced these essays reached a cardinal impasse. There was first and foremost the issue of the extent to which morality can in its fullness only be a Christian morality. Given Roman Catholic commitments to natural law and/or the place of discursive rationality in disclosing the content and character of morality, there was a resistance to the view that the Christian community may possess a decisively more ample appreciation of how to approach life-and-death decision making at both macro and micro levels, including the allocation of resources to critical care. Second, there was also a concern whether aspirations to a universal morality failed to take seriously the claims of local cultures. This last concern raises the interesting question as to whether Christians are (should be) first bound by the content and insight of Christian culture, or whether they first and foremost have (may have, or indeed should have) their lives shaped by their local culture.

This last set of issues backhandedly raises the foundational question as to which if any Christian communities live in the universal illuminating presence of the Holy Spirit so as also to be cultivated by Him and therefore share a moral culture universal to true believing and right-worshipping Christians. This cluster of questions was in various ways confronted by Father Edward Hughes, who recognized a unity of moral insight among the Orthodox, despite their diversity of languages, peoples, and cultural contexts. The discussion again and again addressed what morality should be affirmed by a community united to Christ in the enduring presence of the Holy Spirit. This is, after all, the central issue as to the nature of a Christian morality and bioethics. This issue, however, sets revelation over against reason.

The central challenge in providing an account of the guidance that Roman Catholicism can give to the allocation of resources for health care lies in this foundational controversy: To what extent, if any, may or indeed should a Roman Catholic bioethics be substantively different from secular bioethics? On the one hand, the Roman Catholic commitment to discursive rationality, philosophy, and natural law can support the view that Christian and secular bioethics should be materially equivalent. On the other hand, the Christian life must focus on salvation through Christ, the long-awaited Messiah of Israel and the Son of God. This should carry some special moral implication for how one focuses on death. Again and again during the discussions of the essays that form this volume, it appeared as if the commitment to discursive rationality would deconstruct and evacuate the content of particular Christian moral commitments. It was as if the particularly Christian were a scandal to the claims of universal moral rationality. The result was a tension at the heart of the notion of catholicity that can identify either the whole of right-directed Christian belief or a universality of moral rationality.

A BRIEF INTRODUCTION TO THE CULTURE WARS

Parents are supposed to be impartial. They are expected to love their children equally. If they cannot achieve equality of love, at least they should keep it to themselves. The same can be said for editors of volumes: They are to approach each essay with equal care and consideration. I have tried my best; I have failed. Of all the essays, I love Father James W. Heisig's the most, even when I disagree with much of what he says. The reason is that, even where I believe he has gotten things wrong, he has gotten them wrong in a heuristically very useful way.

First of all, he brings us back to the cluster of core moral theoretical and religious challenges to which I have just alluded: Can there be anything specially and universally Roman Catholic about Roman Catholic moral theology? If so, what and whence is that specificity? In his exploration, Heisig en passant raises decisive philosophical and theological questions of a universal morality, a global bioethics—not just the universalist aspirations of Roman Catholic moral theology. These questions do not lead us to embrace a metaphysical skepticism (i.e., to hold that there is no timeless, content-rich moral truth to be known), but at most to consider an epistemological skepticism (i.e., a recognition that our epistemic condition is such that we are often if not always unable by sound rational argument to choose among alternative moral visions). Of course, this way of putting the matter is mine, not his (Engelhardt 1996). Second, his seems to be the very subtle thesis: The human good is always appreciated in the particular socio-historical contexts within which culture, context, and history shape the moral life. The attempt to articulate the human good in universalist cultural terms leads to moral distortions and impoverishment. Indeed, because of its contextual character, universalist cultural aspirations to a global ethic threaten the very core of the moral life. Putting moral questions in universalist cultural modes that ignore the content-conveying character of the specific will not only misguide us in the moral enterprise and despoil the moral environment. Attempts at such moral universalism may also encourage using answers as tools of power, subjecting one culture and its adherents to another. Heisig reminds us of the dangers of cultural imperialism.

Undoubtedly, I have somewhat misconstrued Heisig's views in the service of heuristic provocation. In any event, he resolutely leads many of the essays to confront a number of ambiguities in the notion "Catholic." For example, does Roman Catholicism disclose a timeless set of philosophical truths, a rich cultural inheritance, or an abiding unity in the Spirit with the true God? Heisig does not really touch on this third point. He invites us instead to confront the question: What, if anything, is morally specific about Roman Catholicism, and in what way? He helps us to take seriously the content-conveying force of culture. No doubt, in all of this I recast Heisig in ways he would resist: Provocateurs always run the risk of being provoked in the name of further discussion.

Heisig recognizes that colonial cultural imperialism has imposed particular senses of health, morality, culture, and religion alien to their colonial subjects, although this sense masquerades under the color of universality. Now mind you, he never cashes in his very important claims about what it would be to have an alternative model of health. After all, concepts of health, like concepts of disease, are complex and rich. Much must be said to give them substance. But that is a different matter. Heisig helps us to ask the cardinal question: How does the particular or specific lens of a culture bind the universally human, whatever that might be, with the individual, whatever that might be? Unlike Seifert and Boyle, who address the problem of anchoring their understanding of tradition in a timeless moral universality secured through discursive reason, and unlike Hughes, who recognizes that Tradition is the encounter over time with the same Spirit, Heisig examines the power of the cultural context. These differences in approach raise questions regarding fundamentally different understandings of religion, moral theology, proper deportment, and catholicity.

THE SPECIFIC MASQUERADING AS THE UNIVERSAL

During three years and at four meetings, the contributors to this volume explored what might appear to be a rather straightforward issue: What can Roman Catholic moral theology teach us about the allocation of scarce medical resources to critical care? Despite the problems just outlined, some concrete guidance was secured. Given manuals galore and reflections aplenty, one might have expected that Roman Catholic moral theology could provide a rich store of guidance drawn from a tradition of reflection on medical issues reaching to the sixteenth century and before.

As was acknowledged above, there was persistent resistance on the part of many of the Roman Catholic authors to the view that Christian morality and bioethics might have a moral content not disclosable by discursive reason. This resistance was to be expected: Roman Catholic moral theology often claims that particular moral commitments from contraception to social justice can in principle be disclosed to the inquiring rational mind of any truly open and persistent thinker. In this sense, Roman Catholic moral theology offers academic fulfillment. God's revelation can in general outline be found not just in Scripture or in oral tradition, but fully fleshed, if not fully clothed, through philosophical investigation, at least if the investigator approaches matters with a mind unsullied by the influence of such base cultures as, for example, may exist in Texas (Engelhardt 1990).

These rationalistic aspirations are brought home to us forcefully by the contributions of Seifert and Boyle. They are sustained by Honnefelder, who argues in a fashion that suggests that there is no great difference or distance between what Roman Catholicism offers and what can reasonably be established. Schotsmans similarly introduces rationally grounded universalist aspirations, albeit in charmingly particular wrappings. He very heuristically engages in the task of defending Belgium as the realization of the good-natured health care system that marries justice, Christianity, and technological excellence.

Here we run aground on the foundational challenge: What purports to be specifically or particularly a characteristic of Roman Catholic moral theology turns out to be purportedly universal and open to all simply as humans. As a consequence, the more one asks to hear about what is specific in Roman Catholic moral theology regarding allocational morality, the more one gets an emphatic answer that would otherwise be quite puzzling: There is nothing specific, there is nothing particular! It is all universal! The universally rational is exactly what is specific about what Roman Catholic moral theology has to offer to the moral challenge of justly allocating scarce medical resources. Every time one presses for a specifically Roman Catholic moral theological suggestion regarding the use of critical care resources, one gets what is almost an indignant reply: "Don't you know, we are by faith committed to reason's ability to disclose morality's content." Roman Catholic morality, at least that relevant to allocational issues, is universally available through discursive reason.

Heisig recognizes that one cannot talk this way without engaging some of the most profound moral conflicts of the age, especially conflicting claims regarding the possibility of a global ethic, the legitimacy of the claims of local cultures to particular axiological insights, and the permissibility of respecting, savoring, and/or nurturing cultural if not moral pluralism. He focuses his appreciation of these challenges through a recognition of cultural imperialism, colonialism, and the virtues of indigenous cultural insights. The issues engaged bear not just on the universality of moral claims, but on the epistemic and metaphysical significance of religion itself. These issues are at the heart of the culture wars: the cultural debates concerning the significance of religion, morality, and tradition in a posttraditional age. These reflections in the end lead to questions such as whether Christ offers to Christians moral insights not available to those who appeal to the Buddha, Confucius, or Muhammad.

Roman Catholic moral theology, even when appealing to universal moral claims grounded in natural law and discursive philosophical argument, nevertheless imports a great deal that is highly specific, culturally freighted, and historically conditioned. As one begins to recognize the particularity of particular notions of moral rationality (e.g., not all recognize the Roman Catholic claims that rational arguments should lead to the conclusion that contraception is morally prohibited), one encounters a cultural rupture. Battle lines open up in a culture war at the root of the moral and theological debates dividing not only Christians from non-Christians, but traditional Christians from posttraditional Christians: different understandings of moral rationality. The divisions engendered by conflicting understandings of moral rationality also lie at the roots of disputes within Roman Catholicism itself and strike at the heart of attempts to articulate the moral theological foundations of proper allocational policy in universalist terms. In particular, as Heisig suggests, why may appropriate or ordinate care not be culturally specific? Why ought the standards for appropriate levels of health care in Asia, Africa, and South America be prima facie the same as those to which Western Europe and North America aspire, rather than as prima facie culturally embedded? Why should there be a uniform standard of excellence, especially in the face of concerns regarding the seductive power of medical technology?

Perhaps these issues are also intended by Heisig in his cryptic reference to "alternative models of health." After all, the diagnosis of disease functions as a warrant for therapeutic interventions. On the one hand, different understandings of human well-being will support or undermine the plausibility of using critical care in particular circumstances. On the other hand, the availability of critical care reshapes how we experience life, illness, disease, and death. Such a commitment involves not just a considerable investment of resources, but also the reinterpretation of care within technologically driven expectations. With its technology and its religions, the West has exported very specific moralities. These moralities have directed the use of high technology, nested in taken-for-granted expectations regarding the goodness of living and dying in highly technologically mediated circumstances. Whose norms should guide? Why should non-Western European and non-North American cultures accept the taken-for-granted technologically constituted expectations regarding critical care medicine developed in the West? Why should they be put in the position of having to excuse themselves from not incorporating the Western culture of technological excellence? I take it that this is among the challenges given to us, albeit cryptically, by Heisig.

The further question then arises of the epistemological and moral theoretical presuppositions that must be engaged to allow space for diverse understandings of "standards of excellence" and of "best care." What, if anything, must be affirmed within the expectations of Roman Catholic moral theology in order to allow moral diversity in the use of medicine, especially high-technology medicine and critical care. Does one need to hold that new values must be engaged at foundational levels or simply that in different cultures technologies will involve different moral and spiritual burdens, some of which can be serious stumbling blocks in the struggle toward salvation? In addition, may it be that Western cultures have grown blind to how high-technology medicine can detract from the journey to salvation? There is much that still must be clarified in these matters.

The question—What can Christians offer as moral guidance in the use of scarce medical resources, especially for critical care?—thus remains without a unanimous answer. If loving one's neighbor rightly depends first on loving the right God wholeheartedly and rightly, then it will be very important first to be sure how and to Whom one is praying, directing one's life, and orienting one's love. If right belief serves the function of liturgical and metaphysical orientation, then one should not at all be astonished that Christian bioethics moves beyond the good to the holy, redefining and relocating the good in the process.

At this point, significant epistemological issues come to the fore. Does one orient oneself first and foremost through sound rational argument? Does one orient oneself within a written and oral tradition? Or does one instead do so first and foremost through union with the Spirit of the true God? At stake once more is the character of the particularly Christian moral knowing that Christians should bring to bear on allocational concerns. The more that moral knowledge is drawn from sound rational argument, the more it literally stands to reason that morality should simply be a universal moral rationality, and that a Christian morality worthy of the name should be equivalent to any morality worthy of the name. The more the Christian character of morality as well as the content of morality is to be found not in universalist moral arguments alone, but rather always appreciated in the thick context of history, society, and place, the less this will be plausible. The answer will have an even different character if the substance of Christian morality is shaped by the experience of the Spirit of God.

This last possibility is a *tertium quid*, which is underscored in the essay of Hughes. If Christianity directs us beyond morality to a God Who is truly transcendent, then Christians may find themselves acting in ways that not only cannot find a justification in reason, but will appear downright unreasonable. The context and substantive content of Christian morality, including that of allocational bioethics, will be derived through grace, not from discursive reason (Engelhardt 2000). For instance, critical care will be useful when it allows an opportunity for repentance, and improper when it is a stumbling block to salvation.

We are returned again to foundational issues regarding morality, religion, culture, and medicine—in particular, to issues of the extent to which Christian morality is universal or particular, and the implications of this for understanding how a Roman Catholic moral theology can guide the allocation of scarce medical resources. Khushf recognizes the issue of where moral particularity is expected when he asks whether there is any more need for a Roman Catholic hospital system than for a Roman Catholic grocery store chain (of course, such a question could only be asked from the perspective of religions not concerned about kosher foods or finding victuals appropriate for periods of fast). All of this returns us to where we began, while still preserving the important progress made. We can better appreciate the core question of where the Christianness of Christian bioethics should make a difference.

My pleading has a Hegelian character: We should resituate our reflections as moments preserved within a larger perspective focused on understanding (1) what particular guidance Roman Catholic moral theology can give to the allocation of resources to critical care, as well as (2) whether such guidance need be uniform or whether it should or may be culture- and condition-specific. We must assess the legitimacy of a global ethics, the place of moral pluralism in specifying such guidance, and most especially the particular commitments of Roman Catholic moral theology regarding the use of resources for critical care. As an important first step in this direction, we have not only the essays in this volume, but also a consensus statement that was first drafted within the same debates that shaped these essays. Our sojourn in coming to terms morally with our new, expensive, and alluring medical technologies has only begun.

NOTES

1. A number of publications have addressed the bioethical issues at stake in critical care. See, e.g., Moskop and Kopelman (1985), and Orlowski (1999). Other books have addressed the issue of critical care as part of their focus; see Bayertz (1996).
2. The history of this distinction in Roman Catholic moral reflections is considerable. At the end of the sixteenth century, the distinction was placed under the rubric of the contrast between ordinary and extraordinary care. For a review of this history, see Cronin (1958). This has been reprinted in Pope John XXIII Center (1989).

BIBLIOGRAPHY

Amundsen, D. W. 1978. The physician's obligation to prolong life: A medical duty without classical roots. *Hastings Center Report* 8: 23–30.

Anderson, G. F., J. Hurd, P. S. Hussey, and M. Jee-Hughes. 2000. Health spending and outcomes: Trends in OECD countries, 1960–1998. *Health Affairs* 19 (3): 150–57.

Basil, Saint. 1962. *Ascetical Works*, trans. by Sister Monica Wagner. Washington, D.C.: Catholic University of America Press.

Bayertz, K., ed. 1996. *Sanctity of Life and Human Dignity.* Dordrecht: Kluwer.

Brody, B. A., and A. Halevy. 1995. Is futility a futile concept? *Journal of Medicine and Philosophy* 2: 123–44.

Cronin, D. A. 1958. *The Moral Law in Regard to the Ordinary and Extraordinary Means of Conserving Life.* Rome: Pontifical Gregorian University.

Engelhardt, H. Tristram, Jr. 1990. Texas: Messages, morals, and myths. *Journal of the American Studies Association of Texas* 21 (October): 33–49.

———. 1996. *The Foundations of Bioethics.* New York: Oxford University Press.

———. 2000. *The Foundations of Christian Bioethics.* Lisse: Swets & Zeitlinger.

Engelhardt, H. T., Jr., and George Khushf. 1995. Futile care for the critically ill patient. *Current Opinion in Critical Care* 1: 329–33.

Halevy, A., and B. A. Brody. 1996. A multi-institutional collaborative policy on medical futility. *Journal of American Medical Association* 276: 571–74.

Hamilton, E., and H. Cairns, ed. 1961. *The Collected Dialogues of Plato.* Princeton, N.J.: Princeton University Press.

Iglehart, J. K. 1990. Canada's health care system faces its problems. *New England Journal of Medicine* 322 (February 22): 562–68.

Knaus, W., D. Wanger, E. Draper, J. Zimmerman, M. Bergner, P. Bastos, C. Sirio, D. Murphy, T. Lotring, and A Damiano. 1991. The APACHE III prognostic system. *Chest* 100 (December 6): 1619–35.

Marmot, M. G., G. D. Smith, S. Stansfeld, C. Patel, F. North, J. Head, I. White, E. Brunner, and A. Foeney. 1991. Health inequalities among British civil servants: The Whitehall II study. *Lancet* 337 (June 8): 1387–93.

Moskop, J. C., and L. Kopelman, eds. 1985. *Ethics and Critical Care Medicine.* Dordrecht: Kluwer.

Orlowski, J., ed. 1999. *Ethics in Critical Care Medicine.* Baltimore: University Publishing Group.

Pope John XXIII Center, ed. 1989. *Conserving Human Life.* Braintree, Mass.: Pope John XXIII Center.

Pope Pius XII. 1957. Allocution "Le Dr. Bruno Haid," November 24, *Acta Apostolicae Sedis* 49; English translation from Address to an International Congress of Anesthesiologists, November 24. *The Pope Speaks* 4 (spring 1958): 395–96.

Society of Critical Care Ethics Committee. 1994. Consensus statement on the triage of critically ill patients. *Journal of American Medical Association* 271 (April 20): 1200–03.

Wildes, K. W., S.J. 1995. *Critical Choices and Critical Care.* Dordrecht: Kluwer.

———. 2000. *Moral Acquaintances.* Notre Dame, Ind.: University of Notre Dame Press.

Facing the Challenges of High-Technology Medicine: Taking the Tradition Seriously

Mark J. Cherry

> To place the hope of one's health in the hands of the doctor is the act of an irrational animal.
> —Saint Basil, "Ascetical Works: The Long Rules"

In the United States, nearly one out of every seven dollars is spent on some form of health care; in 1998, this amounted to approximately 13.6 percent of the gross domestic product (GDP), or $4,178 per capita. By way of comparison, health care in Canada, Germany, Belgium, and Austria in 1998 respectively represented 9.5, 10.6, 8.8, and 8.2 percent of each country's GDP, or approximately $2,312, $2,424, $2,081, and $1,968 per capita (OECD 2000).[1] Of such expenditures, critical care medicine accounts for approximately 15 to 20 percent of all hospital expenses, which in turn amounts to 38 percent of all U.S. health care expenditures (ATS Board of Directors Position Statement 1997). In 1994, intensive care unit (ICU) costs amounted to approximately 1 percent of GDP (roughly $64 billion) (Chalfin, Cohen, and Lambrinos 1995). This increasingly significant investment of personal and social resources into high-technology medicine is driven by very real concerns to ameliorate the physiological collapse brought on by age, accident, injury, and disease.

Critical care medicine provides a heuristic example of the desire to make available an optimal level of care for all who require it, where "optimal" means the highest available standard of care. Technologically sophisticated critical care was developed medically to maintain compromised patients requiring extensive and advanced support of respiration, support of two or more organ systems, and assistance with chronic impairment of one or more organ systems along with intervention for acute reversible failure of additional organ system(s). ICUs focus on two primary categories of patients: (1) those with a high risk of imminent death (e.g., critically ill patients with respiratory failure or heart failure) and (2) those who are potentially at high risk of imminent death (e.g., those admitted for supervision of a high-risk procedure, such as management of cardiac arrhythmias) (Taboada, essay in this volume).

Given its expense, high-technology critical care is primarily a feature of affluent industrial-world societies. Even among affluent nations, however, budgetary retrenchments in the macroallocation of social resources to health care, and within health care to critical care, leads to variations in outcome. For example, when comparing critical care in the United States and the United Kingdom utilizing the Acute Physiology and Chronic Health Evaluation (APACHE) III scoring system, outcomes of intensive care are qualitatively and quantitatively lower in the United Kingdom than in the United States (Pappachan et al. 1999; Wood, Coursin, and Grounds 1999). As Michael Rie points out (in his essay in this volume), these differential outcomes are not due to measurement problems or definitional difficulties; rather, the virtue of such objective, standardized measurements is that they obtain external, objective, third-party critical assessments. Such data allow one to compare outcomes across large populations of ICUs and patients, tracking the quantitative and qualitative vectors of the cost-benefit curve, thereby allowing honest assessment of the benefits and harms of allocating medical and financial resources to critical care.[2]

Consequently, as a matter of morality and public policy it is essential to evaluate when unequal access to critical care is morally permissible and when available standards of health care are unfortunate but not unfair. Must all have equal access to the very best standards of critical care? Is it morally permissible for different countries to have varying standards of critical care? May standards differ within a particular country? From region to region? Or city to city? Or hospital to hospital? Adequately to assess such questions requires the specification of a particular moral context within which one may know truly when to limit access to health care and when to draw back from certain types of treatments.

Here the international, predominately secular, debate has failed adequately to appreciate the depth of such difficulties. In very general terms: secular axiology cannot provide a unique meaningful account of pain, disease, disability, suffering, and death, beyond the firing of synapses, the collapse of human abilities, and the mere end of life. As a result, most contemporary bioethical accounts are remarkably thin. Populated with the jargon of duty and obligation, equality, autonomy, virtue, and beneficence—without careful analysis of the deep theological or moral significance of health care—they are able to encourage us to expand choice, eliminate suffering, and reduce death, but unable authoritatively to determine which choices to make, which kinds of suffering to eliminate, or which deaths to postpone.[3] For example: Is assisting in the suicide of a patient with terminal cancer an act of kindness or of murder? Should very-low-weight, premature neonates be sustained regardless of expense, likelihood of survival, or quality of life? What about patients in a permanently vegetative state? Is reducing the total number of critical care beds a morally permissible means of allocating scarce health care resources? Although it is nearly always possible to order additional tests, surgical interventions, or pharmaceuticals—which will convey at least marginal benefits in terms of additional disease prevention, greater alleviation of suffering, or marginal postponement of death—such expenditures impose ever-expanding financial, moral, social, psychological, and spiritual costs on patients, families, caregivers, and society.

How should one come to terms with such concerns? All health care is provided within the conditions of human finitude. It is false to assume that all can be provided equal care, the very best of care, with physician and patient choice, without rationing, while still managing to control costs.[4] As H. Tristram Engelhardt, Jr., has shown, such a view, however prevalent, fails to face the economic, medical, and moral realities of health care. It represents an ideology, a false consciousness, which all economic indicators and empirical experiences show to be false, but the reality of which few are willing openly to confront (1994,

504–05, 508–09). In much contemporary bioethical reflection, this ideology provides the secular equivalent of orthodox belief; disagreement is to be at least shunned, if not actively persecuted.

Combined with the ever-expanding capacities of medicine, however, as the authors in this volume indicate, such an ideology is proving not merely economically but also morally shortsighted. If human suffering is to have enduring significance, it must be situated within a nest of ontological background assumptions, standards of moral inquiry, and epistemological foundations; it requires a context in which to evaluate essential connotations, as well as to place and integrate understandings. That one would even think to ask "Why?" and hope to receive a coherent, meaningful response requires the specification of a context with particular standards for seeking, understanding, and knowing truly, through which all of reality is mediated (Cherry 1996).[5] Insofar as one is honestly to face the challenges of high-technology medicine together with the limits of human knowledge and abilities, one must come to terms with morally permissible ways in which to limit access to critical care resources.[6] It is this nexus of problems to which the essays in this volume are addressed.

ROMAN CATHOLIC MORAL THEOLOGICAL PERSPECTIVES

The next brace of essays—compassing many of the foundational moral theological viewpoints within contemporary Roman Catholicism, from traditional Catholic moral analysis (Joseph Boyle), to the insights of philosophical personalism (Josef Seifert), to the demands of solidarity (Paul Schotsmans) and human dignity (Ludger Honnefelder)—address this need for moral context. As each argues, where secular bioethics fails appropriately to situate health care within one's life or to give deep meaning to suffering and death, Christian bioethics, and particularly Roman Catholic bioethics, succeeds. It provides insight and meaning to guide the legitimate ways in which social institutions and communities may licitly utilize and, in turn, limit access to scarce medical resources.

Drawing on the significant resources of the natural law tradition, Boyle provides a traditional Roman Catholic moral analysis. Although the Catholic tradition holds that for those who have received God's revelation pursuing health and the means to stay alive should not be of ultimate value, he argues that this does not mean that such natural human concerns are necessarily misguided or that nothing in this life is worth pursuing for its own sake. Rather, the Catholic tradition holds that life and health are among the basic goods of human persons as bodily creatures. As such, they provide legitimate reasons for action that are not reducible to merely instrumental concerns. Health is good bodily functioning, and being alive is a necessary condition for pursuing other goods as well as a part of the personal reality of existence as a human being. This means that life and health are intrinsically valuable and, as such, actions that promote life or protect health are choice-worthy. That an action enhances life or protects health provides a reason sufficient for choosing it; however, it is not necessarily a reason that morally justifies the action. Thus, even affluent societies will be required to make allocation decisions about how to divide public resources to health care. Not all health care that all may want or even may benefit from can or should necessarily be provided. This is in part due to the fact that health care makes open-ended, if not infinite, demands on resources. As Boyle argues, "All who become ill have reason to want effective care, and indeed the best possible care, and that reason persists even if reasonable preventative steps have been used and even after medical treatment has been successfully used" (91–92). Insofar as we can help others in respect to their health, we should.

Yet clinical rationing is clearly called for, he concludes, especially with regard to critical care, because it both is urgently needed to stabilize patients who have suffered trauma or surgery, and is too expensive and burdensome to provide to every patient who might receive some small benefit. It is, therefore, at least permissible for allocation decisions carefully to limit the availability of critical care resources as well as to determine for whom they ought to be made available. Here, Boyle argues, much moral deliberation consists in seeking to expose bias: "Are these favored areas for research and treatment favored because of the private interests of decision makers, researchers, physicians, or the class of patients they serve? Or do they reasonably serve the health interests of the community in ways better than or incomparable with alternative allocation policies?" (92). While all need not be provided with the very best of care, or even necessarily with equal care, social policy concerning limiting access to scare medical resources ought to serve the interests of the community.

Similarly, Seifert argues that the call for universal access to unlimited health care for the prolongation of life is practically unrealizable and morally objectionable as an idolatry of earthly life. Each person is believed to possess absolute dignity, Seifert argues, which implies that individuals have a legitimate sphere of freedom to reject even basic treatment for moral or religious duties. Patients may permissibly refuse excessively risky, expensive, or unusual surgery or other burdensome interventions. It is, therefore, inappropriate to force health care on patients—even beneficial care—without their consent. At the level of social policy, governments should not demand unlimited distribution of public funds for health services. Although health care is an important human good, it would be unacceptable to favor health care to the neglect of other central aspects of human life. Acknowledging unconditional respect for the dignity of each person does not imply that each receive unlimited access to all possible critical care. Rather, careful stewardship of critical care medicine necessarily involves value judgments regarding the proportionate use of health care. Obligations to pursue critical care are not defined solely by the utility of medical interventions, but rather must take into account their feasibility and costs; where "costs" includes financial, physical, psychological, social, moral, and spiritual burdens on patients, families, health care workers, and society.

Whereas particular treatments may be beneficial in themselves, they may still be licitly judged disproportionate and thus nonobligatory, especially when too difficult to obtain, too expensive, or otherwise too burdensome. Moreover, such care may be prohibitively expensive for public health care systems to provide. Although Seifert argues that certain ways of limiting access to medical care are inherently immoral (e.g., superficial secular judgments regarding quality of life), limiting access to the extent to which such care is rendered impossible for economic, scientific, or political reasons—or even if it truly imposes significant burdens on others—is morally legitimate.

Indeed, as Taboada argues, all have, at some point, a moral obligation to accept death. Provided that one does not intend to die, but rather faces a Christian death as an intimate aspect of Christian life, this is neither euthanasia nor suicide. Within Christian morality, Taboada argues, one must accept "(1) a subordination of the person and his acts to God; (2) the existence of a relation between the moral goodness of human acts and eternal life;

(3) the imitation of Christ, Who opens to the person the perspective of perfect love; and (4) the gift of the Holy Spirit, as source and strength of the moral life of Christians" (65). Although one may never intend death, one ought to live one's life and death in imitation of Christ. Christians do not worship life but accept the will of God. Even if available, it is not always morally appropriate to treat patients with aggressive curative care; such is especially inappropriate when either clinically futile or contrary to the patient's wishes. Where secular morality cannot comprehend the importance of a good death for personal salvation, a Christian death, Taboada concludes, requires acceptance of God's will upon us such that we live our deaths as a positive act of giving of ourselves.[7]

Both Honnefelder and Schotsmans consider the inherent dignity of persons foundational to any permissible public health care policy. According to Honnefelder, such dignity reflects a positive human right to health care. This necessarily limits, he argues, the use of the market to distribute health care. Justice must be the distributive mechanism, rather than market efficiency.[8] Where basic rights to health care are concerned, restrictions based on the scarcity of resources can be justified only as the result of triage. If all care cannot be provided, society must create difficult distinctions to screen out those treatments, the loss of which constitutes the lesser evil.

According to Schotsmans, human dignity grounds the principle of solidarity which, he argues, requires that all members of a society be provided with equal access to the very best of care. It is important, however, that he redefines "the best of care" as the amount of care that can be provided equally to all, even if financial feasibility necessitates screening out various treatments and procedures readily available in other parts of the world. Such treatments would never be offered simply because they would not be available. "The best of care means that every individual in society has at least equal access to the highest standard of medical treatment. I understand the 'highest standard' to mean that all services must be made ready so that appropriate medical care may be provided" (132). He addresses problems of scarcity in terms of macroallocation decisions that ensure equal access to the poor and the unemployed. Following the general lines of his argument, insofar as a society cannot afford expensive critical care for all, it may be morally required to adopt a lower standard of care, to which all are held. Centers of excellence that push the envelope of technology will only be morally permissible if equally accessible to all. No one ought to be allowed to purchase better basic health care or even additional life-sustaining critical care with private resources. Here appeal to the values of equality and solidarity appears to trump greater availability of critical care, as well as sustained development of high-technology medicine.

MORAL AND PUBLIC POLICY CHALLENGES

The next three chapters consider the implications of Roman Catholic moral theology regarding the macro-, meso-, and microlevel allocation of critical care medicine. While George Khushf is concerned with the development of institutional guidelines following the general lineaments of Roman Catholic morality, Cathleen Kaveny and Kevin Wildes each develops the implications of distributive justice. Whereas Kaveny views justice, solidarity, and equality as providing significant moral grounds for expanding access to crucial care, Wildes raises important objections to the use of coercive taxation to fund the increasingly extensive demands of health care.

When properly developed within a Christian health care institution, Khushf argues, critical care ought to manifest the integrated approach to the whole person that the church provides. In this way, health care becomes an integral part of the broader witness of Christianity. It thereby leads individuals to theologically grounded ways of living. Health care institutions, he argues, ought to approach the question of limiting access to scarce resources from a sacralizing, rather than secularizing, point of view. Where secular public policy debate focuses on questions of limiting access through economic necessity to medically indicated treatment, within Catholic institutions such policies should be situated within more fundamental reflections and assessments of the central mission and ends of such institutions. Institutional religious values should guide the appropriate distribution of critical care, integrating health care into a broader Christian spiritual outreach: "There should be a culture and practice of care that includes religious values unique to the institution" (172). In short, institutional policy ought always to make it clear that the hospital is a Christian, indeed Roman Catholic, institution addressing both medical and spiritual needs.

Yet, as Kaveny indicates, in seeking to allocate access to scarce resources, one must assess the ways in which various policies reflect to a greater or lesser extent Roman Catholic moral and spiritual commitments. For example: Would it ever be permissible for a patient to be discharged from an ICU in favor of a patient whose need was greater? What preference, if any, should the patient already occupying an ICU bed receive, especially if there are others in greater need who will be denied access? She considers each of the following possibilities: (1) that a patient, once admitted to an ICU bed, be virtually guaranteed to keep it, as long as the care received was not futile, which would protect the patient "against the vicissitudes of her performance on the scales of medical progress, and the competition of others who seek the same attention" (194), (2) that the patient currently in possession of the bed receive little or no preference anytime another patient would benefit more from the good, or (3) that a more objective index for initial admission to the critical care unit—such as a certain minimum or maximum APACHE III score—be used, but then that the patient not be deprived of her bed simply because someone with a better score comes along. Here, "a patient would need to fall below a minimum cutoff score . . . *and* have a score that is substantially lower than a new person presenting for care" (194). Both clinical considerations and moral theological concerns must coincide to determine how best to treat all in an equitable manner.

Independent of such meso- and microallocation questions are macrolevel concerns regarding state appropriation of private resources to purchase critical care for the poor. Although it is clear that ICUs save lives, must all available resources be provided to support critical care? Or is it permissible for individuals, institutions, and societies to allocate resources for other types of goods? As Wildes argues, "the Roman Catholic tradition has long made a distinction between our absolute duties (e.g., not intentionally taking innocent human life) and imperfect duties (e.g., the preservation of human life)."[9] The creation of greater social resources to support equal access to critical care resources for the impecunious necessarily involves more extensive taxation. Yet, "[t]axation policy ought not to stifle the freedom and creativity of individuals" (210). Private property is integral to the creation of important human goods. There must, therefore, be careful balancing between individuals' rights to property and perceived or actual social needs.

Unlike Schotsmans and Honnefelder, Wildes envisages a central role for a market in health care. If individuals are better off, in the sense of having greater access to health care with a market, there ought to be no objection. Indeed, to prohibit such a market could harm the poor, because they would be less well off than with other systems of distribution. Insofar as it is the most efficient producer of goods and services, the market can be seen as the best institution for producing and distributing goods and services.[10] Moreover, especially within developing countries, it might be more rational to focus on waste management and primary care rather than on expanding access to expensive critical care. Such policies will likely lead to significantly more community benefits, even in terms of their direct and indirect effects on health, than investments in critical care. Societies must balance the goods of critical care against other basic human needs, such as primary care, housing, food, and education.

CRITICAL COMMENTARY

When Western Christianity explicitly articulated its notions of proper medical deportment, it had already articulated its own beliefs and culture. Especially among Western Christianity of the High Middle Ages, as exemplified by Thomas Aquinas, these moral understandings were incorporated into Christian theological doctrine. This defended the ability of persons generally to understand the natural law: that there is an objective good for human beings (Aquinas, *ST* I-II, q. 94, a. 2c), which reason can articulate, thus justifying the general canons of moral behavior. Despite significant secularization following the Reformation, Western Christian reflection continued to have considerable influence. There remained in the West the attempt to fashion a rational justification for the general lineaments of Christian culture and moral intuitions, as well as for its fundamental social structures. The key question, however, is whether such a view can be sustained. In our contemporary secular, morally pluralistic society, the moral theological views of Roman Catholicism appear as but one perspective among many.

The next brace of essays considers the moral and theological insights of the Orthodox Jewish, Orthodox Christian, and Protestant Christian religions. Whereas Boyle and Seifert sought after content-full, generally available moral content through reason, and Schotsmans and Honnefelder argued from the inherent dignity of all persons to the importance of solidarity and equal access to critical care, Teodoro Dagi, Edward Hughes, and Dietrich Rössler each develops a more theologically grounded understanding of human nature and of one's obligations regarding the allocation of scarce health care resources. Only after these foundational theological grounds have been articulated and, more important, lived, will one be able to specify individual, institutional, and social obligations regarding access to scarce critical care resources.

For example, as Rie documents, "it is said in Jewish circles that one who saves a life saves a people" (43), which, he argues, captures an absolute respect for human life. However, any attempt to provide the very best care for all, without honest assessment of the economic realities of resource rationing, leads to serious, yet often unacknowledged, scarcity and the potential loss of salvageable patients. The question, then, is what limits—if any—may institutions or societies place on the allocation of scarce resources that would be consistent with the Jewish respect for human life? According to Dagi, when faced with allocation decisions, the canonical Jewish tradition requires that the decision be made along several axes: "[1] immediate and measurable, rather than theoretical, threats to life;

[2] identifiable endangered individuals, [3] specific remedies with predictable effects; [4] maximum number of souls rescued; [and] [5] measures intended to save the life of one individual are not to be compromised in order to rescue another" (230). Are there, then, limits to the obligation to rescue individuals? First, he argues that as a matter of public policy, it is reasonable to pursue the most pressing needs and the most efficient use of resources. Second, limitations may be imposed in particular cases because of the ineffectiveness of the interventions at hand. In neither case, however, is it permissible to ignore the needs of particular individuals because of the demands of public policy, such as abstract appeals to principles of equality or solidarity. In short, although one ought to pursue effective and efficient resource usage, the care provided to specific, named individuals with needs that develop out of a specific threat at a specific moment in time may not be compromised because of a theory of greater or community need.

From the perspective of Orthodox Christianity, Hughes indicates that the Roman Catholic focus—on institutional guidelines, social justice, and political mechanisms for rationing—is theologically shortsighted. Instead, like Dagi, Hughes focuses on personal obligations to patients themselves: those who must function within the health care system, however constructed. Traditional Christianity "concerned primarily with man's relationship with God and tied directly to that with each other, must necessarily value life and individual lives differently. Each life is an opportunity for some individual to enter into relationship with God . . . to try to judge a person's life in the light of his 'functioning' in the physical world without reference to relationships with other people and with his Creator is totally materialistic and, as such, truly inadequate to evaluate what is essentially a spiritual reality" (240). Given this circumstance, he concludes that the Christian community ought to operate hospitals at its own expense, which provide at nominal cost the best of care for all. Such care ought to focus not only on the base physical needs of patients, but on their deeper spiritual needs as well. This is not an appeal for more extensive state-based taxation to coerce compliance with a particular view of just health care for all, nor it is a claim regarding the positive rights of persons for equal access to critical care. Instead, it is the expression of a particular moral obligation that applies directly to Christians and the Christian community. Such care would not, however, focus only on the base physical needs of patients, but also on their deeper spiritual needs.

From a Protestant perspective, Rössler argues, unequal distribution of health care can be seen as morally acceptable. Protestant ethics, he argues, has no special reason to declare preferences in the allocation of scarce medical resources. Although patients may view their particular circumstances and personal suffering as unjust, and thereby as requiring the reallocation of resources to provide for health care, he argues that "Protestant ethics cannot make a practical distinction between misfortune and injustice in view of individual experience. . . . it is not the case that every misfortune is an injustice" (268). It may be true that illness is a misfortune, but it is not thereby an injustice that grounds a claim on the part of the ill to the resources of others. Rather, the insights of Protestant ethics allow the sick individual to perceive the moral and reflective aspects of his situation; to see, to seek, and to accept his fate. Within this fallen world, there is no reason or expectation that one must compensate for all personal misfortunes or disadvantages that are in some way due to "acts of God."

An additional difficulty for sustaining the particularities of the Roman Catholic perspective, as Corinna Delkeskamp-Hayes argues in her essay, is that the Roman Catholic concept of moral theology places Christian morality in a continuum with secular justice, because the general elements of Christian morality are supposedly open to natural reason without any particular belief in God or assistance from the Holy Spirit. The difficulty is that to maintain itself as Christian, Roman Catholics must show that "the Christian moral message—when stated in secularly comprehensible terms so as to render it realizable through secular political structures—neither loses its Christian credentials nor disrupts the integrity of secular political morality" (282). Alternatively, as James Heisig argues in his essay, Catholicism must divest itself of its universalistic claims and recast itself as merely one moral perspective among many. It is, as he says, "a call to purge Catholic tradition of its colonial vestiges and to turn the considerable resources of the church toward the preservation of cultural pluralism and alternative models of social order" (307). Although it is true, as Mary Ann Gardell Cutter documents in her essay, that appeal to reason only captures one aspect of Roman Catholic moral tradition, insofar as the particular content of Catholicism cannot be shown to be uniquely true through reason alone, there will be no reason, absent faith, to hold it to be the only possible moral content. There will then be a real distinction between what Christians may demand of themselves, of what is privately required, and what one will be able with moral authority to impose on others.

CONCLUSION

Opponents of a market in health care nearly always reflect a vision of social justice that calls into question the good fortunes of those who have more opportunities, wealth, and resources to purchase more extensive health care (Engelhardt 1999). Yet, from a general secular perspective, one is not in a position to recognize any particular vision of the good— of the good life for persons—as canonically binding on all. From a general secular perspective, one ought to recognize the guarantee of property rights and free collaboration as essential to human respect and dignity, despite inequalities (see Engelhardt 1996; Nozick 1974). To appropriately situate health care within one's life—as well as to fully appreciate the significance of human suffering, disease, and death—one must move beyond limited secular discourse to the content-full moral visions of the various religious traditions, as such should be brought to bear on bioethical concerns regarding the procurement, distribution, and allocation of health care. Obsession with secular concerns for social solidarity—and equally obscure Christian commitments to charity and altruism—obfuscate fundamental theological concerns for human dignity and sanctification.

However muddied the waters become as societies come to terms with the allocation of scarce health care resources, Christians should not accept secular views on human life, the status of the person, dignity, equality, and social solidarity as settling the issue. It is impossible to provide deep canonical meaning to moral concerns such as "human dignity" or "the sanctity of life" outside the perspective of particular moral and religious communities. As the authors in this volume make clear, arguments regarding the limiting of access to scarce medical resources must be located within the moral intuitions, ontological and political theoretical premises, and special moral concerns of the various religions. It is here that analysis of the procurement and allocation of scarce resources for health care ought to be located.

NOTES

1. These figures represent the international per capita spending on health care of the countries of the contributors to this volume: Joseph Boyle, Canada; Ludger Honnefelder, Dietrich Rössler, and Corinna Delkeskamp-Hayes, Germany; Paul Schotsmans, Belgium; and Josef Seifert, Austria.

2. As critical care resources become more constrained, individual caregivers and institutions must become more diligent regarding the selection of patients who should not receive intensive care, whether too healthy to require such care or too sick for the ICU to offer hope of recovery, and to refuse admission to or to discharge such patients from the ICU. Moreover, greater diligence must be given to tracking patients whose need for intensive care could have been prevented through provision of inexpensive therapeutic interventions. E.g., Rie argues that approximately 80 percent of the readmissions to the ICU for respiratory failure were potentially preventable. In most instances, the need for intensive care was precipitated by the absence or inadequacy of direct care to remove secretions from patients. "Even in secular terms these findings indicate violations of basic human decency as well as the needless waste of resources. This is low quality, low cost, fraudulent sale of health services, which may meet criminal negligence standards" (45). An initial criterion, he concludes, for the moral provision of critical care ought to be careful stewardship of the available resources, which would require providing inexpensive respiratory care beyond the ICU to prevent readmission costs and increased patient mortality.

3. As Hegel points out, determinative moral content requires the specification of a particular context: "Because every action explicitly calls for a particular content and a specific end, while duty as an abstraction entails nothing of the kind, the question arises: what is my duty? As an answer nothing is so far available except: (a) to do the right, and (b) to strive after welfare, one's own welfare, and welfare in universal terms, the welfare of others" (1967 [1821], § 134). Nothing particular follows from the general notions of duty, the right, etc. Even to sort useful information from noise, one must already possess a moral sense, standards of evidence and inference. That is, one must first specify a particular moral content within which to make decisions (see also McKenny 1999, 353).

4. As Kelly documents from the perspective of health care providers, "ordinary care" signifies standard, recognized, or established health care, at the standard of practice, but within the limits of availability (1960, 128–29).

5. Here one might consider the ways in which nonspecific, denominationally neutral religion and generic chaplains have been integrated into the health care services of many hospitals. As Engelhardt documents: "They have been hired to provide spiritual care, but the nature of that care is left strategically under-defined. Were the spiritual care specifically defined in denominational terms, it would take on a particular religious, that is, exclusionary character. But the latter is not the care sought from chaplaincy services by many hospitals. Instead, the chaplain is expected to attend to a patient population drawn from many religions, Christian and non-Christian, as well as those fully unchurched. Ministers who were once ordained in particular religions are reprofessionalized into trans-denominational roles. Institutional expectations reshape their vocation into the role of generic chaplains" (Engelhardt 1998, 32). For an important exception to such nondenominational Christian bioethics, see Engelhardt 2000.

6. In short, although the commandment "Thou shalt not kill" expresses an absolute moral prohibition that shapes Roman Catholic reflection on permissible biomedical interventions and public health care policy, technological expansion of the boundaries of life can blind one to the fact that the imperative is not: "Thou shalt never die": "The horror of

'just letting someone die' stems from a faulty appreciation of what this life is and of what the next life is. Our tenacity in holding to life is dictated by the natural law and strengthened by the commandment, 'Thou shalt not kill.' Yet we have to remember that the natural law and the commandment do not say, 'Thou shalt never die'" (Finney and O'Brien 1956, 260).

7. According to Breshnahan, Catholic moral theology has long urged "(1) that we learn a sober realism about human limits and accept death as a normal event; (2) that we see mere biological survival as not the only good, or even, in given circumstances, the highest good; (3) that we recognize moral ambiguity in our use of high technology and the possibility that cure-oriented treatment may be disproportionate and unreasonable; (4) that we accept the judgments of dying persons about the proportionality of benefits and burdens of treatment, unless such decisions are clearly unreasonable, undeniably suicidal, so doubtfully rational and free; and (5) that we act in accordance with our long moral tradition that supports the moral acceptability, indeed often the moral obligation of using adequate analgesics to relieve suffering in the dying even though we may accelerate the process of dying as an indirect 'side effect'" (1995, 258–59).

8. Similarly, Sulmasy argues that equal access to health care is more important than more efficient distribution or greater access to medical technology: "Even if it were most efficiently distributed via market mechanisms, efficiency and individual liberty ought not to be given moral hegemony over the fundamental respect for human dignity that is required of a just system of health care" (1996, 312).

9. Here one might consider that the duty to aid others in grave temporal need does not usually require that others be assisted in ways that would be of serious inconvenience to oneself. As Jone argues: "In *grave spiritual or temporal need* our neighbor must be helped in as far as this is possible without serious inconvenience to ourselves. Position, justice, or piety may oblige one to make such a sacrifice" (1960, 80). With regard to ordinary need, one must help the impecunious in general from one's superfluous possessions (82). Equal opportunity, property, or even health care are not generally required.

10. As Friedman argues, "the market is, generally speaking, the best set of institutions we know of for producing and distributing things. The more important a good is, the stronger the argument for having it produced by the market. Both barbers and physicians are licensed; both professions have for decades used licensing to keep their numbers down and their salaries up. Government regulation of barbers makes haircuts more expensive; one result, presumably, is that we have fewer haircuts and longer hair. Government regulation of physicians makes medical care more expensive; one result, presumably, is that we have less medical care and shorter lives. Given the choice of deregulating one profession or the other, I would choose the physicians" (1991, 302).

Moreover, it is possible charitably to intend the good of others through for-profit market transactions. Although the virtue of charity is often understood as a benevolent disposition toward others and their welfare, to the relief of suffering, the bestowal of gifts, and other similar actions, Christian charity traditionally focused on the love of others for God. As McHugh and Callan summarize this theological virtue: "Charity refers to divine love, that is, to the love of God for man or the love of man for God. Here, we are considering charity as the virtue by which the creature loves God for His own sake, and others on account of God . . ." (1960, 454). Charity, so understood, is consistent with the market. Among the examples of charity, McHugh and Callan list: "in a wide sense, almsgiving includes selling on credit as a favor to a poor customer; a loan granted at a low rate of interest or without interest, help in securing employment, etc." (495). Assisting others through the market can be a significant act of charity.

BIBLIOGRAPHY

Aquinas, T. 1981. *Summa Theologiae*, trans. by Fathers of the English Dominican Province. Westminster, Md.: Christian Classics.

ATS Board of Directors Position Statement. 1997. Fair allocation of intensive care unit resources. *American Journal of Respiratory Critical Care Medicine* 156: 1282–1301.

Basil, Saint. 1962. Ascetical works: The long rules. In *The Fathers of the Church*, ed. by R. J. Deferrari et al.; trans. by Sister M. M. Wagner, C.S.C. Washington, D.C.: Catholic University of America Press.

Breshnahan, J. 1995. Observations on the rejection of physician-assisted suicide: A Roman Catholic perspective. *Christian Bioethics* 1: 256–84.

Chalfin D. B., I. L. Cohen, and J. Lambrinos. 1995. The economics and cost-effectiveness of critical care medicine. *Intensive Care Medicine* 21: 952–61.

Cherry, M. 1996. Suffering strangers: An historical, metaphysical, and epistemological non-ecumenical interchange. *Christian Bioethics* 2: 253–66.

Engelhardt, H. T., Jr. 1994. Health care reform: A study in moral malfeasance. *Journal of Medicine and Philosophy* 19: 501–16.

———. 1996. *The Foundations of Bioethics*. New York: Oxford University Press.

———. 1998. Generic chaplaincy: Providing spiritual care in a post-Christian age. *Christian Bioethics* 4: 231–38.

———. 1999. The body for fun, beneficence, and profit: A variation on a post-modern theme. In *Persons and Their Bodies: Rights, Responsibilities, Relationships*, ed. by M. J. Cherry. Dordrecht: Kluwer Academic Publishers.

———. 2000. *The Foundations of Christian Bioethics*. Lisse: Swets and Zeitlinger Publishers.

Finney, P., C.M., and P. O'Brien, C.M. 1956. *Moral Problems in Hospital Practice; A Practical Handbook*. Saint Louis: Herder.

Friedman, D. 1991. Should medicine be a commodity? An economist's perspective. In *Rights to Health Care*, ed. by T. J. Bole and W. B. Bondeson. Dordrecht: Kluwer Academic Publishers.

Hegel, G. W. F. 1967 [1821]. *Philosophy of Right*, trans. by T. M. Knox. Oxford: Oxford University Press.

Jone, H. 1960. *Moral Theology*. Westminister, Md.: Newman Press.

Kelly, G. 1960. *Medico-Moral Problems*. Dublin: Clonmore and Reynolds.

McHugh, J., and C. Callan. 1960. *Moral Theology*. New York: Joseph F. Wagner.

McKenny, G. 1999. The integrity of the body: Critical remarks on a persistent theme in bioethics. In *Persons and Their Bodies: Rights, Responsibilities, Relationships*, ed. by M. J. Cherry. Dordrecht: Kluwer Academic Publishers.

Nozick, R. 1974. *Anarchy, State, and Utopia*. New York: Basic Books.

OECD (Organization for Economic Cooperation and Development). 2000. *OECD Health Data 2000*. Paris: OECD.

Pappachan, J. V., B. Millar, E. D. Bennett, and G. B. Smith. 1999. Comparison of

APACHE III outcome from intensive care admission after adjustment for case mix by the APACHE III prognostic system. *Chest* 115 (3): 802–10.

Sulmasy, D. P., O.F.M. 1996. Do the bishops have it right on health care reform? *Christian Bioethics* 2: 309–25.

Wood, K. E., D. B. Coursin, and R. M. Grounds. 1999. Critical care outcomes in the United Kingdom: Sobering wake-up call or stability of the lamppost? *Chest* 115 (3): 614–16.

PART II

A Moral Consensus Statement

Consensus Statement

WORKING GROUP ON ROMAN CATHOLIC APPROACHES TO DETERMINING APPROPRIATE CRITICAL CARE

I. PREFACE

A.   The self-identification of the working group: we are a group of academics from around the world, including theologians, philosophers, physicians, and a lawyer, convened by H. Tristram Engelhardt, Jr. The Roman Catholics among us represent a wide range of Catholic theological opinion. Others in the group represent other Christian and Jewish perspectives and first-hand medical experience of the issues we consider. We have met four times over three years, and have read and discussed each others' contributions to this project, thus creating an interlocking set of essays on determining appropriate critical care.

B.   The subject matter of this project: we are concerned with ethical and religious issues raised by critical care, and most especially with the grounds for limiting access to critical care. We are concerned to explore how and to what extent Roman Catholic moral theology and the broader Catholic worldview, including its spiritual and sacramental view of life, can shed light on these issues. Those who participated in various steps of the drafting of this statement include: Joseph Boyle, Mark J. Cherry, Mary Ann Gardell Cutter, T. Forcht Dagi, Corinna Delkeskamp-Hayes, H. Tristram Engelhardt, Jr., James Heisig, Ludger Honnefelder, Edward Hughes, M. Cathleen Kaveny, George Khushf, Michael Rie, Dietrich Rössler, Josef Seifert, Paulina Taboada, and Kevin Wm. Wildes. Being named in this list does not imply full concurrence with all parts of the statement, as section V B below emphasizes.

II. EPISTEMOLOGICAL ISSUES

A.   Why the focus on critical care?

1.   Critical care has become an icon for current, high-tech, aggressive intervention medicine. The use of high-tech equipment and specially trained personnel seems to promise help even in the most desperate situations, but also predictably causes the painful prolongation of agony for many patients and families.

2.   Critical care is very expensive in comparison to other kinds of health care; a critical care bed is three times as expensive as a normal hospital bed; 15–20

percent of health care costs are directed to critical care. This raises questions of fairness in the use of scarce resources.

3. There are good, evidence-based outcome data in this area. Because of the close monitoring in intensive care units, there is an extensive body of information about the outcomes of critical care for various kinds of patients. Indeed, tracking patients who use ICUs has allowed the development of prognostic assessments which allow evidence-based predictions about the utility of ICU care for various kinds of patients. Consequently, there is a well-established empirical basis for evaluating the potential benefit and burden of critical care in particular cases.

4. Critical care, therefore, provides a sharp focus for moral questions about limiting health care and about coming to terms with evidence-based medicine.

B. Issues of normative epistemology

1. The Roman Catholic moralists involved in our project all accepted that Catholic moral thinking rests on God's particular revelation, culminating in Jesus, and on the moral principles and norms human beings are capable of understanding independently of Divine Revelation, that is, through the natural law.

2. There are as many views among us about the exact boundaries and areas of overlap between these sources of moral knowledge, as there are within the broad Catholic community. In particular, there is some disagreement about the precise authority of the church's teaching office—the magisterium—in interpreting these sources of moral knowledge.

3. Still, participants in the project, both the Catholics and the others, saw within the wide tradition of Catholic moral theology several grounds for agreeing on some general ethical and religious propositions relevant to critical care, as well as some rather specific norms and guidelines.

III. PRINCIPLES

A. Dogmatic: several particular elements of the Roman Catholic worldview, shared in some measure with many other Christians and human beings, have important implications for the care of the very ill and dying generally and for the care of those facing the prospect of death in an intensive care unit. We agree that these particular convictions of Catholics have practical implications to which Catholic hospitals should give priority and for which secular health care facilities should make room. These are:

1. The finitude of human life and the inevitability of death for all of us.

2. The redemptive value of suffering, as awareness of the fallen condition of humankind and as a way to identify with the saving work of Christ and to call forth acts of solidarity and of compassion.

3. The importance of proper preparation for death: there are often obligations to be discharged before death; sacramental and spiritual preparation for death and judgment and eternal life is a grave duty for the ill and for caregivers; the results for those who die can be of ultimate significance.

B. Certain ethical norms, deeply rooted in the Christian moral tradition, have relevance to critical care. These are:

1. The Fifth Comandment, "Thou shalt not kill," is directly relevant to critical care because of the possibility that critical care decisions will be made to end life or precisely to shorten it. It is more broadly relevant to critical care because it underlines to the dignity of each human life.
2. The commandment to love one's neighbor as oneself grounds not only the negative precepts of the decalogue but several positive obligations to help others, including the positive obligation to care for the needy and the ill even when cure is impossible, and the limit of this obligation: never to abandon a patient.
3. The same fundamental moral impulse, grounded in the requirement to love one's neighbors as oneself, requires solidarity at the level of social organization and the use of political authority to support smaller groups and individuals in their response to the demands of solidarity. So, the duties to care and not abandon are duties of communities, including political societies, not only of individuals and families.
4. Given the connection between health and human dignity, solidarity and subsidiarity imply a natural right to health care. Societies capable of organizing to provide for the basic health care of their citizens are obliged to do so. And rich individuals and societies are obliged to help the poor to get basic health care, and poor countries to organize to provide health care to their citizens. But whether or not a society implements a right to health, the need for limiting some kinds of care remains, even though the morally imperative implementation of this right can mitigate the extent of the problem.
5. Some moral considerations in addition to general moral precepts are needed for the guidance of the lives of good people and communities. These considerations are often called practical wisdom or "prudence" in its pre-modern, non-egoistic sense. Although there is much dispute among Catholics about the exact workings of practical wisdom, it deals with issues of proportionality and disproportionality of actions and projects, not in a narrow technical way but against the horizon of a unified Christian life, well lived. That horizon is at least in part shaped by the commitments a Christian makes in response to the particular call of God for his or her life, made in prayerful discernment of God's will. Practical wisdom is needed to deal well with issues caused by the need to limit critical care.

IV. APPLICATIONS

A. The reality of critical care:

1. Critical care takes place in an intensive care unit, but its reality is not that of a place in a hospital, but a set of technologically sophisticated and labor intensive medical services, in particular, monitoring services.
2. Critical care was developed to monitor patients who were being stabilized after surgery or trauma. As such, critical care is an essential component of modern

medicine—a necessary condition for much surgery and a lifesaver for those needing close monitoring. Critical care can be used for other medical purposes. It can, for example, help to extend the life of person who is dying from cancer or congestive heart failure or provide a carefully monitored environment for PVS patients. But critical care was not designed for such purposes and likely would not exist if they were the only purposes it served. Patient-centered and justice-based considerations converge to suggest that critical care services should be restricted to patients who can get medical benefit from the careful monitoring critical care provides.

3. The common culture of critical care, based on sophisticated monitoring equipment and a medical ethos of rapid intervention, exists and is affected by cultural differences around the world and leads to very different levels in quality and quantity of critical care due to economic variations.

B. Some agreed-upon guidelines:

1. There are different levels of social organization at which questions of justice arise. The duty of political society to organize health care in concrete ways so that people's needs are met is important but not sufficient to guarantee good allocation decisions or satisfy the requirements of justice. Allocation decisions within a society's organization of health care, for example, in hospital systems or clinically within hospitals and departments, are required. Worldwide issues of justice, difficult as they are to formulate and address, must also be addressed.

2. Medical treatment, including that which makes use of evidence-based medicine, is distinct from and not as morally basic as basic care. The former can be terminated for patient based reasons, futility, or justice-based reasons. The latter may never be completely terminated; that would be abandonment of a needy human being.

3. Decisions to limit access to critical care must attend to the plurality of values affected by these decisions. A Christian hierarchy of values that respects the dignity of each person's life but does not absolutize the value of extending life at the cost of other important values, for example, those listed in section III A above.

4. Among the considerations relevant to decisions to refuse, withhold, or limit medical treatments are the riskiness of the procedures, the pain and suffering they involve, and the costs broadly understood—expense and use of resources, including the time and effort of trained personnel.

5. Futility is not a helpful category in approaching decisions to limit critical care. Strict futility would exclude very few from critical care or other medical treatment; when the notion is expanded so as to allow it to function as a criterion of exclusion, it ceases to designate futility but instead refers to value judgments that should be clearly stated for what they are.

6. The use of externally imposed constraints on the medically appropriate use of critical care facilities is wrong. For example, insurance-driven or bureaucrati-

cally created time limits on the use of intensive care units are wrong. It should be possible to keep people in intensive care as long as it is therapeutically beneficial and to remove them when it is clear that it is not beneficial or only disproportionately so.

7. Just allocation policies must be based on publicly accessible and contestable procedures. Health care facilities and physicians owe it to patients and their families clearly to state such policies.

V. FURTHER WORK

A.   Two areas in which we agree further work is required:

1. There are questions which health care institutions need to address: Catholic institutions must face starkly the possible conflicts between the culture of intensive care and the obligations to prepare for death. Other institutions must attend more fully to the fact that their patients often have religious concerns for which institutional space must be made.

2. The questions raised by the international and intercultural dimensions of critical care are very difficult. On the one hand, Catholics hold that natural law provides some universal precepts. Among them is the imperative to share the benefits of our way of life. On the other hand, we recognize that the technological and cultural forms in which most of us live are of contingent and particular value. We are for the most part modern Western Europeans and North Americans who cannot speak for humanity and can pretend to do so only most offensively.

B.   An area where disagreement exists among us:

1. The forty-year-long debates among Roman Catholic moralists focused on proportionalism and double effect are represented among the Catholic moralists in this working group, and have not been settled among us by our discussions about limiting critical care. These disagreements concerning basic moral concepts are likely to mark differences in the interpretation of the Fifth Commandment and of its application in casuistry. Although we did not find important areas of the specific issue of limiting critical care to be affected by these differences, the suspicion remains that there are many particular cases of withholding and limiting treatment where the disagreements on Catholic moral theory would lead to contrary judgments.

PART III

The Challenges of Critical Care: High Technology, Rising Costs, and Guarded Promises

Respect for Human Life in the World of Intensive Care Units: Secular and Reform Jewish Reflections on the Roman Catholic View

Michael A. Rie

In this volume, Roman Catholic scholars attempt to synthesize those features of Catholic theology that might impart a distinct vision of resource allocation in critical care settings. In the twentieth century, critical care medicine and intensive care units were the site of significant technological and medical progress. Economic resource allocation and consumption issues developed in parallel with such short- and long-term prognostic possibilities for the prolongation of life. For example, as early as 1957 Pope Pius XII was asked to explicate a Catholic moral position regarding the use of critical care technology for individuals with severe brain injuries. Secular ethics has also struggled with these and similar problems. Indeed, physicians generally have been confronted with such questions for some time (see, e.g., LeMaire 1996; Lanken, Terry, and Osborne 1997; Osborne and Patterson 1996; Society of Critical Care Medicine Ethics Committee 1997).

The authors of this volume have come to a general consensus regarding the implications of Roman Catholic moral theology for the allocation of critical care resources. As a non-Christian, non–Roman Catholic, it appears to me that Catholics hold "respect for human life" to be a central principle. Jews hold a similar principle and share a common heritage. Whereas Catholic theology appears to support the view that all human life is sacred, it is said in Jewish circles that one who saves a life saves a people. Such principles come under serious challenge, however, in intensive care units (ICUs), where accepting the sacredness of all human life as an absolute principle may lead, contradictorily, to the loss of salvageable human life through less than optimal care for all. Attempting to provide the very best of care for all, without any honest assessment of resource rationing, leads to serious, yet often unacknowledged, scarcity and the loss of salvageable patients. This circumstance underlies my reflections in this chapter.

Although high-technology critical care is a feature of affluent societies, critical care takes on a very different character in the world of poor nations. Even among rich nations, there is a variability of outcomes from intensive care incident to the ability of such countries to supply greater or lesser resources to critical care (Pappachan et al. 1999; Wood, Coursin, and Grounds 1999). The United Kingdom, for example, expends much less money per capita for critical care services than the United States. When the same objective measurement system is applied to the severity of illness in British ICUs and U.S. ICUs, Pappachan and Wood and colleagues each puzzle regarding why the outcomes of intensive care are qualitatively and quantitatively lower in the United Kingdom than in the United States. Rather than acknowledging the declining quality of care associated with the allocation of fewer resources, each group of authors (having studied the entire Southwest of England) wonders whether such differences in life expectancy and quality of life are due to measurement problems or definitional problems in the United Kingdom versus the United States. Yet, the virtue of an objective system of measurement (such as the Acute Physiology and Chronic Health Evaluation, or APACHE III scoring system) is that it obtains external, third-party, standardized measurements, rather than the subjective measurements of those who evaluate their own performance. Use of objective measurements allows one to compare outcomes across large populations of ICUs and classes of patients. Such prognostic scoring systems are scientifically powerful instruments for determining when we are on the proximal declining vector of a cost-benefit curve. Altering scoring criteria by location or country obfuscates critical data and supports the misallocation of funds, which costs lives.

Physicians, who care for critically ill patients, believe that when they are able to help people substantively to recover from serious illness and to take up independent healthy lives, it is a societal injustice and a violation of professional moral integrity for salvageable people to die, while dying patients continue to receive equal or greater quantities of communal resources. Whether one is Catholic, Jewish, or devoutly secular, individuals demand miraculous cures. They want to prolong human life, even if only for a short time, provided that patients are not intolerably suffering. The moral importance of such prognostic data for Catholic theology is clear: If all are to be treated equally and if all human life is precious, it is morally inappropriate for salvageable human life to be lost in the breach of medical mediocrity, while scarce resources are spent on the short-term prolongation of life for the dying.

Here, central conceptual concerns include concepts of wellness and health as the end point of any health insurance system. Managed care principles with their emphasis on inexpensive but effective preventative medicine ought to find a home in the Catholic view of the social community. Yet, people will be born, live, and die even if we allocate all of our resources to prevention (see, e.g., Aaron and Schwartz 1990; Berk and Monheit 1992; Millman and Robertson Actuaries 1994). Indeed, the banner of prevention has often been a distraction, because the care of more than 90 percent of the population consumes less than 10 percent of the available financial and technology resources within the U.S. system. Because there are currently no adequate systems for measuring the consequences of translocating resources to prevention from therapeutic uses in hospitals and ICUs, I have urged the further development of objective measurement science with regard to negative outcome assessment for the ICU (Rie 1997). This measurement has been termed Continuous Quality Decrement (CQD) or Negative Outcomes Measurement Benchmarking. One purpose of this essay is to give a discrete example of this science and to demonstrate that it requires a large-scale investment in objective external standardized measurement systems performed upon health institutions and health providers. It is generally assumed that providers ought to perform quality assurance and accountability measurements (see Kaiser Conference 1997). Yet, in the United States, there are no quality standards established by the U.S. government to indicate when hospitals and physicians perform with sufficient competence to justify the receipt of tax dollars for patient care. Instead of medical standards of care, legal accountability has centered around whether there has been fraudulent submission of bills, duplicate requests for payment, undocumented service delivery, and so on. I contend that quality assurance must include standards for assessing declining quality of care, especially when quality of care degrades without either notification to or consent from those receiving such care. If people could know what financial inputs were necessary to achieve the desired outputs from a health care system, they would then be free to choose those levels of care they wish to purchase, as well as those levels that should be shunned as unworthy of purchase. This would create the basis for an honest market for health care. In the absence of such information, providers and payers are free to make all kinds of assertions which cannot be independently and externally verified. This is equally true for national health care systems with centralized resource control.

My purpose here is twofold. First, I give a discrete example of CQD measures that can be derived from prognostic scoring methods. My example does not rely directly on ICU care; rather, recent epidemiology supports the conclusion that inexpensive, low-quality, basic care of hospital patients results in the return of patients, who were initially at low risk of death, to the ICU. Such patients are dying with increasing frequency, at great financial expenditure, due to the lack of quality inexpensive prevention care. Even in secular terms, these findings indicate violations of basic human decency as well as the needless waste of resources. This is low-quality, low-cost, fraudulent sale of health services, which may meet criminal negligence standards.

Second, I offer an account of "Jewishness" with respect to appropriate resource allocation in circumstances in which one knows, or should have known, that resource constriction without adequate outcomes assessment in health care would lead to serious moral violations. The Union of American Hebrew Congregations Bioethics Program Guide VII, titled "Allocation of Scarce Medical Resources as a Basic Foundation of Jewish Thinking Regarding Resource Allocation in the Jewish Tradition," provides insight into content-full Jewish morality. This document was produced in 1994 and is available through the Union of American Hebrew Congregations (UAHC 1994). It is more of a set of serious reflections than a concrete policy proposal.

In the section titled "Allocation of Scarce Resources," Rabbi Richard F. Address of Philadelphia states:

> The mood that then emerges from our tradition seems to follow several currents. We understand that one life is equal to the next and that one may not say that mine is more or less important than any other life. Thus we cannot take steps to actively destroy another life for our benefit. We understand that in certain situations choices must be made regarding allocation of resources especially in critical illness situations. Doing nothing and allowing people to die when some can be saved is not a Jewish value. As to whom to choose, "it must be on purely medical grounds, select-

ing the one who has a better chance of benefiting from the remedy." The mood of our tradition then underscores the fundamental value of life, its quality, and the principle that in deciding whom to allocate scarce resources, the choice is to be made based upon which person would receive the greatest benefit from those resources. (UAHC 1994)

I take this view to be central to a sense of "Reform Jewishness" as a critical care physician. If the institutional epidemiology shows that this principle is being violated, then all elements of the system conspire to be disrespectful of human life, at least in terms of the faith tradition that I understand and know.

This fundamental nature of "Jewishness" permits reflective Jewish physicians and nurses to understand that certain activities in our health care system reach levels of performance with demonstrated mediocrity, as well as negative or declining performance outcomes, systematically increasing death rates of salvageable patients. I argue that this constitutes "a crime against humanity," which Reform Jewish physicians are morally required to oppose. The tradition should provide independent guidance to physicians apart from the potential criminal nature of "secular quality fraud." The duty to allocate resources to preserve human life based on verifiable medical criteria ought to be understood as a religious imperative. Should I fail to follow such a system, then I fail to act as a faithful Reform Jewish physician (UAHC 1994).[1]

MANAGED CARE SOCIAL RESEARCH WITHOUT CONSENT: THE NUREMBERG CODE OF ETHICS, JEWISHNESS, AND CATHOLICNESS

Since World War II, Jews around the world have reexamined their faith with regard to the Holocaust. One of the byproducts of the Holocaust was the review of medical research conducted on prisoners in concentration camps, human rights abuses of prisoners, and the extent to which such activities constituted crimes against humanity. Much of the relevant information has been culled into a conference volume (Annas and Grodin 1992). The concepts which led to the Nuremberg Code were that to experiment or to conduct research activities upon either research subjects or medical patients without informed consent was an internationally recognized immoral act. This code eventually entered the structure of funding for medical research and other types of serious research in nonmedical fields involving human subjects.

It has been pointed out (Rie 1995a, 1995b, 1997; Engelhardt and Rie 1986, 1992; 1999, 367–79) that it is possible to conceptualize a measurement of CQD as an assessment of objective negative outcomes. CQD has been defined as the inverse of Continuous Quality Improvement (CQI), generally acknowledged in industry and health care. Though some types of decrements may be unavoidable, when quality declines in significant magnitude the circumstance warrants moral and religious reflection. It is not the purpose of this paper to establish that level of decrement. However, insofar as systematic mediocrity leads to statistically significant increases in the death of salvageable individuals, especially those who could have been saved at low cost, then there must be systemwide accountability. Such an account ought to be reflected in moral theology. The death of salvageable patients through inattentive health care policy is a form of care that faithful Catholics should avoid. Indeed, as I will argue, such systematic mediocrity constitutes per se violation of the Nuremberg Code of Ethics, since it is an example of de facto nonconsensual human experimentation leading to immoral outcomes in health care.

Given Roman Catholic understandings of the infinite value of human life, it is morally illicit to incur deaths though "quality fraud" whether from private greed or governmental policy. As I have pointed out under the banner of the "Schindler-Wiesenthal Dilemma" (Rie 1995a, 1995b), as resources become constricted, a tremendous moral dilemma arises for individual caregivers, and health care institutions, to select patients who should not receive care or to limit the amount of time that patients receive care. In the absence of honest confrontation with the first two options, resource scarcity forces the move to a general mediocritization of the care given. Should excessive preventable death of salvageable patients become a statistically significant and demonstrated outcome of such resource attrition, then Catholic moral theology would have the opportunity to articulate that some forms of care would not be requisite in this life for a faithful Catholic to find salvation with Jesus in the next life. Of course the societal context of basic health care needs might preclude any Catholic view or might favor limited critical care.

For the Jew, life is infinitely precious. But to what extent should Jews, Catholics, or anybody impoverish themselves, or their community, to acquire more marginal care at higher costs either at the very end of life or which will only extend life for a brief period? Providing all such care would require a religious community to impoverish itself unless it adequately dealt with the issue of resource allocation. For Jews, it would be a direct violation of Yahweh's Commandments to Moses to fail to continue to procreate the Jewish community, Jewish thought, and Jewish morality to successor generations ad infinitum. Thus, mindless consumption of resources for health care, especially critical care, and its overall drain on community resources, can be seen as a direct violation of the Jewish tradition. It is clear on moral grounds that Reform Jews ought not to subscribe to such expenditures.[2]

Recent reports indicate (Rie and Glessner 1999a, 1999b) a high incidence of readmission to the ICU of patients who should not have required readmission, but for whom medical mediocrity directly contributed to physiological difficulties, and thus the need for critical care. This study looked only at patients previously admitted with what is termed "low risk death and low risk monitor" readmission status. A low-risk monitor readmission in APACHE terminology is a patient who is predicted only to need acute monitoring care without major therapeutic intervention. A low-risk-of-death patient is one for whom there is a risk-stratified death prediction of less than 10 percent at the time of initial ICU admission. Following these patients, the data revealed approximately a 10 percent rate of readmission to ICU occurs when on a risk-stratified basis it should have been less than 5 percent. Further analysis of respiratory readmissions indicated that of the patients readmitted for respiratory failure, about 80 percent of the failures were potentially preventable, and in most instances the readmission was due seemingly to absence or inadequacy of direct care involving removal of secretions from patients to prevent respiratory failure and death. Upon reassessment, when these patients were readmitted to the ICU, their morbidity and mortality scores had significantly increased. Indeed, their mortality was significantly out of proportion to what would have been predicted had these patients been an original ICU admission (see also Chen et al. 1997; Cullen et al. 1995; Leape et al. 1995). In addition, the data indicated that a more cost-effective stewardship of resources results if more respiratory care is given beyond the ICU to prevent readmission costs and increased patient mortality (see, e.g., Institute for Healthcare Improvement 1997). Some will argue that this simply means that hospitals should readjust the efficiency of how they deploy their budgets. This assertion is open to question if the entire system is under financial stringency to cut its resources across the board because of an overall stricture of funding. The ability scientifically to disclose CQDs provides the evidence base for "Negative Outcomes Quality Assessment." At the same time, it provides a moral "prosecutorial database" in a longer historical framework for those who have conspired systematically to lower the level of care to people as a matter of financial managed care. In short, this circumstance constitutes social experimentation without public disclosure or individual informed consent. This is an example of quality fraud in medical outcomes.

As I indicate what I consider to be crimes against humanity in health resource allocation, I take as my example the life and research of a famous Jewish scholar, Shimon Dubnow. Dubnow was a historian who lived in Eastern Europe in the first part of the twentieth century and who wrote a definitive history of the years 1939–40. He had previously been a professor in Berlin in the 1920s and had returned to Eastern Europe. He chose to stay in Eastern Europe even though he had the opportunity to leave with the arrival of German occupation at the beginning of World War II. He was not a Zionist, and actually wanted to preserve the Jewish culture in Eastern Europe. He stayed in the ghetto in Riga and was finally killed by his former graduate student, Johann Siebert, who was the director of the Gestapo in Riga. As he was slaughtered together with the chief rabbi of Riga for infuriating the Gestapo director, his final words were reportedly: "Jews, remember, remember [in Yiddish: *Schreibt un verschreibt*], write down everything." This adage has become a testament that every survivor and every Jew wanted to follow so as to become a witness. In Dubnow's case, he infuriated the Gestapo director by writing down the precise number of Jews and others who had been slaughtered in the forests outside of Riga when Siebert arrogantly proclaimed this to him. According to the account of Elie Wiesel, the slaughter of Dubnow occurred when he took out a piece of paper and asked again what the precise number of people slaughtered in the forest might be and wrote it down. Dubnow was then asked whether he was still a humanist who believed in the human species and he answered yes, whereupon he and the rabbi were killed (Wiesel 1992).

The message from Dubnow is that one must always document the truth. I add to the burden of the Catholic theologians the issue of defining Catholic immorality regarding the care of sick people. Clearly, any physician devoted to the care of the sick will be most concerned about diminishing the quality of care given to patients. Paulina Taboada makes a valiant step in her essay in this volume, stating simply that as physicians, if we are unable to offer that standard of care which we would normally be able to provide in critical care, it would be better to provide it to lesser numbers but to maintain the standard. We should not diminish the general standard and promote mediocrity as our new de facto degenerate professional integrity. If physicians permit themselves to practice a mediocre standard of medicine, even as the de facto result of insufficient resources, we become historical coconspirators to the denigration of the infinite value of human life, which is a violation of both Jewish and Catholic morality.

Although Kevin Wildes in his essay addresses the issue of the limits of moral taxation for health care and gives us an overview of where the Catholic moral tradition might address broader health policy issues, as a physician I am unable to comment on this broad vision. This essay situates itself along the lines of the ways in which resource insufficiency, together with dishonesty, promotes medical mediocrity, including moral pains and conflicts for those who care for the sick, and the challenges such difficulties pose to religious tradition. The thesis continues to be that a society that has insufficient resources to meet Promethean standards of care and does not acknowledge that circumstance with respect to the relative outcomes of its critical care system, is a false bearer of respect for human life. I agree with Wildes that Catholic, Jewish, or secular thought might favor less critical care under a wide variety of resource considerations. This certainly does not create a religious mandate to spend more than we have to spend. If the central bodies of theological thinking and articulation cannot provide direction for physicians, nurses, and other health care professionals, then at least those providers should not become coconspirators in the dishonest and unacknowledged continual quality decline within health systems. Unfortunately, here most religious traditions, including Roman Catholicism, are silent. If we are unable to affect the public disclosure of resource allocation, either through diminished number or quality of services, then, consistent with the spirit of Dubnow, we must become documentors of the truth and provide written witness so that it will find resolution at a later date. At least in Jewish history, there is long patience. We must arm ourselves with the truth and witness to that truth while the religious traditions in which we live accommodate and come to accept resource allocation in critical care medicine.

In the United States, there is general belief that there has been a failure to disclose quality outcome measures under systems of managed health care. There is further public concern that accountability for resource attrition mischief can be correlated with human injury and that those who have diminished resources in either private or public insurance should be held liable because they did not inform patients of the diminishing quality of care or of the likely outcomes of such care. At what point is the systematic injury of a population, absent a specific public rationing policy, a form of overt disrespect for human life, according to Catholics? What is at issue is a moral understanding of the respect for human life as it applies to organizational distribution of resources within a health insurance plan. Regardless of one's religious tradition, it is unlikely that individuals will want excessive preventable death through sloppy care. This progressive radicalization in our society is closely tied to "unvirtuous market mechanisms" unleashed through morally vacuous managed care policies in the United States. This is not to imply that managed care itself is without significant merit in Catholic social policy. What is at issue is the role of some guiding morality that would underlie organizational distribution. If secular pluralism lacks the moral fiber to bind distributional policy, then religious traditions may provide significant service by defining the limit conditions of the respect for human life. For example, one should not adopt the absoluteness of human life as a preeminent value that trumps all other values. Expending scarce resources for the marginal prolongation of human life is unjustified. It wastes resources and tacitly allows other, more salvageable patients to die. Allocation decisions may be difficult but the tacit slaughter of the salvageable should not be countenanced by men and women who wish to live in a peaceable democracy (de Tocqueville 1991). In short, it is in countering the horrors of mindless mediocrity, as well as the empty version of respect for human life as a preeminent trumping value, where the Catholic tradition might exercise its greatest health policy capabilities in a pluralistic democracy. The same would apply to Jewish bioethics.

Communities should not become impoverished to save human lives, even if they must devote considerable resources to saving human lives, while preserving their resources for other purposes which also have value. Having said as much, there exists the problem of how different visions of the good life, the good society, and the good death in religious ethics or secular ethics can allow for the existence of peaceable, pluralist communities. Catholicism should be cautious in universalizing health care standards without also addressing ways to increase resources to meet more basic needs. The changing economic circumstances of societies challenge rigid moral views, at least in critical care medicine, about what is obtainable and what becomes shear hypocrisy of health care delivery. Although we all might agree that we should spend money for basic health care and nutrition, vaccinations, and the like, those of us who care for patients at the other end of life's spectrum seek direction beyond chaos theory and de facto commitments to mediocrity by nonpolicy resolution.

CONCLUSION

Although readers will find metaphors concerning the Nuremberg Code of Ethics, crimes against humanity, and managed health care to be on the bioethical frontier, I have provided evidence to indicate that these issues are not merely rhetorical, but in fact continually confront us. The moral crime of "quality fraud" is not that all should receive excellent care, since that is not possible. The Oregon Health Plan (Strosberg et al. 1992) appropriately understood this circumstance, while the rest of the world continues to commit to mediocrity of equal care and de facto passive extermination of salvageable patients. Allocation must be faced openly and honestly so that individuals know what sort of care they are purchasing and what to expect from their health care system. The Catholic tradition that considers all souls equal in the Heaven of God, should reconsider the moral foundation of respect for human life in ICU in this life and the next. Catholics and Jews should welcome a Catholic view that this volume may inspire. There is no doubt for this author that we must expand our intellectual horizon at the theological, medical, and ethical interface, so that we may cull the most creative thoughts in this volume. If bad things are really happening, then all must see them. Moral and legal punishments shall arise for those who champion corporate systematic mediocrity without disclosure. Absent open and honest consideration, perhaps there will be "secularized holy war."

NOTES

1. Reform and Orthodox Jewish views in this area diverge.
2. It is unclear where Orthodox Jewry will be on this subject.

BIBLIOGRAPHY

Aaron, H., and W. B. Schwartz. 1990. Rationing health care: The choice before us. *Science* 247: 418–22.

Annas, G. T., and M. A. Grodin. 1992. *The Nazi Doctors and the Nuremberg Code.* New York: Oxford University Press.

Berk, L., and A. C. Monheit. 1992. The concentrations of health expenditures: An update. *Health Affairs* 11 (4): 145–49.

Chen, L. M., C. M. Martin, W. Sibbald, and S. Keenan. 1997. Patients readmitted to the intensive care unit (ICU) during the same hospitalization. A multi-center cohort study. *Critical Care Medicine* (Supplement) 25 (1): A83.

Cullen, D. J., D. W. Bates, S. D. Small, J. Cooper, A. Nemeskal, and L. Leape. 1995. The incident reporting system does not detect adverse drug events. *Joint Commission Journal of Quality Improvement* 21: 541–48.

de Tocqueville, A. 1991. *Democracy in America,* trans. by George Lawrence, ed. by J. P. Mayer. San Bernardino, Calif.: Borgo Press.

Engelhardt, H. T., and M. A. Rie. 1986. Intensive care units, scarce resources and conflicting principles of justice. *Journal of the American Medical Association* 253: 1159–64.

———. 1992. Selling virtue: Ethics as a profit maximizing strategy in healthcare delivery. *Journal of Health and Social Policy* 4 (1): 27–35.

———. 1999. Luxury critical care, pluralistic standards and respect for moral diversity. In *Ethics and Critical Care Medicine,* ed. by J. Orlowski. Hagerstown, Md.: University Publishing Group.

Institute for Healthcare Improvement. 1997. Breakthrough Series: Reducing Costs and Improving Outcomes in Adult Intensive Care. Boston.

Kaiser Conference. 1997. Kaiser conference proceedings: Quality in a changing system: Challenges in measuring quality. *Health Affairs* 16 (3): 6–277.

Lanken, P. N., P. B. Terry, and M. Osborne. 1997. Ethics and allocating intensive care resources. *New Horizons* 5 (1): 38–50.

Leape, L. L., D. Bates, D. Cullen, J. Cooper, H. Demonaco, T. Gallivan, R. Hallisey, J. Ives, N. Laird, and G. Laffel. 1995. Systems analysis of adverse drug events. *Journal of the American Medical Association* 274 (1): 35–43.

LeMaire, F. 1996. Managed care evaluation and ethics in US medicine: What lessons can Europe learn? *Current Opinion in Critical Care* 2: 311–12.

Millman and Robertson Actuaries. 1994. *Health Management Guidelines.* Seattle: Millman U.S.A.

Osborne, M., and J. Patterson. 1996. Ethical allocation of ICU resources: A view from the USA. *Intensive Care Medicine* 22: 1009–14.

Pappachan, J. V., B. B. Millar, E. D. Bennett, and G. B. Smith. 1999. Comparison of outcome from intensive care admission after adjustment for case mix by the APACHE III prognostic system. *Chest* 115 (3): 802–10.

Rie, M. A. 1995a. From managed care torts to corporate fraud class actions: Declining quality accountability and free market quality assurance. Paper presented at American Society Law Medical Ethics meeting, September, Boston.

———. 1995b. The Oregonian ICU: Multitiered monetarized morality in health insurance law. *Journal of Law, Medicine, and Ethics* 23 (2): 149–66.

————. 1997. Rationing critical care services in the United States. *Current Opinion in Critical Care* 3: 329–33.

Rie, M. A., and T. Glessner. 1999a. APACHE III risk stratified ICU readmissions for respiratory distress. *Anesthesiology,* Supplement 91 (3A): A309.

————. 1999b. Best cost and best value budgeting for ICU respiratory readmissions. *Anesthesiology* 91 (3A): A289.

Society of Critical Care Medicine Ethics Committee. 1997. Consensus statement regarding futile and other possibly inadvisable treatments. *Critical Care Medicine* 25: 887–91.

Strosberg M., J. M. Weiner, R. Baker, and I. Fein. 1992. *Rationing America's Healthcare: The Oregon Plan and Beyond.* Washington, D.C.: Brookings Institution Press.

UAHC (Union of American Hebrew Congregations) Bioethics Committee. 1994. *Program Guide VII: Allocation of Scarce Medical Resources.* Philadelphia: UAHC.

Wiesel, Elie. 1992. Quoted in introduction to *The Nazi doctors and the Nuremburg Code: Human Rights in Human Experimentation,* ed. by G. J. Annas and M. A. Grodin. New York: Oxford University Press.

Wood K. E., D. B. Coursin, and R. M. Grounds. 1999. Critical care outcomes in the United Kingdom: Sobering wake-up call or stability of the lamppost? *Chest* 115 (3): 614–16.

What Is Appropriate Intensive Care? A Roman Catholic Perspective

Paulina Taboada

In this era of medical progress—which Hans Jonas characterized as dominated by the logic of the "technological imperative" (1979)—questions concerning moral criteria suitable for determining what constitutes appropriate use of biomedical technology have become extremely relevant. Moreover, with the development of advanced life-support technology in intensive care units (ICUs) in the past few decades, the urgency of a practical answer to this question is becoming more and more evident. Medical efforts in ICUs, although motivated by the legitimate desire to offer every opportunity for survival, in some cases may only briefly prolong life and lead to increased suffering both for patients and their families. Furthermore, treatment in ICUs involves a significant investment of medical resources, expending an important part of the gross national product for most countries around the world (Scheiber, Poullier, and Greenwald 1994). Thus, the issue raises important clinical, ethical, financial, and political questions.

Since the famous Quinlan case (*Quinlan* 1976) many attempts to identify moral and legal criteria for defining the appropriate use of high-technology medicine have been undertaken. Nevertheless, the question is far from being definitely settled. Because decisions to withhold or withdraw life-supporting measures in ICUs often result in the patient's death, reaching the proper degree of moral certainty about their legitimacy becomes extremely important. In fact, a careful distinction between those interventions that have a real chance to benefit the patient, those that lead to an artificial prolongation of agony, and those that in fact represent an acceleration of an unavoidable death is necessary. Drawing this distinction in concrete situations is sometimes very difficult. The necessity of finding substantive criteria delimiting the range of ethically sound decisions is evident.

As a Catholic medical doctor and philosopher, who works at a teaching hospital of the Pontifical University in Chile, I was invited to contribute to this volume to reflect on the specific contributions of Roman Catholic moral teachings to this issue. In order to do so, I will use the traditional sources of Catholicism: the Gospel, the Catechism of the Catholic Church, and some of the official documents of the magisterium, such as encyclicals and pastoral letters. I do not intend to deal with the epistemological questions regarding the validity or universality of these sources (see Seifert's essay in this volume), nor with questions concerning allocation decisions and the right of individuals to receive intensive care as a matter of social justice (see the essays in this volume by Boyle, Kaveny, and Wildes). Rather, I focus on the patient-centered decision-making process (microethics) and on the ways in which the above-mentioned sources are able to shed light for the practice of intensive medicine today. Thus, in the following I shall (1) describe the peculiarities of the medical services provided in ICUs and the kinds of patients that may benefit from them; (2) raise the particular moral dilemmas related with this type of medical care; and (3) draw some moral principles from the Roman Catholic tradition that have practical implications for orienting the praxis of high-technology medicine.

WHAT IS SPECIAL ABOUT INTENSIVE CARE?

Specialized units in which expert medical, nursing, and technical staff were provided with equipment for monitoring and immediate lifesaving interventions evolved in parallel with advances in invasive surgical and medical procedures. Accordingly, "the development of ICUs may be traced to the postoperative recovery units, thence to the respiratory care units, subsequently to shock and trauma units, and finally to units that provide comprehensive cardiopulmonary support for both medical and surgical patients with immediate life-threatening respiratory and/or cardiac impairment" (Weil, von Planta, and Rackow 1989, 1). Intensive care has been defined as "a service for patients with potentially recoverable conditions who can benefit from more detailed observation and invasive treatment than can safely be provided in general wards or high dependency areas" (Smith and Nielsen 1999, 1544). It is, therefore, usually reserved for patients with potential or established organ failure. The most commonly supported organ is the lung, but facilities also exist for the diagnosis, prevention, and treatment of other organ dysfunctions. Thus, intensive care is appropriate for patients requiring or likely to require advanced respiratory support, patients requiring support of two or more organ systems, and patients with chronic impairment of one or more organ systems who also require support for an acute reversible failure of another organ. Patients requiring intensive care may suffer from a wide range of medical conditions. Despite this wide variety, they can be grouped into two main categories: (1) those in actual high risk of imminent death (i.e., critically ill patients with respiratory failure, heart failure, etc.) and (2) those potentially at high risk of imminent death (e.g., patients admitted to an ICU in order to have a potentially dangerous procedure performed, such as management of cardiac arrythmias).

As with any other treatment, the decision to offer a patient intensive care should be based on *potential benefit*. Hence, patients who are *too well* to benefit from this particular kind of treatment or those with *no hope of recovering* should not be admitted to an ICU. Nevertheless, it is important to keep in mind that patients should be admitted to intensive care before their condition reaches a point beyond which recovery is impossible. Therefore, early referral is particularly important. If referral is delayed until the patient's life is clearly at risk, the chances of full recovery are jeopardized. Contrarily, early referral improves chances of recovery, reduces the potential for organ dysfunction, may reduce the length of stay in intensive care as well as in the hospital, and may thereby also reduce the costs of treatment.

Nevertheless, these potential benefits of early ICU admission need to be weighed against associated risks. Indeed, life-supporting interventions and the very confinement of patients to ICUs are not without risk. Critically ill patients are known to be immuno-suppressed, and therefore are subject to iatrogenic infections as complications of invasive interventions. We cannot escape the fact that the benefits of invasive monitoring and interventions are at the cost of significant risks and complications. Moreover, the risks associated with ICU interventions that might seem legitimate for a given clinical condition may not be so for another. Given these circumstances, there is an increasing awareness of the potential misuse of critical care interventions and of the need to define adequate selection criteria.

In recent years, intensive care doctors have made substantial efforts to establish criteria for the identification of patients who may significantly benefit from early intensive care admission. Smith and Nielsen (1999), for instance, propose a list of eleven exclusively empirical ICU admission criteria, such as threatened airway, respiratory or cardiac arrest, or a sudden fall in the level of consciousness. Kilner (1990), instead, identified five different kinds of criteria: medical benefit, imminent death, likelihood of benefit, length of benefit, and quality of benefit. After analyzing their pros and cons, Kilner concludes that only the first three can be retained as ethically acceptable. His conclusion suggests the necessity of complementing merely technical ICU admission criteria with ethical reflection. In other words, to determine who may benefit from intensive medicine, we need to understand what is truly good for the person, considered as a psycho-physical whole, rather than merely the potential physiological effects of ICU interventions on patients. This presupposes an understanding of personhood and true human values.

In the following, I shall refer to two human values that are especially at stake in ICUs. The proposed characterization of ICU patients includes, namely, at least two important elements: the *potential health benefits* associated with particular *risks* (derived from the clinical condition or its treatment) and *imminence of death*. Accordingly, the primary moral dilemmas involved in ICU decisions that I address in the following are: (1) questions concerning the content, extension, and limits of our moral duty to pursue health, as confronted with the risks inherent in certain medical interventions; and (2) questions regarding the adequate attitude for facing imminent death, according to Roman Catholic tradition.

THE MORAL DUTY TO PURSUE PROPORTIONATE HEALTH CARE

According to the Catholic tradition, life and health represent basic human goods that allow persons further fulfillment of vital goals (vocation). They represent morally relevant values that deserve a proper "*value-answer*" (von Hildebrand 1952, 1980). Hence, a fundamental moral intuition tells us about the existence of a moral obligation to preserve life and health. Nevertheless, it is also evident that nobody is obliged to use all available medical interventions, but rather only those offering a reasonable benefit-risk ratio. A more difficult question is whether one can refuse medical interventions in spite of their potential benefits or accept treatments for which the risks are still very high or not yet well known, as is sometimes the case with ICU interventions. These situations confront us with questions concerning the limits of our moral obligation to pursue health.

The Principle of Therapeutic Proportionality

In an attempt to distinguish morally obligatory from morally nonobligatory medical interventions, a conceptual distinction between "ordinary" and "extraordinary" means has been proposed by Roman Catholic tradition since 1957. The content of this traditional Roman Catholic teaching is presently better known as the *principle of therapeutic proportionality* (Pontifical Council for Pastoral Assistance to Health Care Workers [Charter] 1995, n. 64). This principle states that there is a moral obligation to provide patients with those treatments that fulfill a *relation of due proportion* between the means employed and the end pursued. Medical interventions in situations in which this relation does not hold are considered "disproportionate" (referred to above as "extraordinary") and are regarded as morally nonobligatory.

A superficial reading of this principle may raise a sensation of vagueness. What is the precise meaning of a *relation of due proportion*? Are there any objective criteria for verifying its fulfillment? *The Charter for Health Care Workers* of the Pontifical Council for Pastoral Assistance to Health Care Workers specifies the evaluative criteria for such proportionality judgments:

> To verify and establish whether there is due proportion in a particular case, the means should be well evaluated by comparing the type of therapy, the degree of difficulty and risk involved, the necessary expenses, and the possibility of application, with the result that can be expected, taking into account the conditions of patients and their physical and moral powers. (Charter, n. 64)

A first striking point is the fact that proportionality judgments refer to particular clinical situations. Nevertheless, to say that these kinds of judgments are relative to individual situations is not the same as saying that they are merely subjective. To be legitimate, such judgments need to be grounded in objective states of affairs regarding the clinical condition and the present state of medical art. The certainty of the clinical diagnosis, the utility or futility of a given therapy, the benefits and risks presently known for the different therapeutic alternatives, the accuracy of the prognosis, and so on are all important criteria for judging the proportionality of medical interventions.

The need for quantitative methodology in evaluating medical activities is becoming increasingly appreciated, as reflected in the development of evidence-based medicine in recent years (Evidence-Based Medicine Working Group 1992). I consider the application of this methodology a useful tool for evaluating ethically relevant clinical information. Nevertheless, when stressing the importance of considering quantitative (statistical) information in judging therapeutic proportionality, I do not intend to affirm that it is possible to *derive a moral ought from a "probability-value"* (i.e., to conclude that a moral obligation can be sufficiently grounded in statistical probabilities). To state this would mean identifying statistics with ethics. This would represent a modern version of the *naturalistic fallacy,* already refuted by Moore (1959).[1] Rather, it seems prudent to ground our decisions in the most accurate possible knowledge of the objective state of affairs, especially in critical situations, such as those associated with ICU admissions. The need to place empirically derived clinical information in a larger decision-making framework—one that explicitly acknowledges the role of moral values in clinical decision making—is evident.

Quantitative and Qualitative Aspects of Therapeutic Proportionality

The idea of proportionality in medical care does not belong only to Roman Catholic tradition. Plato, in the *Republic,* emphasized the inappropriateness of medical efforts that result only in the prolongation of suffering.

> Asclepius . . . taught medicine for those who were healthy in their nature but were suffering from a specific disease; he rid them of it . . . then ordered them to live as usual. . . . For those, however, whose bodies were always in a state of inner sickness he did not attempt to prescribe a regimen . . . to make their life a prolonged misery. . . . Medicine was not intended for them and they should not be treated even if they were richer than Midas. (Plato 1981, 76–77)

The conception of the goal of medicine as helping an organism that is healthy in its nature, but affected by a reversible disease, is an important heritage of Greek medicine. Greek physicians learned to recognize those situations in which a disease represented an obstacle to the realization of an otherwise healthy nature, from those situations in which nature was sick, leading human existence to its natural end. Thus, death was not considered a failure of medicine, but as the natural end of human life. Also, Hippocratic medicine invites physicians to acknowledge when medical efforts will most probably fail:

> Whenever therefore a man suffers from an ill, which is too strong for the means at disposal of medicine, he surely must not even expect that it can be overcome by medicine. (Hippocratic Corpus 1977, 6–7)

In modern terms, the perception of medical *futility* derived from the Hippocratic Corpus might be considered a *probabilistic* notion. Hippocrates rejected efforts that were probabilistically unlikely to achieve a cure. Plato, instead, supported a *qualitative* concept of medical futility, objecting to those therapies that resulted in "lives not worth being lived." Thus, both quantitative and qualitative aspects of medical futility are recognized in the most ancient traditions. Both quantitative and qualitative aspects relate to a single underlying notion: The result is not commensurate to the effort. This is precisely the content of the principle of therapeutic proportionality, as taught by the Roman Catholic Church: Medical treatments that do not fulfill a *relation of due proportion* between means and results are considered *disproportionate* and, therefore, morally nonobligatory.

Although both quantitative and qualitative aspects are tightly interconnected and cannot be easily isolated in particular situations, it might be methodologically helpful both for physicians and patients (or their surrogates) to consider these aspects separately. It is important to establish which aspects of the proportionality judgment belong mainly to physicians, in virtue of their technical expertise, and which to patients and their proxies, in virtue of their autonomy. In the following, I shall briefly introduce some considerations that have been helpful in evaluating therapeutic proportionality according to the experience of our Ethics Committee at the Clinical Hospital of the Catholic University of Chile.

Elements Involved in Therapeutic Proportionality

I will list these elements under the headings of "means" and "results," although I am aware that these distinctions have merely heuristic value. It is clear that the proportionality of the means can only be judged with reference to the intended results.

Considerations Regarding the Means

Certainty of clinical diagnosis. It might seem obvious, but before even asking whether a given medical intervention is proportionate, one has ideally to reach a reasonable degree of certainty about the clinical diagnosis. As stated in the *Charter for Health Care Workers*: "Guided by this integrally human and properly Christian view of sickness, health care workers should seek, first and foremost, to observe illness and analyze it in the patient. . . . A condition for any treatment is the previous and exact identification of the symptoms and causes of the illness" (Charter, n. 56). Hence, the process of clarifying the diagnosis is commonly considered "an action to promote health" (n. 58) and, therefore, morally good.

Nevertheless, I know from my own clinical experience that certifying medical diagnosis is not always easy. For clinicians, there are situations in which the ethical dilemmas emerge precisely from having to make delicate therapeutic decisions without being able to reach reasonable diagnostic certainty. This is often the case in critical care, where the need to support the patient's vital functions may, at least initially, take priority over establishing the diagnosis. For example, patients with life-threatening shock need immediate treatment rather than diagnosis of the cause, as the principles of management are the same whether shock results from massive myocardial infarction or a gastrointestinal bleed. Similarly, although the actual management may differ, the principles of treating other life-threatening organ failures (e.g., respiratory failure or coma) do not depend on the precise diagnosis.

But it is important to distinguish these situations from those others in which physicians start doubting the proportionality of undertaking concrete diagnostic or therapeutic interventions without having first sufficiently clarified the clinical condition, allowing themselves to be guided by the vague intuition of an ominous prognosis. Not infrequently, the analysis of our Ethics Committee ends up showing the moral relevance of undertaking some further efforts to clarify the diagnosis and prognosis of a given clinical condition before advancing any judgment regarding proportionality of treatment. The application of formal rules of evidence for evaluating the clinical literature, as proposed by evidence-based medicine, combined with sound clinical intuition and experience, therefore is a preliminary condition for any proportionality judgment.

Therapeutic utility or futility. As stated above, "patients have a right to any treatment from which they can draw salutary benefit" (Charter, n. 63). The moral obligation to implement useful treatments refers not only to curative but also to palliative care. Nevertheless, defining therapeutic utility is not an easy task. This concept has been widely explored in the medical literature in the past several years. Schneiderman and his associates, for instance, propose a patient-benefit-centered definition of medical futility (1998; Schneiderman, Faber-Langendoen, and Jecker 1994; Schneiderman, Jecker, and Jonsen 1990, 1996). This definition is based on a distinction between *benefits* and *effects*. According to Schneiderman, "in judging futility, physicians must distinguish between an *effect*, which is limited to some part of the patient's body, and a *benefit*, which appreciably improves the person as a whole. Treatment that fails to provide the latter, whether or not it achieves the former, is 'futile'" (Schneiderman, Jecker, and Jonsen 1990, 949). Schneiderman concludes that physicians are morally obliged to implement only those medical interventions likely to achieve clinical benefits, but they are not obliged to offer those measures that enhance physiological effects, although such treatment may be morally allowed on compassionate grounds.

Although Schneiderman's distinction between benefits and effects might be useful to a certain extent, it is not as clear as it might a priori appear. In my opinion, Schneiderman's conception of clinical futility entails the danger of subjectivism. He excessively emphasizes conscious experience as a condition for defining medical utility. Indeed, the subjective experience of the benefits of a given therapy is not a necessary condition for its objective utility, as shown, for instance, in the case of diabetes mellitus therapy. Schneiderman's distinction between benefits and effects also disregards the fact that restoring health is not the only legitimate goal of medical interventions. Preserving or enhancing the patient's comfort and general well-being, preventing further diseases or complications of a given disease, and so on, are also desirable goals of medical interventions.

Schneiderman's notion of medical futility includes both quantitative and qualitative components. The quantitative portion of his definition stipulates that physicians should regard a treatment as futile if empirical data show that the treatment has less than 1 chance in 100 to benefit the patient. Every clinician knows that it is almost impossible to attain such a degree of certainty in medical practice. The qualitative portion of the definition establishes that if a treatment merely preserves permanent unconsciousness or cannot end dependence on life-supporting therapies, physicians should consider the treatment futile. A similar conception of futility is proposed by Caplan, who states: "Medical futility must be understood as referring to both the probability and the desirability of attaining a particular diagnostic, therapeutic, or palliative goal" (1996, 688).

I agree with the conception of medical futility as involving both quantitative and qualitative dimensions. Nevertheless, with Christensen (1992), I would rather propose a distinction between absolute, statistical, and disproportionate futility. *Absolute futility* refers to treatments that are completely ineffective interventions in physiological terms. Because there is general agreement that physicians are not obliged to implement absolutely futile measures, the limitation of such therapy does not pose moral dilemmas. *Statistical futility* expresses the low probability of a specific measure to achieve a given goal. This information in itself does not say anything about the moral obligation to implement such a measure. Nevertheless, it represents morally relevant clinical information that needs to be considered in judging its proportionality. The expression *disproportionate futility* qualifies a value-laden decision to abstain from a certain medical intervention, in spite of its low statistical probability of achieving a beneficial therapeutic goal, because it is not justified in a given situation due to the sufferings, risks, costs, and so on, it implies for the patient or his family.

This distinction enables the identification of those dimensions of medical futility limited to the evidence-based probability of attaining a given goal from other dimensions related to value judgments. Simplifying a very complex decision-making process, one could say that the statistical component of the utility judgments belongs primarily to the domain of physicians in virtue of their technical expertise, whereas the value-laden component referring to the desirability of achieving a given goal—or to the convenience of taking some risks and burdens associated with a specific medical intervention—necessarily involves exercising the virtue of prudence both for physicians and patients.

Benefits and risks of therapeutic alternatives. Each medical intervention involves certain risks. The moral obligation to pursue health includes the duty to undergo only "proportionate risks" (Charter, nn. 60, 65). Considerations regarding quantitative and qualitative aspects of risk estimation, analogous to those stated above, should be introduced here and applied to each of the therapeutic alternatives. The experience of our Ethics Committee shows that physicians often focus their attention only on a limited number of alternatives. Our analysis of the proportionality of risks has been facilitated when we actively include all the therapeutic alternatives known for a given condition. Evidence-based medicine provides valuable information here as well.

Nevertheless, in the particular case of ICUs, it is not always possible to ground our judgments on rigorous experiments or large randomized, controlled trials to evaluate the benefits and risks of therapies. Thus, doctors delivering intensive care often have to decide which patients can benefit most without the availability of such data, because it would be unethical randomly to allocate severely ill patients to receive intensive care or general ward care. The alternative is to use observational methods that study the outcomes of care that patients receive as part of their standard treatment in the ICU or of new therapies. Nevertheless, before inferences can be drawn about the outcomes of such treatments, the characteristics of the patients admitted to intensive care have to be taken into account—a process known as "adjusting for case mix."

Under such circumstances, more than achieving certainties, one has to try to reduce uncertainties. The ethical agreement is that the implementation of experimental treatments, for which the risks are still high or not yet completely known, may be morally allowed but is not obligatory. "In the absence of other remedies, it is licit to have the recourse, with the consent of the patient, to the means made available by the most advanced medicine, even if they are still at an experimental stage and not without some risk" (Charter, n. 65). Nevertheless, it may also be

> licit to be satisfied with the normal means offered by medicine. No one can be obliged, therefore, to have the recourse to a type of remedy which, although already in use, is still not without dangers or is too onerous. This refusal is not the equivalent of suicide. Rather, it may signify either simple acceptance of the human condition, or the wish to avoid putting into effect a remedy disproportionate to the results that can be hoped for, or the desire not to place too great a burden on the family or on society. (Charter, n. 65)

This statement leads us logically to the consideration of a further element of therapeutic proportionality.

Burdens. The above-mentioned charter states that there is a moral obligation to implement those *possible* attentions "from which [patients] can draw salutary benefit."

> It is licit to interrupt the application of such means when the results disappoint the hopes placed in them, because there is no longer due proportion between the investment of instruments and personnel and the foreseeable results or because the techniques used subject the patient to suffering and discomfort greater than the benefits to be obtained. (Charter, n. 65)

Thus, the moral obligation to pursue proportionate health care is not defined by the strict utility of certain medical interventions, but also by their feasibility and costs. Nevertheless, the expression "costs" has to be understood in a broad sense, including not only financial aspects, but also other kinds of burdens to patients, families, and health care workers. These burdens may be physical, psychological, financial, social, or even spiritual. Hence, a given therapy might be defined as beneficial and yet still judged as disproportionate, when too difficult to obtain, too expensive, too burdensome, and so on. In such qualified cases, the moral obligation to use such a treatment may be suspended. This can be a common situation in developing countries, where medical resources are not always available, raising further ethical dilemmas related to the problem of social justice and solidarity in the allocation of health resources around the world.

The just allocation of scarce medical resources is a serious concern for both industrial and developing countries. Moreover, developing countries need to be particularly efficient in this respect, in order to ensure social justice. There is a broad consensus about the necessity of major reform in health care systems. Besides fundamental moral issues related to the goals of medicine, there are also financial aspects supporting the urgent need for such reform. It is well known that expenditures on health care represent an increasing part of the gross national product for most countries. Hence, such health care reform has to face important issues of priority and equity. Nevertheless, in the search for moral criteria orienting a just distribution of limited health resources, it is important to keep in mind that "the physician's primary commitment is to the patient"(American College of Physicians 1992, 948). Thus, the physician should not argue on grounds of distributive justice in order to justify individual decisions to limit care. The very nature of the patient-physician relationship does not allow physicians to make unilateral decisions based on financial costs.

Considerations Regarding the Results

Accuracy of prognosis. The ability objectively to estimate a patient's probability of death is a relatively new area of clinical research. Systems to analyze severity of disease have been used in critical care since 1981, when the Acute Physiology and Chronic Health Evaluation (APACHE) scoring system was introduced (Knaus et al. 1981). This system is based on weightings of the most important clinical variables and has proved to be useful in evaluating in hospital mortality of patients in ICUs. After it, other similar systems have been proposed.[2] Applying these scores, ICU doctors are able to predict the potential benefits a given patient could receive from critical care.

Intuitively, one expects that clarifying a patient's prognosis will help clinicians as well as patients in decision making. Nevertheless, this intuition has yet to be empirically proven. Although empirically based risk evaluation systems for ICU patients, like APACHE and others, have been demonstrated to be useful in clinical research on new therapies, they have been much less successful in reducing the uncertainty of daily clinical decision making. Recently, important large-scale studies have been undertaken to explore whether feedback of empirical probabilities to clinicians would result in improving the accuracy of their subjective probability estimates or in facilitating their decision making. The Study to Understand Prognosis and Preferences of Outcomes and Risks of Treatments (SUPPORT) introduced a new prognostic system, applicable not only to ICU patients, as were previous systems, but also to otherwise severely ill patients (SUPPORT 1995).[3] This prognostic model was designed to predict patient death probability in the near future. For cases in which the probability of death was nearly certain, limiting medical interventions, even life-supporting measures in the ICU, is morally legitimate. Nevertheless, despite an intense interdisciplinary effort to make this prognostic information available both for physicians and patients, the SUPPORT intervention did not prove to be effective in facilitating decisions to limit care.

Because intuition still suggests that improving the accuracy of prognosis and patient-physician communication should facilitate clinical decisions, especially decisions to limit care, questions concerning reasons for the apparent failure of SUPPORT arise. A possible explanation of this finding is that the quantitative component of the prognosis, as expressed by probabilities, needs to be related to a given situation. The uncertainty about the clinical evolution of a particular case, over against statistical assessments, is an important source of moral dilemmas in clinical decision making. It is also important to keep in mind that mortality represents only one of the possible prognoses. Yet, so far, we do not have good predictive models for clinical outcomes other than death. These predictions rely presently mainly on clinical intuition and experience, representing a further source of uncertainty and moral dilemmas in decisions to limit care.

Quality of life. In making decisions about the proportionality of care, patients and health care workers often take into account the current and projected quality of life. The neurological condition of the patient frequently plays a decisive role in this process. In the context of the present analysis, I do not intend to go into the debate on the role of quality-of-life judgments in medicine. I just want to prevent the real danger of giving excessive weight to quality-of-life judgments in establishing the proportionality of certain therapies. Any assessment of quality of life necessarily includes value judgments, which may easily lead to the segregation of particular groups of patients whose appropriate treatments could be systematically denied. Therefore, it may be important to remember that, from a Roman Catholic perspective, sanctity of life always has precedence over quality of life. Accordingly, proportionally beneficial treatments can never be denied to patients only on the grounds of a prediction of a bad quality of life. Otherwise, a hidden euthanistic mentality could be introduced. "The Christian knows by faith that sickness and suffering share in the salvific efficacy of the Redeemer's cross" (Charter, n. 54). Christ always gave special attention to the weakest, the poorest, and the abandoned. His attitude exemplifies a logic that goes precisely in the opposite direction of the logic dominating contemporary welfare societies.

Therapeutic Proportionality and Proportionalism

Having listed the elements involved in judgments regarding therapeutic proportionality, it is necessary to mention the concrete way in which these elements should be taken into account in particular situations. To prevent misunderstandings regarding the compatibility of the principle of therapeutic proportionality with more general moral orientations of the Catholic Church, a distinction between this conception and ethical *proportionalism* needs to be made. It is important to understand the essential difference between both positions, because it is well known that the Catholic tradition recommends the former, while repeatedly criticizing the latter, most recently in John Paul II's encyclical *Veritatis Splendor* (*VS*).

Taking into account the positive and negative foreseeable consequences of our actions is doubtless a constitutive part of moral judgment. Thus, not having considered predictable negative effects of our actions does not excuse our moral responsibility for them. The clarity with which consequentialism understands this aspect of morality is certainly one of the great merits of this position. Its fault consists in suggesting that maximizing the positive and minimizing the negative results of our actions constitutes the very essence of morality. Nevertheless, the moment in which we balance the consequences of our actions is certainly an important moment in moral reasoning, but not necessarily the main one. The careful consideration of the nature (species) of the action and of the intention of the acting person are also important determinants of the morality of this act.[4] Accordingly, Catholic tradition affirms the existence of some kind (species) of actions that by their very nature are never susceptible of being ordered toward the good (so-called *intrinsece malum*), regardless of the intention of the agent, or the particular circumstances or their possible positive consequences (*VS*, 79–80 ff.).

Thus, when determining what constitutes proportionate health care in general, and appropriate intensive care in particular, one has to keep always in mind that the most basic principle-orienting medical practice, according to the Roman Catholic tradition, is that nobody is allowed intentionally to kill or otherwise injure the integrity of an innocent person. This moral norm derives from the Fifth Commandment and has its positive expression in the love precept (see the essay by Boyle in this volume). Thus, within the Catholic tradition, determination of the paths of action in which "the results are worth the efforts" presupposes that one excludes from the very beginning any option involving intrinsically bad actions. Hence, there is a fundamental difference between the Roman Catholic understanding of therapeutic proportionality and *proportionalism*. Weighing the results of our actions cannot be limited to a balance of their extrinsic consequences (physical, psychological, social, or financial). One must also take into account whether or not the act itself represents a subordination of the person to God's will (an appropriate value-answer) and an imitation of Christ's example. It is only with regard to the existence of higher, transcendental values, which the person is invited to respect, and taking also into account the assistance of the Holy Spirit, that it is possible to judge an action as morally obligatory (proportionate), in spite of its extreme difficulty or the existence of apparently negative consequences for the person. This consideration has important implications for the moral life of Christians, because it is in each single action where the person reinforces or deconstructs his fundamental attitude toward God and the good.

In other words, the ways in which different elements involved in therapeutic proportionality have to be weighted in a given situation must be guided by the virtue of prudence in trying to discern God's will. The concept of prudence as understood by this religious tradition does not correspond to the present secular conception of prudence. As Wildes states:

> Prudence, in contemporary philosophy, has come to mean the notion of rational self-interest. However, within the Roman Catholic tradition prudence has been a cardinal virtue which judges not according to rational self-interest but according to the presence of, and the response to, the Holy Spirit. The medieval understanding of prudence . . . was not moral wisdom but the ability to be practically wise . . . the exercise of right choice in particular cases, in light of moral universal knowledge. . . . For St. Thomas . . . prudence was the knowledge of what should be done and avoided and it guided reasoning about what ought to be done. The prudent man, in the world of medieval casuistry, had a Christian sense about how one ought to act. This moral sense shaped his judgment. Lacking absolute standards of ordinary and extraordinary care, the tradition has relied on prudential judgment: the judgment that seeks to discern God's will. (1995, 110–11)

In extreme situations, judging medical interventions as disproportionate may be equivalent to recognizing an imminent and unavoidable death. As Pope John Paul II affirms: "Facing death, the enigma of human condition becomes supreme. . . . In front of the mystery of death one stands impotent; human certainties vacillate" (1992, 1). This may explain the particular difficulty of decisions to limit care in ICUs. The advances in life-supporting technology have been such that vital functions can be sustained for long periods under circumstances where survival or restoration of function is not possible any more. Quoting Pope Pius XII, Engelhardt (in his essay in this volume) introduces the notion of "moral danger" in reference to the use of advanced technology oriented to an artificial prolongation of human life. Insofar as attempts to use high-technology health care involve a distortion of the moral life and the idolatry of mere physical survival, then one would have established grounds for regarding some extraordinary or disproportionate care as morally dangerous to Christians.

THE MORAL DUTY TO ACCEPT DEATH

Indeed, the Roman Catholic Church affirms that "[artificially prolonged agony] is contrary to the dignity of the dying person and to the moral obligation of accepting death" (Charter, n. 119). In other words, for Catholics there is a *moral duty to accept death*. Hence, answering questions about what constitutes an appropriate use of life-supporting technology in ICUs from a Roman Catholic perspective presupposes an understanding of the Christian attitude toward imminent death and the meaning of the so-called good Christian death.

In the Declaration on Euthanasia (1980), the Catholic Church proposes that the "right to die with serenity, with human and Christian dignity" is a constitutive part of the right to live. So, at the end of life the right to life becomes specified as a right to "die with dignity." It is well known that, in contradistinction to the way in which most proponents of euthanasia and medically assisted suicide understand the expression "dying with dignity," Catholic faith absolutely excludes the possibility of intentionally taking one's own life or helping others to do so. But it also excludes the so-called *medicalization of death*, arguing that this is "contrary to the dignity of the dying person and to the moral duty to accept death" (Charter, n. 119). Thus, while defending the right to "die with dignity," Catholics refer to a "right to live one's own death in a human and Christian way"(Charter, n. 119).

Dying as an Actus Humanus, *and the "Good Christian Death"*

Catholic faith considers death as the "salary of fault" (Romans 6:23). Nevertheless, for those dying in God's grace, death is regarded as a participation in Christ's death and Resurrection (*Catechism of the Catholic Church* 1994, 1006, 1009). Hence, the Catholic conception of death presupposes an understanding of dying as an *actus humanus* and not merely as an *actus homini.*[5] In other words, from a Catholic perspective death cannot be regarded as something happening to us (mere passivity). On the contrary, dying is considered an act that our free will is able to sanction: we are free to accept or to reject it. This means that our attitude toward the inevitability of death corresponds to a free choice. We are not able to choose whether or not we want to die, but we are free to choose an attitude of acceptance or rebellion. Accordingly, we can die a *good* or a *bad* death, in the moral sense of the expression.

To understand what counts as a *good Christian death*, one must first identify the specific contents of Christian morality and apply them to the act of dying. John Paul II (*VS*, n. 28) summarizes the essential contents of Christian morality in the following four points: (1) a subordination of the person and his acts to God; (2) the existence of a relation between the moral goodness of human acts and eternal life; (3) the imitation of Christ, Who opens to the person the perspective of perfect love; and (4) the gift of the Holy Spirit, as source and strength of the moral life of Christians. Applying these contents to the act of dying, one realizes, first, that subordinating oneself and the act of dying to God means to accept that only God is the "Lord of life and death." This excludes each act—whether action or omission—that intentionally causes or accelerates death. Second, accepting the existence of a relation between a good death and eternal life presupposes the idea that dying has to be regarded a meritorious act. So, dying a *good death* is the culmination of a *good life*. This notion is linked with the third point, namely, the assertion that it is the imitation of Christ that opens a perspective toward the understanding of death as an act of perfect love. Here the fourth aspect—namely, the necessity of the assistance and strength of the Holy Spirit for the full moral life of Christians—becomes evident. It provides the necessary clue to an affirmation of the possibility of living Christian moral commitments, in spite of our natural weakness and inner divisions, even in the supreme moment of death.

If the imitation of Christ reveals the meaning of dying as an act of perfect love, then we will have to look at His example. The Gospel has beautiful images showing the inner struggles Christ had to live through before being able to give Himself into the hands of His Father. Not even for Christ Himself was death something easy to accept. The structure of His seven words at the Cross (Luke 23:33–46; John 19:25–30) provides insight into the meaning of dying well. His first three words express the necessity of dying, shedding light

on the persons surrounding Him. There, He first asks for forgiveness for those who cruci-
fied Him; second, opens the doors of salvation to one of His fellows; and third, offers His
Mother as one of His most precious gifts to humankind. His way of dying gives perfect tes-
timony of His constant way of living and His doctrine: forgetting Himself and giving Himself to the good of others, even of those who present themselves as His enemies. After these
three, we can read two further words. They describe His sufferings at this supreme hour:
His tremendous loneliness and thirst. Finally, the last two words, spoken immediately before His death, describe the total peace inhabiting His soul. After experiencing the most
radical loneliness, He was able to come back to the dialogue with His Father, a dialogue that
was always the very center of His life.

Jesus' entire life and especially His passion is morally normative for Christians.
Christ's example tells us that death can be lived as the supreme act of human transcendence:
love. If someone dies young, such as at the age of thirty-three, we typically describe this as a
premature and unfortunate death. Nevertheless, Christ considered His life fulfilled. He
died when everything was done—everything was fulfilled (John 19:30). His death is an example of the possibility of transforming death into a supreme manifestation of love at any
time in our lives. But it is not possible to transform the act of dying into a free act of love if
we live it as something happening to us against our will. The inner attitude required from
us corresponds to the fifth of the emotional reactions of patients facing death described by
Kübler-Ross (1969), an attitude that not all her patients were able to reach.[6] It is this attitude of inner acceptance of God's will upon us that allows us to live our death as a positive
act of giving of ourselves (*actus humanus*).

Contemporary Health Care Standards Regarding Death

I believe that these reflections on the meaning of the "good Christian death" have
important practical consequences for reorienting our current standards of practicing critical care. Death is not primarily a medical or scientific event. Death has deep cultural,
moral, and religious meaning. One's view of what counts as death, or what counts as a
good death, is doubtless deeply influenced by the moral commitments that one holds.
Thus, cultural, moral, and religious views of death shape how it is understood and determine what is considered to be appropriate behavior, both for the dying person and his family, as well as for the caring personnel. But, health care is a cooperative enterprise that
brings together people from different cultural and religious backgrounds. In the hospital,
one dies surrounded by people who have very different views of the meanings of a good life
and a good death.

The orientation toward cure characterizing contemporary medicine encourages aggressive treatment, even if clinically inappropriate or contrary to the patient's wishes, in order to avoid any perception of undertreatment. To be involved in such a cultural trend, or
in its opposite (i.e., the growing acceptance of the practice of euthanasia and physician-assisted suicide) may impose grave moral dilemmas on dying persons: not "allowing" them to
die in ways they consider morally appropriate. "Let me die my own death and not the death
of physicians," said R. M. Rilke, one of my favorite poets, facing the diagnosis of leukemia
at the end of his life. His statement reflects both the desire to "master" his own death—to
live it as an *actus humanus*—and a reaction against what he considers the current medical

culture. If a Christian intends to take seriously his moral duty to accept death, he cannot avoid the question of whether contemporary health care standards will really allow him to die a *"good Christian death."*

The findings of SUPPORT (1995) provide some empirical data necessary to address this question.[7] According to SUPPORT, in the United States[8] (at least at the five leading medical institutions involved in the study) nearly 40 percent of patients spent at least ten days in intensive care before death. According to family reports, about half of those who where able to communicate during their last three days of life were in serious pain. The study documented great discrepancies between patients' desires and their actual treatment. For instance, in 80 percent of cases, physicians misunderstood patients' preferences regarding cardiopulmonary resuscitation (CPR). For half the patients, who had wanted CPR to be withheld, their physicians never wrote a do-not-resuscitate order.

The results of SUPPORT suggest that medical efforts to prolong life too often merely prolong dying, even against the explicit desires of patients. Although the study did not address the particular reasons why patients and their families rejected certain life-supporting measures, its results suggest that contemporary health care standards are not sensitive enough to the moral and religious dimensions that should shape our attitudes toward life and death. Health care workers too often fall into the temptation of using all available technology in order to avoid imminent death. They seem to have special difficulties in accepting human finitude and death.

TOWARD A PERSONALISTIC VIRTUE-ETHICS FOR CRITICAL CARE

In an era of medical progress, in which the "technological imperative" (Jonas 1979) suggests that everything that is technologically possible is also ethically legitimate or, even more, ethically mandatory, the criteria for deciding what constitutes an appropriate use of high-technology medicine cannot be driven from the logic of strict physiological utility. In caring for critically ill persons, the logic of dominion, characterizing the process of technological progress, needs to be replaced by a "personalistic" logic.[9] The physician's duty to "maintain the dignity of the person and [to] respect the uniqueness of each person," the American College of Physicians Ethics Manual states (1992, 948), involves both the moral duty to implement proportionate life-supporting measures and the moral obligation to accept death. The above-mentioned peculiar characteristics of ICU patients demands from health care workers, even more explicitly than in other areas of medicine, some fundamental moral attitudes or virtues to secure the ethical dimension of the person's life and death. I will summarize these basic attitudes as an unconditional respect for the dignity of each person and the acceptance of human finitude.

In order to discover what constitutes an appropriate use of life-supporting technology in ICUs, "a physician shall be dedicated to providing competent medical services with compassion and respect for human dignity" (American Medical Association 1981, 1). I think that this statement, summarizing three key attitudes for the praxis of medicine in general, needs to be specifically emphasized for intensive medicine. In other words, the appropriate use of high-technology medicine demands, at least, these three basic virtues: (1) medical expertise, (2) compassion, and (3) respect for the dignity of the person, even in situations of extreme debility and suffering. Moreover, I would like to suggest that it is precisely a compassionate attitude that allows recognition of the concrete ways in which medical expertise can be used truly to respect the dignity of each person, especially in situations of imminent risk of death.

The term "compassion" is today commonly understood as synonymous with pity. This is not the way in which I use "compassion." With Dougherty and Purtilo, I define it as

> the virtue by which we have a sympathetic consciousness of sharing the distress and suffering of another person and on that basis are inclined to offer assistance in alleviating and/or living through that suffering. Hence, there are two key elements in defining compassion: 1) an ability and willingness to enter into another's situation deeply enough to gain knowledge of the person's experience of suffering; and 2) a virtue characterized by the desire to alleviate the person's suffering or, if that is not possible, to be support by living through it vicariously. (1995, 427)

Compassion, understood as a moral virtue, is thus directed primarily to the person and secondarily to his sufferings. Because it entails the willingness effectively to alleviate a person's suffering, it demands that one possess the corresponding expertise or "know-how." And it is evident that human suffering has many different sources. From this perspective, medical interventions able to benefit critically ill persons cannot be narrowly understood as those having the potential to produce certain physiological effects on the person's body, which is doubtless an important goal of critical care. The medical commitment toward a suffering person reaches far more than his body. In the context of ICUs, a peculiar source of human suffering is the person's natural fear of imminent death, derived either from the clinical condition itself or from the risks related to life-supporting technologies. Thus, health care workers should develop a special sensitivity toward these aspects, permitting their patients to reflect on their moral duty to accept death and to receive the necessary psychological and spiritual assistance. This will require, among other things, being aware of the importance of preserving the patient's state of consciousness, as long as clinical conditions and therapeutic goals allow.

If it is true that compassion is primarily directed to the person in virtue of his sufferings, and only secondarily to his sufferings, then we can draw two further practical conclusions. Whenever life-supporting interventions are judged proportionate, the respect due to the dignity of each person will require us to implement such measures in spite of the potential risks and sufferings. Conversely, in situations of extreme and prolonged suffering, a truly compassionate attitude will prevent health care providers from being tempted to accelerate death in order to alleviate their patient's suffering. On the contrary, a compassionate attitude may disclose for health care providers the ways in which their competent medical knowledge can be best used to palliate sufferings so as truly to respect each person's dignity, even in the events surrounding an unavoidable death.

According to this personalistic approach, the core of moral reasoning is derived from the fact that the proper addressee for a person as a subject of moral action is not duty as duty, or law as law, but a concrete, real person, who, in virtue of his dignity and ontologic structure, defines for every other person the field of his moral duty. We discover and fulfill ourselves as persons only when we affirm others as persons. Whenever we betray the respect due to another person, we simultaneously betray ourselves. In other words, our responsibility toward others converges with the responsibility toward ourselves. "Persona est affirmanda propter seipsam et propter dignitatem suam" (Styczen 1981). Such unconditional respect for the dignity of each human person, as God's image, is at the foundation of Christian ethics.

CONCLUSION

I have suggested that, according to Roman Catholic tradition, individual decisions determining what constitutes an appropriate use of high-technology medicine necessarily involve value judgments related to moral obligations to pursue proportionate health care (also referred to as "ordinary means") and the duty to accept death. Such decisions should be grounded in objective states of affairs regarding both the nature of a given clinical condition and the present state of medical art. The virtue of prudence, understood as practical wisdom trying to discern God's will, plays a key role in disclosing the way in which the different elements involved in therapeutic proportionality have to be weighted in individual situations. There are also other fundamental moral attitudes that should orient the contemporary praxis of critical care—which I have summarized as unconditional respect for the dignity of each person—even in situations of extreme weakness, and the acceptance of human finitude. Such a personalistic approach to health care in general, and to critical care in particular, provides clues for overcoming the contemporary logic of the so-called technological imperative.

Although my previous reflections refer mainly to the process of individual decision making (microethics), I think that they may have some implications for institutional ethics and even for macroethics (see the essay in this volume by Khushf). Engelhardt (also in this volume) proposes that critical care should not be held to the same standards of excellence in all countries or even necessarily in all regions of any particular country. He argues that although morality is universal, the economic and medical resources of a particular country or region will be important factors for determining what critical care ought to be provided and under what circumstances. He concludes that it may, therefore, be morally permissible that there are variations in access to and differences in standards of critical care from country to country and within any country.

Although differences in resources will certainly lead to variations in availability and standards of critical care, I think that it is extremely important to establish minimum standards of excellence, under which it will be better not to have an ICU at all. If the services provided by an ICU are "mediocre," then it is quite probable that patients will not survive or will need to stay longer. In the first case, one could say that no real medical intervention was offered to that patient, according to the present state of medical progress. In the second case, prolonged ICU hospitalization will result in an artificially augmented occupation rate, which will prevent other patients from ICU admission. This will result in increasing the number of uncovered ICU requests, generating an "unvirtuous circle" (see the essay by Rie in this volume). Thus, for a given community, it may be fair to have smaller ICUs, which effectively satisfy the present standards of excellence, than bigger mediocre ICUs, which cannot offer real chances of overcoming clinical conditions for which the present state of medical art has reasonable probabilities of success.

Estimating a population's present need for ICU services presupposes some criteria for identifying those patients who may benefit from life-supporting measures, independent of the actual possibility of satisfying such need. Determining the gap between the estimated need and the actual ICU size will provide important information for hospital directors, politicians, lawmakers, and others. They must honestly face complex problems related to social priorities, according to that community's budget and its moral responsibility toward other aspects of the common good besides intensive care (see the essays in this volume by Boyle, Kaveny, and Wildes).

It becomes clear that the decision to have an ICU cannot be simply justified on the basis of the availability of eligible patients and suitable personnel and facilities. Further moral criteria related to distributive justice and solidarity need to be considered. Such decisions also presuppose "political will." Therefore, if despite the perceived need and feasibility of implementing an ICU, the administrative authority decides that financial resources cannot be allocated, the individual members of the hospital are not morally responsible toward the community for not providing this kind of assistance. But "the principle of distributive justice demands that we seek the morally correct distribution of benefits and burdens in society" (American College of Physicians 1992, 947).

NOTES

1. Moore states: " I shall deal with theories which owe their prevalence to the supposition that good can be defined by reference to a *natural object* . . . and I give it but one name, the naturalistic fallacy. . . . This method consists in substituting for 'good' some one property of a natural object or of a collection of natural objects; and in thus replacing Ethics by some one of the natural sciences" (1959, 39–40).

2. In 1984, Le Gall et al. showed that an abbreviated version of the original APACHE score performed with similar effectiveness. This system, known as the Simplified Acute Physiology Score (SAPS), has been broadly used, especially in France and many European countries. Using a different approach, based on the selection of the most influential variables by logistic regression, Teres, Brown, and Lemeshow (1982) developed a model to estimate the probability of mortality for ICU patients. This model evolved into the Mortality Probability Model (MPM) in 1985 (Lemeshow et al. 1985). In 1985, a new version of APACHE, known as APACHE II, was published (Knaus et al. 1985). Recently, new versions of these three systems have been released: APACHE III, SAPS II, and MPM II. It has been demonstrated that these new versions of the severity of disease evaluation systems perform better than their older counterparts (Castella et al. 1995). They are used today around the world to determine a patient's prognosis in ICUs.

3. The Study to Understand Prognosis and Preferences of Outcomes and Risks of Treatments (SUPPORT) and the Hospitalized Elderly Longitudinal Project (HELP) have primarily sought to understand and improve decision making for seriously ill and for elderly hospitalized patients. Both studies included very sick and elderly persons, many of whom died during the follow-up period, but who were not in an intensive care unit, as different from former prognostic models. HELP was intended only to describe the largely unexamined experience of elderly hospitalized persons. However, SUPPORT

also studied an intervention, improved prognostic and subjective information and efforts of specially trained nurse specialists, to enhance communication and accelerate decision making.

4. Scholastic philosophy affirms that the moral value of our free acts depends on the nature of its object (also known as *moral species or "finis proximus operis"*), the intention of the agent *(finis operantis)* and the circumstances (Aquinas 1981, *ST* I–II, q. 18–21).

5. I refer here to the classical moral distinction between *physical* and *moral* acts, which is also expressed by the terms *actus homini* and *actus humanus* (Wojtyla 1980). The *physical* realization of an act *(actus homini)* does not necessarily coincide with the realization of a *moral* act. Only an action in which human freedom is exercised *(actus humanus)* can be morally qualified.

6. The five stages of the emotional reactions of patients facing death described by this author are: anger, denial and isolation, pact or negotiation, depression, and acceptance.

7. The SUPPORT intervention targeted improvement in the following five areas: (1) time before orders against resuscitation, (2) agreement between physician and patient about orders against resuscitation, (3) time in the ICU, in a coma, or on a ventilator before death, (4) alleviation of pain, and (5) use of resources. Despite intense efforts directed to improve communication, the results of SUPPORT have been disappointing: The intervention was ineffective in improving any of these five aspects.

8. I am not aware of the existence of studies like SUPPORT performed in my country or other countries around the world. Nevertheless, my personal perception is that the situation in my country does not differ substantially from the one described for the United States.

9. "Persona est affirmanda propter seipsam et propter dignitatem suam" (Styczen 1981).

BIBLIOGRAPHY

American College of Physicians. 1992. American College of Physicians ethics manual, 3d ed. *Annals of Internal Medicine* 117: 947–60.

American Medical Association. 1981. *Principles of Medical Ethics.* Chicago: American Medical Association.

Aquinas, Saint Thomas. 1981. *Summa Theologiae,* trans. by Fathers of the English Dominican Province. Westminster, Md.: Christian Classics.

Caplan, A. 1996. Odds and ends: Trust and the debate over medical futility. *Annals of Internal Medicine* 125: 688–89.

Castella, X., A. Artigas, J. Bion, and A. Kari. 1995. A comparison of severity of illness scoring systems for intensive care unit patients: Results of a multicenter, multinational study. *Critical Care Medicine* 23: 1327–35.

Catechism of the Catholic Church. 1994. Ligouri, Mo.: Ligouri Publications.

Christensen, K. 1992. Applying the concept of futility at the bedside. *Cambridge Quarterly of Healthcare Ethics* 1: 239–48.

Congregation for the Doctrine of the Faith. 1980. Vatican declaration on euthanasia. *Acta Apostolica Sedis* 72: 547–49.

Dougherty, C., and R. Purtilo. 1995. Physicians' duty of compassion. *Cambridge Quarterly of Healthcare Ethics* 4: 426–33.

Evidence-Based Medicine Working Group. 1992. Evidence-based medicine. A new approach to teaching the practice of medicine. *Journal of the American Medical Association* 268 (17): 2420–25.

Hippocratic Corpus. 1977. The art. In *Ethics in Medicine: Historical Perspectives and Contemporary Concerns*, ed. by S. J. Reiser, A. J. Dick, and W. J. Curran. Cambridge, Mass.: MIT Press.

John Paul II. 1992. To participants at the international congress on care for the dying person. *OssRom* March 18, n. 1.

———. 1993. Veritatis Splendor. In *Encíclicas de Juan Pablo II*, Madrid: Edibesa.

Jonas, H. 1979. *Das Prinzip Verantwortung. Versuch einer Ethik für die technologische Zivilisation.* Frankfurt: Insel Verlag.

Kilner, J. F. 1990. *Who Lives? Who Dies?* New Haven, Conn.: Yale University Press.

Knaus, W. A., E. A. Draper, D. P. Wagner, and J. Zimmerman. 1985. APACHE II: A severity of disease classification system. *Critical Care Medicine* 13: 818–29.

Knaus, W. A., D. P. Wagner, E. A. Draper, J. Zimmerman, M. Bergner, P. Bastos, C. Sirio, D. Murphy, T. Lotring, and A. Damiano. 1991. The APACHE III prognostic system. Risk prediction of hospital mortality for critically ill hospitalized adults. *Chest* 100: 1619–36.

Knaus, W. A., J. E. Zimmerman, D. P. Wagner, E. Draper, and D. Lawrence. 1981. APACHE—acute physiology and chronic health evaluation: A physiologically based classification system. *Critical Care Medicine* 9: 591–97.

Kübler-Ross, E. 1969. *Sobre la muerte y los moribundos.* Barcelona: Grijalbo.

Le Gall, J., P. Loirat, A. Alperovith, P. Glaser, C. Granthil, D. Mathieu, P. Mercier, R. Thomas, and D. Villers. 1984. A simplified acute physiologic score for ICU patients. *Critical Care Medicine* 12: 975–77.

Lemeshow, S., D. Teres, H. Pastides, J. Avrunin, and J. Steingrub. 1985. A method for predicting survival and mortality of ICU patients using objectively derived weights. *Critical Care Medicine* 13: 519–25.

Moore, G. E. 1959. *Principia Ethica.* New York: Cambridge University Press.

Plato. 1981. *Republic,* trans. by G. M. Grube. Indianapolis: Hackett.

Pontifical Council for Pastoral Assistance to Health Care Workers. 1995. *Charter for Health Care Workers.* Vatican City: Vatican Press.

Quinlan, In Re. 1976. 70 NJ 10, 355 A2d 647 (1976), cert denied, 429 US 922.

Scheiber, G. J., J. P. Poullier, and L. M. Greenwald. 1994. Health system performance in OECD countries, 1980–1982. *Health Affairs* 13: 100–112.

Schneiderman, L. 1998. Commentary: Bringing clarity to the futility debate: Are the cases wrong? *Cambridge Quarterly of Healthcare Ethics* 7: 269–78.

Schneiderman, L., K. Faber-Langendoen, and N. Jecker. 1994. Beyond futility to an ethics of care. *American Journal of Medicine* 96: 110–14.

Schneiderman, L., N. Jecker, and A. Jonsen. 1990. Medical futility: Its meaning and ethical implications. *Annals of Internal Medicine* 112: 949–54.

———. 1996. Medical futility: Response to critiques. *Annals of Internal Medicine* 125: 669–74.

Smith, G., and M. Nielsen. 1999. ABC of intensive care. Criteria for admission. *British Medical Journal* 318: 1544–47.

Styczen, T. 1981. *The ABC of Ethics*. Unpublished manuscript, Catholic University of Lublin, Lublin.

SUPPORT (Study to Understand Prognosis and Preferences of Outcomes and Risks of Treatments). 1995. *Journal of the American Medical Association* 274: 1591–98.

Teres, D., R. B. Brown, and S. Lemeshow. 1982. Predicting mortality of intensive care patients. The importance of coma. *Critical Care Medicine* 10: 86–95.

von Hildebrand, D. 1952. *Christian Ethics*. New York: David McKay Company.

———. 1980. *Moralia*. Regensburg: Kohlhammer.

Weil, M., M. von Planta, and E. Rackow. 1989. Critical care medicine: Introduction and historical perspective. In *Textbook of Critical Care*, 2d ed., ed. by W. Shoemaker. Philadelphia: W. B. Saunders.

Wildes, K. W. 1995. Conserving life and conserving means: Lead us not into temptation. In *Critical Choices and Critical Care*, ed. by K. Wildes. Dordrecht: Kluwer Academic Publishers.

Wojtyla, K. 1980. *The Acting Person*. Dordrecht: Reidel.

PART IV

Moral Theological Perspectives

Limiting Access to Health Care:
A Traditional Roman Catholic
Analysis

Joseph Boyle

The Roman Catholic moral tradition has had much to say about withholding and otherwise limiting medical treatments, including those needed to keep a person alive. Many both within and outside the Roman Catholic community have found the discussion of these matters by Catholic authorities and scholars to be helpful. This is true even when the tradition fails to generate responses that are fully determinate or completely compelling, as is clear from the enduring interest in the Catholic discussion of ordinary and extraordinary ways of treating patients. Most Catholic teaching and scholarship concerning withholding treatment have focused on the scope of health care decisions by individuals and their families, as well as on the corresponding rights and duties of health care professionals. As in other areas of moral perplexity, the tradition has been concerned to identify correctly those participants in various kinds of health care decisions who rightly have the final say. Of course, all decisions by authorities should be shaped by general moral principles and precepts. The framework for these particular authoritative decisions is set by the implications of the Fifth Commandment (Thou shalt not kill), so that decisions to limit life-sustaining treatment that are morally identical to choices to end life are excluded from the range of choices authorities may make.

Traditional Roman Catholic views on withholding medical treatment certainly seem able to deal with the questions raised by the apparent need to limit the care that health care professionals and institutions make available to patients, and in particular the need to limit some patients' access to intensive care units. This is a new question about limiting medical treatment; its answer, as I hope to show below, is not simply an implication of the traditional doctrine on withholding treatment. To answer that new question, the resources of the traditional doctrine must be supplemented by the theory of public authority and of human rights embedded in Catholic social teaching.

Therefore, in my contribution to this volume, I will seek in the first section to summarize the Catholic teaching on withholding treatments, so as to bring its light to bear on the aspects of the new question that it can readily illuminate. Although this teaching does not by itself settle the new question about limiting access to treatments such as intensive care units, it does help to reveal the distinctive character of this new problem by providing a point of comparison. For the traditional teaching is patient-centered in a way that public allocation decisions cannot be. In the second section, I suggest how considerations from Catholic social teaching are necessary to provide a moral analysis of allocation decisions in general. I will argue that church teaching concerning the role of authority in social choice implies a moral justification of reasonable public decisions to deal with medical scarcity. Public coordination is needed to supplement individual service to objectives that individuals are morally bound to serve if they can but that cannot be adequately secured by a multitude of individual initiatives. The teaching about welfare rights points to norms for carrying out this allocation in a fair manner. In the third section, I will argue that combining elements of the traditional moral theology of withholding treatment with the implications of Catholic social teaching concerning social authority and scarcity provides a basis for a systematic analysis of the issues raised by the need to limit the treatment offered to patients.

This systematic analysis is not sufficient to generate detailed directives for all who must make decisions in this area; rather, it is meant to highlight the considerations relevant for morally assessing the full range of moral issues that decision makers must address. So my analysis is meant to address an ethical problem that faces all those having responsibility for allocation decisions in modern health care. I shall not address the further challenges to witness to Gospel values, a challenge Catholic health care institutions face when this problem is only more or less properly handled in the wider secular health care system. Nor shall I address the problems individual Christians face when institutional responses either fail to respond fully to people's needs, or even exacerbate their problems by creating sinful social structures.

The approach I will take is that of traditional Catholic moral analysis. The reasoning involved in this approach is the application of general moral considerations to situations sufficiently complex to require careful analysis to reveal their moral character. This reasoning aims to expose the factors in morally opaque situations that make them difficult to assess morally. Isolating such factors allows assessment to proceed by allowing judgments as to their moral relevance—for example, that some coercive conditions make possible a choice in response to them that is a very different choice than people would make absent such coercion. The person who hands over his wallet at gunpoint is making a different choice than in an ordinary transaction.[1]

My approach takes seriously the teaching of the church and treats respectfully the methods, reasoning, and consensus of scholars working within the Catholic moral tradition. My rationale for such an approach is that, like many Catholic moralists, I believe that Catholic moral teaching reveals God's will, and plainly states easily accessible moral truths, which are nevertheless often obscured or set aside. But it is not my purpose here to address directly the questions about the philosophical credibility of natural law, or the theological questions about the nature of the alleged supernatural warrants for Catholic moral teaching and the body of moral theology that authentically explains and applies this teaching. Rather, my central purpose is to apply to one new and difficult problem the substantial body of moral doctrine that exists in the Catholic tradition. Whatever others may think about the deep questions of moral theory and theology that such an undertaking raises, I proceed as I do, hoping that what I say—if it is a correct development of the tradition—may persuade some, give pause to others, and more generally contribute to the broader discussion of the problems being discussed in this volume.

My analysis is likely to fail to persuade many who do not accept the authorities and norms of inquiry of the Catholic tradition, and even some who do accept them. That failure will not argue against the soundness of my analysis; indeed, failure to persuade even those who accept these authorities on such complex and new matters is to be expected.[2] Still, the capacity of such analysis to illumine the moral issues for some who do not accept Catholic authorities or norms of moral inquiry provides a basis for hoping that reasoning and discussion can at least sometimes help resolve difficult moral problems and that the tradition is sufficiently resilient to withstand postmodern relativism.

LIMITING TREATMENT IN THE CATHOLIC TRADITION

Specific Catholic norms for directing health care decisions are usually recognized as implications of two things: larger normative themes, such as the Christian meaning of life and death, as well as more fundamental moral principles, such as the second of the summary commandments on love. Before stating these specific norms, therefore, I will briefly say something about the relevant themes and principles.

The Place of Health Care in a Good Life

The Catholic tradition holds that, for those who have received God's revelation, pursuing health and the means to stay alive should not be of ultimate human value; only God's Kingdom and the goods of persons, just insofar as they are members of this Kingdom, are of ultimate value. Indeed, for a mature Christian, the pursuit of any human good is likely to be harmful and wrong if not integrated into his or her allegiance to the Kingdom of God. This situating of human value within the revealed plan of God, does not, however, mean that natural human concerns are necessarily misguided or that nothing in life really is worth pursuing for its own sake. Catholics regard the good things of this life not as ladders to God's Kingdom, which drop away when the Kingdom is fully realized, but rather as elements of the Kingdom that are purified and fully realized in it.[3] Indeed, the Catholic tradition pushes in the direction of holding that life and health are among the basic goods of human persons as bodily creatures; that is, they provide legitimate reasons for action that are neither simply instrumental to other human concerns nor reducible to what people happen to want.

This last claim can be articulated as follows. Health is good bodily functioning and is the perfection of our being alive just as animals (Lee 1998, 135–42). Being alive is not only a necessary condition for pursuing other goods but is part of the personal reality of a human being. This means that life and health are intrinsically good; that is, whenever an action in view promotes or protects life or health, that action is so far forth choice-worthy: that it protects or enhances life or health provides a reason sufficient for doing it, though not necessarily a reason that morally justifies doing it.

The Catholic acceptance of the inherent value of human bodily life is shown clearly in the church's evaluation of death. The death of Jesus is understood as a bad thing in itself; something from which God brought good, but an evil nevertheless. By blessing Jesus's complete obedience even in the face of death with the gift of bodily resurrection, not only for Jesus individually but for all those joined to him by Baptism and Holy Communion, God surely reveals that death is bad and bodily life good. Death is the last enemy to be overcome, and Jesus's repugnance at His own anticipated death, shared by many who followed Him in martyrdom, reveals its evil.

Similarly, Jesus's actions in regard to ill health and disease reveal them also to be human evils. Jesus often healed people as a sign of His divine authority and as an anticipation of the Kingdom whose imminent arrival He preached. Of course, if Jesus had wanted to be a physician, He could have healed everyone; but, given the purposes for which He healed and His evident compassion for those He helped, it is hard to understand these actions except as supposing the evil of ill health and disease. Moreover, the suffering and pain that accompany death, disease, and ill health are also regarded by the tradition as part of the evil of bodily debility, at least insofar as they do more than provide information about our unhealthy condition.

In short, the Catholic tradition implies the view that life and health are goods valuable in themselves because of their constitutive relation to humans as bodily creatures, and that their opposites, death and disease, are, just as such, bad. They are redeemable evils to be sure, and not as such moral evils, but evils nonetheless.[4]

The intrinsic goodness of any good we may seek does not imply the moral goodness of any and all actions done for its sake. Such actions may violate other responsibilities one has to other people and goods: Intrinsic goodness means desirability as an end, not as a means to something further; it does not mean either most desirable, all things considered, or morally obligatory. So although one always has a reason for an action that promotes or protects the good of life or health, one may have reasons, even conclusive ones, to forgo that action or to act differently to serve other goods instead. Thus, although intrinsically good, the goods of life and health do not always trump considerations based on other human goods.

Indeed, the Catholic tradition is well aware of the temptations involved in seeking doctors' help. It recognizes a variety of ways in which one can wrongly choose actions for the sake of life and health.

Most often, one chooses wrongly for the sake of these goods when the strong emotions connected with staying alive and feeling well are allowed to block the appropriate consideration of other goods and of other moral considerations. Most of us, most of the time, hate the thought of our own dying or that of those we love. We also find abhorrent the pain and debility of illness. That repugnance can motivate a refusal to consider whether the effort to stay or keep alive or to maintain good and pain-free bodily functioning is appropriate, given all the responsibilities one has to God, others, and oneself as determined by one's personal vocation.

Jesus and most of His martyrs found death repugnant, but refused to let that repugnance prevent their doing their duty, even when they saw clearly that it would get them killed. Similarly, the lifestyles of many holy missionaries and ascetics were not controlled by the natural desire and good reasons supporting a healthy life, and they were even less concerned about merely feeling good.

Still, inasmuch as life and health are goods of the human person, the possibility of failure with respect to them can arise not only from excessive concern about them, but also from a lack of proper concern to promote and protect them. In the absence of the strong emotions surrounding serious illness or debility and the prospect of death, it is easy to overlook the good reasons that suggest or call for action for the sake of life and health. So neglecting health is a real temptation, and the virtue of temperance helps people, among other things, to organize their characters so as to resist this sort of negligence.

But even more clearly and radically, there is the temptation not sufficiently to regard and respect these goods when normal functioning is greatly compromised or when death is at hand. In these cases, the distorting emotional tendency often is to ignore and avoid the suffering of the disabled, and in the case of the dying simply to get the suffering—that of the dying person and that of family members and caregivers—over with. In this context, it seems to me that the church has distinguished two things that are often hard to distinguish: (1) accepting God's will and uniting one's suffering and death with that of the Lord, on the one hand; and (2) failing courageously to respect life and live it as fully as one can as it comes to its often unpleasant end, on the other.

Specific Moral Norms Directing Health Care Decisions

Within the Catholic tradition, perhaps the most salient norm relevant to health care decisions is that intentionally killing an innocent person is always gravely wrong. This norm prohibits euthanasia and suicide, including euthanasia or suicide by omission, that is, the withholding of any treatment, medical or otherwise, with a view toward ending life. Aside from its strong presence within the entire postmedieval tradition, as a reading of the Fifth Commandment of the Mosaic Decalogue, this norm seems an immediate and sure implication of respect for the good of human life assessed in light of the second of the love commandments. Similarly, acts and omissions done with the intent to harm health are absolutely prohibited. Both these prohibitions have been refined in their application by the tradition's practice of casuistry, particularly the casuistry of double effect.

Prohibitions against intentional killing and other, lesser intentional attacks on bodily well-being, do not by themselves provide the moral guidance needed to avoid either negligence with respect to or excessive concern with these goods. But the norms needed for this guidance have been understood as compatible with the Fifth Commandment.

The standards by which a person determines whether choices affecting these goods are negligent, excessively solicitous for them, or fully rational and upright plainly are based on a multitude of moral considerations. There are cases in which actions undertaken for the sake of life or health have negative side effects bearing on these very goods sufficient to justify the judgment that these actions are to be forgone because they are excessive. Treatments involving continuing, debilitating pain or significant incapacitation of normal biological function might be excessive in this way.[5] But more commonly, even when the negative side effects of actions for the sake of life and health include damage to these goods, it is their impact on other goods of a person's life that provides the basis for such judgments.

But here the basis for the judgment that the treatment is disproportionate or excessive becomes difficult to articulate. There is no single pattern within which human goods are promoted, respected, and protected in all good lives. A standard is needed that is both less general and more individual than the basic moral principles, such as the love commandments, and still morally relevant, rationally expressible, and applicable to the goods whose pursuit constitutes a person's life. Something like the life plan of a morally good person seems to provide the needed standard. For not all good people need live according to the same pattern of life, but all good people have a set of morally upright commitments, by virtue of which their lives are organized and given moral identity.

The personal vocation by which each person responds to God's call to live well by making a unique contribution to His Kingdom is the Christian form of this moral ideal. It provides a basis, in addition to the requirements of general moral norms and principles, for determining what is reasonable and appropriate in one's actions, relationships, and projects.

The position of truthfulness and integrity, fairness and piety within a good person's life is largely settled by general moral norms alone; one cannot lie, treat others unfairly, or ignore one's creaturely status before God without violating universal moral norms. But these norms do not settle the particular people one will commit oneself to, the particular forms of religious piety one will adopt, or the particular form of life in which one will realize one's potentialities and relate to others. Nor do general norms settle the position within a good person's life of other goods, such as learning, skill, life, and health. People who think of their lives vocationally will recognize their abilities as gifts to be used well and the needs of others as opportunities for service. Responsible commitments will be made as one seeks a way of life that will use one's abilities to serve real human goods. Those commitments generate responsibilities to definite people, and living out those responsibilities structures a moral life. The structure is not rigid because one's abilities and opportunities develop and change; moreover, one's responsibilities to others make very variable demands during the course of one's life.

Thus, not all are required to be scholars, or to be craftsmen or artists up to the level of their skill, or to choose the healthiest lifestyle. But for most people, one or more of these goods will have a central and determinative position in their lives such that failure to look after it is wrong. Scholars morally must get the facts and theory as right as they can, and owe considerable personal commitment to such efforts. Parents of young children must take care of their own health as part of their parental role.

The standard provided by one's personal vocation is plainly relevant to a person's use of health care resources.[6] Indeed, it provides a way to understand the traditional ideas of "proportionate" or "ordinary" medical treatments. When one's use of health care involves violating no moral responsibility common to all and comports better with one's personal vocation than not using it would, it is proportionate or ordinary, otherwise not.

My proposed conception of an ordinary treatment makes clear why ordinary treatments are, as the tradition held, morally obligatory, and not simply by stipulation: There is no generally applicable reason to forgo them, and they fit with the more specific, morally defined orientation of a person's life. One can think of cases in which the general moral considerations will require treatment for some person, or in which one's vocation simply requires it. These too are ordinary, proportionate treatments, but with an additional reason to accept the treatment.

Similarly, actions for the sake of life and health will be "disproportionate" or "extraordinary" when they are in some significant way incompatible with carrying out the decision maker's personal vocation. This is not as far from the traditional way of putting it as may appear. For it involves only a further defining of the tradition's idea of a grave burden in terms of one's personal vocation.

This may appear to define the idea of a grave burden too weakly. For in the tradition a grave burden must be something serious enough to justify refusing medical treatment needed to stay alive. But I believe this definition of a grave burden is not too weak for the task. The life and death decisions it must justify are not choices precisely to end life, because these are prohibited by the Fifth Commandment, but choices about whether actions to keep oneself alive are justified. That justification cannot be made by deductions from moral principle because, in addition to the absolute prohibitions of killing and harming bodily life, the general norms are vague and in need of a basis for determining an action's fit in a given person's life. The organized set of commitments making up a person's unique vocation provides a relevant basis for determining that kind of fit. And the tradition provides no generally stated alternatives to this account, but proceeds casuistically, relying on clear cases of what is or is not proportionate. My account explains why these cases are clear.

Those commitments will be transformed in various ways by serious illness or by the need to care for a seriously ill family member. Sickness can radically change one's capacities and the possibilities to carry on the projects that were central to one's vocation before sickness. So the relevant understanding of one's vocation is not that defined prior to and independent of the condition of illness; one's vocation is not a large-scale project, but a cooperative, responsive venture in which one is faithful to commitments made but open to using one's de facto resources to continue shaping a good life. The sickness or injury of oneself or of one for whom one has responsibility are not chosen but given (even if one bears responsibility for causing them). As a given, sickness or injury becomes an element of one's vocation insofar as it calls for one to cope responsibly and to reorder the rest of one's life so as to continue, in this altered set of circumstances, to do what one can responsibly to live.

There are two further reasons for accepting my vocational definition of ordinary and extraordinary treatments. The first is that this account allows a clear focus on an issue the tradition has tended to ignore, namely, impermissible treatments. As far as I know, the tradition has not been much interested in impermissible treatments; it was much more interested in sorting out those treatments people were morally bound to use and those they were morally free to use or reject. Of course, this discussion was framed by the assumption that there were certain moral absolutes, such as the Fifth Commandment, which excluded some things—for example, abortions, euthanasia and some mutilations—as medical options.

This focus of the tradition does not, however, imply that the only impermissible treatments for a given person are those excluded by universal moral precepts such as the Fifth Commandment. For it seems reasonable that, in addition to the traditional limits set by such general moral standards, there should be some medical options that are impermissible for a given person to use because of that person's unique set of responsibilities. Plainly, the application of very general moral principles to the particularities of a health care decision can reveal it to be wrong. The otherwise reasonable use of medical resources would be impermissible for someone if his or her use of them were unfair to others, or if it put him or her into an occasion of sin without an adequate reason. Similarly, forgoing a health care regime that would make it impossible to carry out important aspects of one's personal vocation seems obligatory, not simply permissible.

In short, the tradition, as I read it, has something clear to say about why some treatments are morally required and why others are not morally required. Its approach has implications for impermissible treatments, but those have largely remained tacit in the tradition. The vocational account of the tradition allows these implications to be articulated.

The second aspect of the tradition illuminated by the vocational account of ordinary and extraordinary treatments is its understanding of the special authority of the competent patient in medical decision making. This conception is the basis for the Catholic account of the right of competent patients to refuse medical treatment. Physicians and other health care professionals are not as such in a position to judge what fits or does not fit with a person's overall responsibilities in life. The potential patient, therefore, is the final authority concerning what medical treatments he or she will accept. The modern idea of autonomy, that control of one's life is good, regardless of what one does with it, also justifies patient authority over health care decisions. But the Catholic rationale for this authority is distinct from and indeed incompatible with this modern idea of autonomy.

When people are incapable of participating in the deliberation and choice of their own medical care, the decisions are appropriately left to those whose vocations include responsibility for those incapacitated or immature people, ordinarily but not necessarily family members. In such cases, personal vocation again provides the final standard for determining what care is appropriately accepted or rejected, but the personal vocation that is relevant here is that of the decision maker who is responsible for the patient, and not the patient himself or herself. For the immature patient has not formed an autonomous life that vocational commitments might structure morally, and the formerly competent patient cannot act to integrate current decisions into his or her established vocational commitment. Moreover, the person responsible for a noncompetent patient must face the implications of his or her efforts to care for the patient for his or her other responsibilities. So taking responsibility for such a patient becomes part of the responsible person's vocation, however much the patient's illness might disrupt the caregiver's prior life plans. For this reason, the noncompetent patient's vocational commitments and overall welfare are part of what is morally determinative in treatment decisions. But the final decision is that of another person, and aspects of the responsible person's vocation can make claims that limit what can be done for the noncompetent dependent. For example, issues of fairness can very quickly emerge on the domestic level when the cost of care for elderly family members conflicts with the need to provide education for the younger members of the family. Plainly, this situation allows for a conflict of interest on the part of those responsible for incompetent people. But considerations other than the noncompetent patient's welfare can be relevant to treatment decisions, and the temptations raised by that fact are minimized by noting that the entire deliberation should be carried out in light of all the obligations of the responsible party.

Should Physicians Refuse to Offer Futile Treatments?

Formulations of the doctrine of ordinary and extraordinary treatments by many twentieth-century theologians have included, along with the requirement that a grave burden be present, an additional consideration sufficient by itself to justify the withholding of medical treatment—namely, futility. So, by introducing this additional consideration, medical treatments are to be ordinary only if they offer a reasonable hope of benefit (Ashley and O'Rourke 1997, 420). Surely, however, the very description of a real case of futile treatment includes a reason for judging that it would be wrong to use it, not merely permissible to forgo it. For if a treatment promises no benefit whatsoever, then the actions constituting the treatment cannot be undertaken for the goods, such as health, that medicine ordinarily serves. It is unclear what purpose such actions are meant to serve. Perhaps they are in some way really aimed at the medical goals to which they are judged completely unrelated; perhaps they are meant to make patients or families feel better. Whatever motivational possibilities exist here, it does appear that such actions are for the sake of merely apparent goods, and that by itself is sufficient to judge them unreasonable and so wrong. Furthermore, given that such actions are wrong because they serve no real human good, it is impossible to justify any harmful side effects of such actions. So whatever costs strictly futile treatments impose on anyone at all, and there surely are some such costs, at least the use of time and effort of all involved, which could be used instead for beneficial activities, are without rational justification.

Now it certainly appears that what is true of futility when the likelihood of benefit is thought to be literally nonexistent is also true of futility defined in terms of very low likelihood of benefit: for example, procedures done on dying persons that at best will extend their lives a day or two while in no way facilitating their functioning or making them more comfortable. It certainly also appears that the features of strictly futile treatments that render them impermissible to use also characterize many other choices to use very unlikely and unpromising medical treatments. However, when the futile treatment has some small promise of success, it seems possible that one might have a reason to choose it that does not involve the moral flaws invariably present in the futile treatment of the strictest kind. But that possibility does not prevent the development of a medical consensus that some treatments are so unpromising and unlikely to be medically successful that they should not generally be offered to patients.

These generalities are not meant to disguise the difficulties involved in sorting out kinds of treatment that should not be offered to patients because they are so unpromising from kinds of treatment that are risky and unpromising but nevertheless fall within a patient's discretion about what risks and other burdens he or she should accept. As far as I know, the needed casuistry has not been carried out.[7]

The primary persons bound by the obligation not to use the kinds of futile treatments distinguished in the preceding paragraphs are those who must make the decision to use or forgo such treatment. Upon coming to believe as a result of medical study and consultation that the treatment in question is futile, the competent patient or the designated proxy ought to reject its use. One should not waste resources on oneself or on those one loves to no good end, and one should not cause those for whom one has responsibility to suffer for no good purpose.

However, it seems that physicians have a responsibility here that is not simply to respect patient judgment and preference. For in these cases, the physician has a duty not to provide futile treatment, because such treatment does not help the patient in the ways physicians should, and may cause the patient unjustified harm.

On the Catholic account, stated, as far as I know, most clearly by Pius XII, physicians cannot treat patients against their express will, and physicians cannot do to patients things that are impermissible for patients themselves to do (Boyle 1981, 86–87). This last norm is plainly introduced to apply to procedures prohibited by general moral norms like the Fifth Commandment, but it seems to me to have application in the matter of strictly futile treatment as well. If it is wrong for patients and their families to seek certain kinds of treatments, and if the ground for the wrongness is something within a physician's competence to recognize as wrong, then it is wrong for the physician to provide the treatment. That seems to me to be the case with respect to futile treatments: Strict futility is something physicians can recognize in their role as physicians. Moreover, a physician can see clearly the implications of judgments of futility for physician and patient responsibility without assuming that the physician has knowledge of or authority over the patient's entire life.

Physicians and other health care professionals are seldom in a position to assess the soundness of most reasons people give for refusing treatments or for preferring treatments different from those preferred by the physician. For that reason, physicians must respect refusals of treatment and make an effort to provide a range of reasonable treatment options for patients. However, physicians should not offer options that they believe are outside the medical profession's scientific consensus as to what should be offered to patients. Physicians are not slaves of patient desire but are professionals who should help patients on the basis of a body of scientific knowledge.

Concerns about the integrity of physicians and health care institutions are part of the reason why futile treatments should be refused. And concerns about the fair use of resources are another part of that reason, because scarce medical resources are being used. My argument, however, is that there is a failure to serve the patient, as a physician should, when patient or family insistence is permitted to trump a tested medical judgment that a treatment is futile or medically inappropriate for some other reason.

I suggest, in short, that physicians morally ought to refuse to cooperate with patient requests for treatments that medical consensus judges strictly futile or so unlikely to benefit as to warrant a similar verdict. Adequately informed patients and families will request futile treatments only if they are acting wrongly and asking physicians to do so as well. Acceding to such requests helps no one and turns health care providers into slaves, as it were, to patient and family desire. Note that the primary ground I am suggesting for physician and institutional refusal of truly futile treatments is not the economic impact of such treatments on other people and not the integrity of health care and its practitioners understood as something separable from service to patients. Rather, the ground for such refusals is the traditional concern for the patient's true good as something physicians can promote. Like quackery, futile treatment cannot do that.

This development of several aspects of the traditional teaching about withholding medical treatment suggests that physicians have a duty not to provide strictly futile treatments. But noting this limit of patient autonomy and detailing the logic of a traditional position that excludes some treatments as impermissible sketches only a small part of the response to what has become a significant problem of costs (Halevy, Neal, and Brody 1996, 100–104). Clarity about strict futility and about patient-centered refusals of such treatments is needed to address this larger question, but is not sufficient to answer it. It is worth considering what further progress toward answering the moral questions raised by the economics of limited resources can be made by reflecting on the Catholic moral tradition.

The Limits of Domestic Fairness
Morally good medical decision making by patients or their proxies takes into account the likely effects of their decisions on all those affected by them. The tradition, however, has for good reason directed the attention of decision makers to the effects on the person treated and on those most immediately affected—in particular, family members and similar care pro-

viders. For decision making about health care based on a competent person's judgment about its fit with his or her vocation or by another person having responsibility for a noncompetent person as part of his or her vocation will naturally focus on those one is especially called to serve in one's vocation, and for most of us that is primarily those near and dear.

Still, loving neighbor as self, as explicated by Christ, requires that our moral reflection consider a wider range of people, potentially anybody affected by our actions. In particular, if (1) our own use of medical resources for ourselves and those near and dear deprives of these resources others who need them as urgently as we do, and (2) we have no reason, except an emotional attachment to ourselves or those near and dear, for using them ourselves rather than leaving them for the other needy, then our use is unfair to them and so is not only disproportionate but impermissible.

The apparent stringency of this application of the Golden Rule (which is embodied in the second love commandment) evaporates when the limits of the cases to which it applies are noticed. In particular, it usually is reasonable to favor those near and dear, given our intimate association with them in living, our obligations to them and opportunity to help them. Still, there are cases where a person deliberates about spending a sum of money on health care that could be spent to address some other equally or more rationally compelling human need. Such cases often arise in a domestic context: The health needs of a family member or neighbor make demands incompatible with the real needs of others in the immediate community in which responsible parties have obligations. So this stringent implication of the Golden Rule does have real application in a limited, domestic sphere.

But it is difficult to see how this stringent norm, as applied to individual decision makers, gets applied in the larger system of government- and insurance-company-supported heath care. How can a person's accepting health care for self or others to which he or she is entitled by natural right or contract negatively affect others? The system within which such a person operates may be unjust to many people, a sinful social structure. But how do the decisions about what health care to accept or refuse by any person operating within it harm or help those not treated fairly by the system? Of course, a person can act politically to make a socialized system (such as Canada's, with which I am familiar) more equitable and far-reaching; and a person can make a conscientious choice to buy a smaller health care package for himself and his family so as to have more to share with the needy. But the individual health care decisions of patients and families within the health care systems now existing do not as such seem to be harmful or unfair to other people.

Part of the reason is that such individual decisions are uncoordinated and do not as such have any tendency to affect the operation of the system. Domestic decisions about health care, in short, ought to consider questions of fairness in the use of health care resources, but in most cases in which the negative impact is on those outside the reach of domestic considerations there is little individuals making health care decisions can do to bring about a more equitable distribution of health care resources.

THE SOCIAL NATURE OF HEALTH CARE AND CATHOLIC SOCIAL TEACHING

The scarcity of medical resources that affects domestic decisions about limiting health care seems to function differently in moral thinking than does the scarcity of medical resources of the entire community for which a health care system exists. In the former case, the issues are easily formulated in terms of what is proportionate, disproportionate, or impermissible. The decision is made by those who must suffer its consequences.

In systemic scarcity, by contrast, someone in authority in a community or institutional system must decide that some resources will be directed to meeting certain needs of community members, and as a result become unavailable to meet other needs of all or some in the community. Such decisions must be made in abstraction from the interests in the denied resources of those denied them. In the extreme case of allocating health care resources, medical options promising real and vital benefit will be denied to some people. Although the authoritative decisions should be fair, they cannot take account of such personal considerations as emerge when vocationally based decisions assess fairness in the context of all the goods of all the people involved. In short, the considerations that justify health care authorities in making allocation decisions in which resources are directed toward some at the expense of others cannot include a detailed consideration of what makes medical treatments gravely burdensome or impermissible for individuals and families. For in systemic allocation decisions, the issue is fairness in using the resources; decision makers cannot and should not consider fairness enriched by the factors that emerge in responsible domestic decision making.

I think that these factors—the need for action by social authority, the authority's need to set aside personalized consideration of the interests of those denied treatment, and the fact that real benefits might need to be denied—explain why thinking about allocating health care, taken as a limited social resource, is so distasteful. The limiting of useful care implied in allocations required by the existence of need in excess of resources is obnoxious, because it necessarily recognizes but abstracts from the fact that those denied the care may reasonably need it. That is, the care is denied not for their sake, but to allocate a scarce resource, recognizing that some denied the care are likely to need and want it. By contrast, in domestic decisions about limiting treatment, the interests of the patient are always considered, even if they are not always decisive, and the interests of the immediate community of which the patient is part are also considered by proxies. Thus these are hard questions, in part because those who must decide cannot make the welfare of individual patients the foremost consideration. Even the broadly defined welfare of patients and families—the whole good of the person that emerges in the context of reflection on one's full set of vocational responsibilities—cannot be a central consideration here. In the nature of the case, the issue is to decide how fairly to distribute a scarce resource, even if that distribution has as a side effect some harm to the welfare of some potential patients.

Authority and Subsidiarity in Catholic Social Thought

Obnoxious though such decisions may be, the Catholic tradition does not condemn them as necessarily wrong, but implicitly recognizes that under certain circumstances they may be justified. One purpose of authority in Catholic social teaching is to coordinate the actions of individuals so they can cooperate for common goods. The need for the kind of social choice authority makes possible is especially urgent when moral problems emerge that cannot be solved by the uncoordinated actions of even the most conscientious individuals and small communities.

The fair use of health care resources is a problem that cannot be solved by purely individual initiative. That is because health care is organized and paid for through a complex social system that frames and limits the impact of individual health care decisions. This is true not only of communities with socialized medicine, but also of those that rely on insurance and an array of public and private, for-profit and nonprofit institutions to deliver and pay for health care.

One might, of course, lament the level of social organization that now characterizes health care in industrial countries. But these systems serve life and health, and make possible a greater realization of these goods, both in terms of the persons reached by modern health care and the extent of the benefits provided to those who are served. Catholic social teaching recognizes these advantages of the socialization (which may or may not include significant politicization) of modern health care as of modern life generally. So the challenge is to establish and use appropriate authority to guarantee that the health care system properly and fairly serves human need. Plainly, in a situation of scarcity of health care resources, that authority may face the obnoxious decision of denying some forms of health care to some people who need them.

The reasoning in the preceding paragraphs is often understood as an implication of the principle of subsidiarity. In Catholic teaching, this principle is understood as protecting from inappropriate interference by political society the legitimate initiatives of individuals, families, voluntary associations, and other incomplete societies. But as the word itself suggests, the principle articulates the proper relationship between larger, more powerful communities and smaller, less powerful communities and individuals as being a helping or assisting relationship between former and latter. Thus, the principle also requires the authoritative intervention of larger communities when necessary to help individuals and smaller communities respond properly to the requirements of the human good. That is what justifies political coordination of individual actions incapable by themselves of fairly serving the goods of life and health by means of the vast array of techniques now available.

The Right to Health Care

This side of subsidiarity is understood in the tradition to justify political society in the enforcement of some moral responsibilities, for example, through redistributive taxation. The strong affirmation in Catholic social teaching of significant welfare rights, including the right to health care, rests upon this helping function of political society. The responsibility for such things as life and health, as well as for education and opportunities for fulfilling lives, lies primarily with families, individuals, and voluntary associations. But these individuals and groups are often unable to secure these goods for themselves without public support, and are more often unable to provide them to others (as the Golden Rule demands, when this is possible) without the coordination of social action by community authority, including political authority.

As was suggested above, Catholic social thought is reasonably interpreted as holding that the socialization of health care into a socially regulated and subsidized system is justified by the service this system is able to provide people in pursuing responsibly the goods of life and health, and in fulfilling their prepolitical obligations to provide neighborly assistance to the ill and disabled they can help. This rationale is not overturned by the fact that the organization of health care into a socially regulated system raises moral questions that would not arise if health care remained a more thoroughly private, domestic matter. Appropriate social authority is needed to coordinate the actions of the system to address moral questions, particularly questions of fairness that conscientious individual decision cannot effectively handle. Because of the impact of good and ill health on the lives of people and communities bound together in political society, it seems that political authority has an irreducible role in dealing with these questions of fairness. Thus, I understand the right to health care to be the justified claim of the members of a society on their society to benefit fairly from the socially regulated use of the organized social reality of health care to address human need.

It is worth noting that the justification of welfare entitlements as an implication of subsidiarity that is exemplified in the reasoning of the last paragraph concerning the right to health care has some practical and not simply justificatory implications. Modern welfare rights presuppose levels of social organization and functional diversification that make coordinated social action serve human goods more efficiently than individual or neighborly initiatives can serve them. The underlying obligation to help others exists in all societies, because the most basic principle from which this obligation is derived—that is, the principle formulated by Christians as the twofold love commandment—applies universally. But meaningful welfare rights cannot exist in all societies. Similarly, welfare rights can exist only in societies wealthy enough to sustain redistributive taxation without removing from people the discretion over their lives that is a more basic condition of their serving the relevant human goods than the resources made available by taxation.[8]

This has two implications. First, there is a limit to the extent political society may impose on citizens in pursuit of its subsidiarity functions. Second, the right to health care cannot be understood as a kind of decent minimum which by providing for all the citizens and leaders of wealthy countries can judge that they have done what fairness requires. For the basic moral norm underlying modern welfare rights is that we must help our neighbors as we are able (because we are to love them as we love ourselves). A justified public scheme of taxation for welfare rights must be limited to respect individual discretion over life. So what we can do is limited. But that variable limit does not mean that we would not be obliged to help more if we could. Many of us have not fulfilled our duty in this area, even after the tax collector has had his way with us.

Welfare rights thus understood are rights people have as members of a polity. The moral principle underlying rights, love of neighbor, extends beyond political boundaries and encompasses all we are able to reach. But the social organization of health care is significantly national in scope, and the reach of the coordination of the political and other authorities in this system is often limited by borders and other limits of political authority. Thus, considerations about the relative lack of health care by many around the world do not provide much help for those thinking about how to allocate the resources of the system for which they are responsible. For these decisions are not likely to affect how much is available for those outside the system.

Finally, it should be noted that it is the socialization of health care and the common human responsibility to be fair as applied to decision makers in the health care system that are morally decisive here. Even if the right to health care were not acknowledged, or if it is only inadequately recognized and enforced, the health care system would remain a quasi-public system, and those with authority over it would have to face allocation decisions as fairly as they could. Allocation of resources such as intensive care is morally difficult in a system that accepts fully the church's idea of welfare rights. But it is also a problem for fair-minded decision makers in any health care system.

ALLOCATION DECISIONS: POLITICAL AND CLINICAL

There are several areas of fundamental public concern that call for significant public support and organization: domestic justice and the legal system, defense, education, sanitation and health care, transportation, communications, and so on. Taken as a whole, these areas of public concern, to the extent they fall within public decision making, make demands most societies cannot fully meet. Perhaps some of these areas make demands that are finite; for example, there is only so much garbage and sewage to dispose of, and even if disposing of it in optimum ways is expensive, the expense is limited. But other areas of public concern seem to make demands that are quite open ended, if not infinite; for example, health care.[9] Thus, taken as a whole, the set of social demands on resources, broadly understood, creates a condition of scarcity—if not in principle, then at least in the world as it is. That is, even the wealthiest modern polities lack the resources to do everything worth doing. The result is a need to allocate social resources among the various areas of social concern.

Such social decisions, usually now taken by legislative bodies, do not appear to be settled by moral principle in such a way that only one allocation pattern is morally acceptable. Only in situations of crisis, such as wars or natural disasters, is there even a rough and ready ordering of social priorities that allows for allocation closely based on moral principle. Otherwise, there seem to be reasonable alternatives not settled by moral principle. However, various biases and special interests can unreasonably skew such decisions, and an essential part of public deliberation about them is exposing biases and special interests that may favor some without serving the common good or possibly even harming it. So, in spite of the possibility of morally skewed results at this level of decision making, such decisions can be morally good; and when they are not, they can be remedied politically.

It is obvious that politics sometimes establishes sinful social structures, by, for example, unreasonably favoring the interests of veterans or of powerful business organizations, such as insurance companies. Immorality at this level, however, does not mean that those who make decisions within the allocation schemes thus established must be acting wrongly. The cooperation with evil by such decision makers need not intend that evil. Rather, any support that such decision makers give to the evildoing of others need only involve acceptance of it as a side effect of their trying to be as fair as the situation allows.[10] It is possible to be fair and otherwise reasonable in dealing with a resource that is more scarce than it need be on account of human immorality.

There is a further level for allocation decisions about health care resources. Allocation decisions about how to divide the resources a society devotes to health care among various needs for care are likely to be necessary even in affluent societies. This is partly due to the fact that health care makes open ended, if not infinite, demands on resources. All who become ill have reason to want effective care, and indeed the best possible care, and that reason persists even if reasonable preventative steps have been used and even after medical treatment has been successfully used.

Perhaps more can be said here than at the most general level of political allocation about reasonable general allocation of resources. For here, at least, a single human good is at stake, health, whose relation to such political concerns as equality of opportunity appears to have some determinateness. Thus entry-level care, diagnosis, and emergency care (including pain control) are of such basic interest to so many people that they seem to deserve priority within health care, simply as a matter of what is most elementary to the realization of the good of health. Similarly, those things, like inoculations, nutrition, and childhood diagnosis and treatment, and other things needed for most people to get a good start in life appear to have moral priority over more exotic medical treatments. Still, here, as in the case of general political allocation, much of the moral deliberation will consist in seeking to expose bias: are these favored areas for research and treatment favored because of the private interests of decision makers, researchers, physicians, or the class of patients they serve? Or do they reasonably serve the health interests of the community in ways better than or incomparable with alternative allocation policies?

It is sometimes thought that age is a legitimate consideration in this kind of allocation decision, that is, that it is right to exclude the elderly in rationing some treatments. This seems to me unjust, and the arguments in its favor unsound (Boyle 1992, 147–57).[11] One's claim on a fair share of health care resources is not forfeited merely because one is getting old; one's duty to help others with respect to health is plainly not limited by their age. If we can help others with respect to their health, we should. If we cannot, because we lack the resources, then our duty does not apply.

Thus, the refusal to use age as a criterion for rationing is not inconsistent with my claim that the use of available health care resources for clearly more urgent things might preclude their being any left to give some kinds of help to certain people who happen to be elderly. In this case, age is not as such a criterion for allocation, and the negative result for elderly people is a side effect of an allocation based on other considerations.

A more difficult set of social decisions about allocating health care emerges at the level of clinical decision making. By clinical decision making concerning health resource allocation, I mean making decisions in the clinical setting to offer to some patients and to deny to others treatments that prior allocation decisions have made available—but not sufficiently to help all patients who could profit from their use.

Such a decision is needed when a crisis arises because of disaster or temporary excessive demand on a facility, such as an emergency room. It seems to me that the moral issues concerning rationing in such situations are well understood and uncomplicated. If, however, health care facilities such as emergency rooms are compelled regularly to ration their service with the bad result that some people in urgent need are denied immediate pain control, diagnosis, and treatment, then the allocation of resources that leads to such chronic shortages seems indefensible: There has been a failure to provide some care that all have reason to expect, and that in part justifies the health care system as a socialized institution.

Clinical rationing is also required when there is reason to make a medical service available for some patients but also to deny it to some who might get some benefit from it. The reality of critical care calls for this kind of clinical rationing, because (1) this service is urgently needed to monitor and stabilize patients who have suffered trauma or surgery, but (2) is too expensive and burdensome for general use by patients who might get some small benefit from it. In such situations, clinical judgments are needed to decide which patients will receive the service and which will not.

As noted above, well-founded and tested judgments that treatment, such as critical care, is futile are not likely to be of much help in addressing allocation issues raised by a health care system. Furthermore, these judgments are not primarily grounds for allocation decisions but for patient-centered refusals of inappropriate treatment. Of course, in those cases where an expensive and scarce treatment such as critical care is futile, the patient-centered considerations and concerns about fair and efficient use of the treatment converge in supporting the refusal to offer the treatment.

However, other less stringent judgments that such treatment is "futile," where the benefit of the treatment is thought to be either real but slight or unlikely but genuinely possible, are appropriate grounds for clinical allocation decisions and are likely to have wide application. The reasoning is that: (1) the resource is scarce and must be efficiently used; (2) use for patients who are unlikely to benefit at all or likely to benefit very little is unfair to those who might better use the resource; so, (3) it may reasonably be denied to such patients. This reasoning applies not only where the benefit is so slight as to be negligible, but also where medical treatments promise real benefit, but benefit slight in comparison with other social needs for resources.

In the specific case of critical care, it appears that outcome studies now allow confident predictions of the benefits intensive care can provide to patients in various conditions. Clinical judgments that benefits will be slight or unlikely can therefore be made with confidence, and members of the class of patients unlikely to benefit significantly from intensive care can be identified (Knaus, Wagner, and Lynn 1991, 389–94; Knaus et al. 1991, 1619–25). So the patients to whom the argument in the previous paragraph applies can be identified clinically; similarly, patients for whom such treatments are strictly futile can also be identified.

The clinical judgments needed to identify which patients fall into the category of people unlikely to benefit greatly from such medical treatment may create a conflict of interest for physicians. Physicians seem duty bound by virtue of their professional obligations toward their patients to act only in their interests, and certainly not to refuse to offer helpful treatments because of the impact on other people. At the very least, therefore, it seems to me that physicians should not, as the helpers of the patients they serve, function as gatekeepers to medical treatment or as triage officers. If those functions must be fulfilled, then others, or physicians at arms' length or with significant procedural caution and oversight, should carry them out (Society of Critical Care Medicine Ethics Committee 1994, 1201).

To sum up: It seems that, according to the reasoning and principles accepted within the Catholic moral tradition, patients or their proxies can refuse medical treatment out of domestic concern for the scarcity of medical resources; and that, analogously but for different reasons, various kinds of social choice by governmental and health planning authorities can justly limit the availability of some medical options. Needless to say, this does not mean that individual or public decisions can be morally good if they deny or refuse treatment precisely in order to shorten or end human life. Physicians should refuse strictly futile treatments on traditional, professional grounds. More broadly futile treatments can be fairly denied to some whose benefit is likely to be small or uncertain, even as these same resources are maintained and developed for the substantial benefit of other patients. The possible conflicts of interest and other possibilities for unfairness that this judgment allows do not seem insuperable.

NOTES

1. This is casuistical reasoning, but not of the sort that begins with paradigm cases and excludes general moral considerations. Paradigm cases, that is, cases characterized in a way that makes clear what is to be done, are important in all kinds of casuistical reasoning. But the casuistry of the Catholic moral tradition assumes that the moral character of the situations that make up paradigm cases is grounded in moral norms and ultimately in the general principles of the natural law. The comparisons and contrasts of doubtful to morally perspicuous cases reveal, on the Catholic conception of casuistry, diverse implications of these general principles.

2. See Aquinas, *Summa Theologiae,* 1a–2ae, question 94, article 4; question 100, article 2. In these discussions, Aquinas makes clear that in addition to principles known to all and their immediate implications, such as the precepts of the Decalogue, which presumably should be known to all, there are the more detailed implications of moral principle in which the full array of moral circumstances are considered. These are difficult and knowable only to the learned.

3. Although elements of this view have been held by Christians for a long time, it is only recently common Catholic teaching; see Vatican Council II, *Gaudium et Spes, Pastoral Constitution on the Church in the Modern World,* paragraphs 38–39.

4. For a contrary Christian view, see the essay in this volume by the Very Reverend Edward Hughes.

5. In her essay in this volume, Taboada usefully details the narrowly medical considerations Catholic teaching allows as relevant to decisions to limit treatment.

6. The use of the notion of a person's unique personal vocation as a standard for settling moral questions which cannot be settled by the application of universal moral norms has been developed by Grisez, in works in which I have collaborated. See his *The Way of the Lord Jesus: Volume 2: Living A Christian Life* (1993a, especially 77–130; and as applied specifically to health care, 519–45).

7. For useful discussions of the various kinds of futility see Engelhardt and Khushf (1995, 329–33); and Halevy and Brody (1996, 571–74).

8. See my article, "Catholic social justice and health care entitlement packages" (1996, 282–92). On the manualists' analysis of the limits of taxation, see the essay by Wildes in this volume.

9. Efforts to rationalize health care so as to make it as efficient as possible, e.g., managed care, are morally required in the context of scarce medical resources. But seeking efficiency is not rationing. If used to avoid facing the necessity for rationing, such measures become grotesque. For an example, see the essay by Kaveny in this volume, which discusses how the length of a patient's stay in an intensive care unit is inappropriately used to measure the value of the care given.

10. See Grisez for an account of the Catholic moral tradition's understanding of cooperation with evil (1997, 871–97).

11. See my "Should age make a difference in health care entitlement?" (1992, 147–57).

BIBLIOGRAPHY

Aquinas, Thomas. 1981. *Summa Theologiae*, trans. by Fathers of the English Dominican Province. Westminster, Md.: Christian Classics.

Ashley, B., and K. O'Rourke. 1997. *Health Care Ethics: A Theological Analysis*, 4th ed. Washington, D.C.: Georgetown University Press.

Boyle, J. 1981. The patient/physician relationship. In *Moral Responsibility in Prolonging Life Decisions*, ed. by D. McCarthy and A. Moraczewski, O.P. Saint Louis: Pope John Center.

————. 1992. Should age make a difference in health care entitlement? In *The Dependent Elderly: Autonomy, Justice and Quality of Care*, ed. by L. Gormally. Cambridge: Cambridge University Press.

————. 1996. Catholic social justice and health care entitlement packages. *Christian Bioethics* 2: 282–92.

Engelhardt, H. T., Jr., and G. Khushf. 1995. Futile care for the critically ill patient. *Current Opinion in Critical Care* 1: 329–33.

Flannery, A. 1986. *Vatican Council II*. Northport, N.Y.: Costello Publishing.

Grisez, G. 1993. *The Way of the Lord Jesus: Volume 2: Living A Christian Life*. Quincy, Ill.: Franciscan Press.

————. 1997. *The Way of the Lord Jesus: Volume 3: Difficult Moral Questions*. Quincy, Ill: Franciscan Press.

Halevy, A., and B. A. Brody. 1996. The city of Houston city-wide task force on medical futility. *Journal of the American Medical Association* 276: 571–74.

Halevy, A., R. C. Neal, and B. Brody. 1996. The low frequency of futility in an adult intensive care unit. *Archives of Internal Medicine* 156: 100–104.

Knaus, W. A., D. Wagner, E. Draper, J. Zimmerman, M. Bergner, P. Bastos, C. Sirio, D. Murphy, T. Lotring, and A. Damiano. 1991. The APACHE III prognostic system: Risk prediction of hospital mortality for critically ill hospitalized adults. *Chest* 100: 1619–25.

Knaus, W. A., D. P. Wagner, and J. Lynn. 1991. Short term mortality predictions for critically ill hospitalized adults: Science and ethics. *Science* 254: 389–94.

Lee, P. 1998. Human beings are animals. In *Natural Law and Moral Inquiry: Ethics, Metaphysics, and Politics in the Work of Germain Grisez*, ed. by Robert George. Washington, D.C.: Georgetown University Press.

Society of Critical Care Medicine Ethics Committee. 1994. Consensus statement on the triage of critically ill patients. *Journal of the American Medical Association* 271: 1201.

Toward a Personalistic Ethics of Limiting Access to Medical Treatment: Philosophical and Catholic Positions

Josef Seifert

THE VALUE AND DIGNITY OF EACH PERSON AS THE FOUNDATION OF PHILOSOPHICAL AND CATHOLIC BIOETHICS

All philosophical, and certainly all Christian and Catholic, reflections on medical ethics ought to take as their starting point the unique dignity and value of the human person, regardless of age, physical or mental ability, race, or gender. Although almost all human beings, philosophers, and adherents of any religion possess some grasp of this dignity, there are countless degrees of experiential as well as of philosophical and theological clarity and depth with which the dignity of the human person can be perceived and theoretically understood. To summarize: Each person—whether man, woman, unborn child, or dying grandparent—possesses a higher and more sublime value, "dignity," which demands, morally speaking, "absolute respect." Such respect is not due to any nonpersonal entity, including animals. The qualitative content of dignity can only be grasped when we keep before our minds persons and the four roots of their dignity to be discussed below. The value of each person is an objective value of incomparable depth, which characterizes the person qua person and makes it absolutely and intrinsically wrong to trample upon this dignity in actions and crimes, such as those committed at Auschwitz. This same dignity constitutes the moral relevance of persons in intensive care units (ICUs), requiring many acts while absolutely forbidding others.

One might speak here of "negative absolutes" when dealing with the described absolute imperatives. Yet one should recognize the primacy of not harming or violating human dignity by certain actions as a positive absolute, one in the service of a positive value. Only the sublime positive value of human dignity can explain that it is absolutely forbidden to attack it. These moral absolutes, which forbid certain acts under all circumstances, throw into relief the positive value of human dignity. These moral absolutes require such a high positive respect for human life that actions directed against it are absolutely forbidden.[1]

Considerations of the depth of human dignity stated in the book of Genesis and emphasized in the Jewish-Rabbinic tradition lead to the Catholic contribution to this bioethical discussion. The Catholic faith, or simply the full Christian faith, adds to secular (as well as to many religious) notions of personal dignity and value, significant or even revolutionary new dimensions—yet dimensions that never constitute a break with, or a contradiction of, those genuine elements of truth which we discover by our reason, as opposed to many errors and prejudices that secular reason entertains, which are of course profoundly contradicted by the Christian vision. In short, Christianity clashes profoundly with "this world."

Compatibility and Union between Faith and Reason (Philosophy)

First, and of great importance, the Catholic Church has always recognized the possibility of natural and philosophical knowledge of human dignity. It rejects not only through faith but also for philosophical reasons the kind of skepticism and postmodern value-nihilism that H. T. Engelhardt, Jr., in his procedural libertarianism, holds to be inevitable for the secular philosopher, after the alleged collapse of the effort of modernity to found a "canonical content" of ethics by rational knowledge.[2] From such a position it follows that the moral demands flowing from personal dignity, inasmuch as they are accessible to human reason, do not apply only to a private ethics for moral strangers in a public world but to that public world itself. From this position, it follows that there are not two ethical systems, as Engelhardt suggests in *The Foundations of Bioethics,* one for Christians and another for the public world, which would allow such acts as infanticide. Rather, there is but one single ethics, some of whose contents human reason can grasp, even though other dimensions disclose themselves only through true faith. This circumstance has profound consequences for the treatment of human persons in ICUs.

The term "canonical" has at least three very different meanings: (1) being objective, (2) being open to rational knowledge, and (3) being authoritative for and in the public political-legal order of a pluralistic society.[3] If all knowability and public relevance of content-full human rights and moral imperatives were denied, for the public world nothing would remain but principles of noncoerciveness, informed consent, and tolerance. Even these include content-full values not recognized by all. Moreover, any radical division between philosophical and religious ethics appears to lead to a more fideistic standpoint than that of the Protestant reformers Luther or Calvin, who recognized in many respects the ability of reason to grasp some canonical content in ethics as well as some metaphysical truths, such as the existence of God or the spirituality and immortality of the soul.[4]

The Catholic Church disagrees profoundly with such a despair of reason and philosophical knowledge, as well as with such a radically fideistic position. The church insists on the validity and universality of rational knowledge and on a rationally knowable, moral, and prepositive legal "natural law"—although this knowledge is clearly recognized, by many Catholic thinkers and magisterial church documents, to be imperfect and threatened in sinful man. Evidence for this high regard and affirmation of the rational knowledge of man are various biblically based Catholic dogmas and other teachings that assert the powers of rational knowledge.[5] Nevertheless, the powers of rational knowledge, particularly of ethical knowledge, were, according to Catholic teaching, very negatively affected, though by no means completely destroyed, by the fall of man. Therefore, human reason, in order to distinguish its authentic and true ethical intuitions from its sophistical arguments and frequent blindness, stands in need of a divine and ecclesiastic teaching authority. One can apply here the three reasons for which, according to Saint Thomas Aquinas, God revealed not only those truths that human reason cannot know about God, but also His own existence and many other truths necessary for man and his salvation that human reason also can know:[6] (1) so that those dimensions of the natural moral law that can only be known by a few with the help of reason can be known by all; (2) so that what these few discover only after many and arduous reflections of human reason can be known with ease by every child who accepts in faith the Bible and the Catechism; and (3) so that what can be known by the reason of even the greatest minds only with some admixture of error can be known by all of us without being obscured by errors. One could add to those: (4) so that through the purification of the soul by a Christian life of virtue the intellect can be purified and freed from the countless sources of ethical value blindness.[7]

The dignity of the person is, according to Catholicism and rational philosophy, not solely recognized in religion. The Roman Jurists saw and described it by their saying that "man is a sacred thing to man" (*homo homini res sacra est*). Of this unspeakable dignity, Epictetus finds magnificent words in his *Diatribes* and Cicero in his *De Legibus*[8] and *De Re Publica*.[9] One could mention numerous others, including Confucius, Buddha, and Gandhi. Many pagan philosophers speak of it with utmost fervor and saw it, unfortunately, more clearly than many Christians who slaughtered each other in religious wars. Christians and Catholics ought to affirm this dignity of the person far more clearly than pagans—and even more deeply than believing Jews and Muslims, to whom the extent of human dignity believed in by Christians, who accept Christ's incarnation, passion, and resurrection, seems to be unreachable and to involve a scandal against the absoluteness of God, whom they believe could not have descended from heaven or possess so deep a love for us human persons that He would deliver His only incarnate Son for us to the most excruciating passion and crucifixion.

Let us reflect briefly on those sources and dimensions of human dignity that are in principle understood by all of us. Human dignity, inasmuch as it is accessible to human reason, is objectively grounded in the existence, life, and nature of the human person and possesses fourfold roots and dimensions.[10] This dignity has its primary source (1) in the very nature and existence of a person, even when he is persistently unconscious; (2) in his conscious awakened state, in which the distinguishing features of personhood become actualized and experienced; (3) in his fulfilling his vocation by becoming morally and in other ways good; and (4) in his status or dignity acquired by office, talents, grace, and other gifts and relations, which do not originally rest in the person himself but constitute some *être apprivoisé*, some "being tamed," to use Saint-Exupery's graceful expression when describing in *The Little Prince* the prince's relation to his rose and the fox. Here this expression stands for the entirety of dignity that is the fruit of gifts and graces not rooted simply in human nature as such. Consider briefly the fourfold roots of personal dignity.[11]

Dignitas Humanae Substantiae et Vitae[12]

The most basic, though not the most sublime, level of human dignity is that which inalienably belongs to the person in virtue of just being and living as a person. This value and source of human dignity is unfortunately often lost sight of in our contemporary world,[13] which has had enormous effects in discussions of abortion, euthanasia, infanticide, and the appropriate use of critical care units. In these, the recognition of the first source of human dignity will lead to treating persons also in their permanently unconscious, or the so-called brain dead,[14] state with full respect, continuing their basic life support, and so on. It is among the most significant tasks for philosophy today to refound an understanding of the substantial character of the person as individual substance of spiritual nature preceding all actualizations of his powers, and of the dignity founded on this level of personal being as such (Seifert 1989b). The inalienable *dignitas humanae substantiae* belongs—one can argue when one recognizes the character of the person as *substantial entity* that stands in being in its own right (Seifert 1997a, 81–105)—to every human being. Biological human life cannot be divorced from the intrinsic dignity of a person's existence and substantial being (Seifert 1993b, chap. 3).

To hold such a view of the person as an individual substance of rational nature, as the condition of the possibility of rational acts that cannot arise from nowhere and presuppose a substantial subject as their bearer and ground, can be defended on pure philosophical grounds and developed in the direction of a personalistic metaphysics of the person (Seifert 1989b; 1994, 57–75; 1997a, 81–105). However, such a view, in contrast to a Lockean or Humean or other antisubstantial notion of personhood, also appears to be part of Catholic faith and is presupposed in the Trinitarian and Christological dogmas, as well as in such clear moral teachings as the rejection of euthanasia and abortion in all cases:[15] "Human life is sacred and inviolable at every moment of its existence, including the initial phase which precedes birth" (John Paul II 1995, n. 61).[16]

The Dignity of Rational Conscious Life

Personal dignity is related both to the being and life and to the consciousness of persons. As Robert Spaemann pointed out, the very notions of the inalienable dignity and human rights of persons, which were originally introduced to justify the existence of *universal* human values and rights as well as of a human dignity proper to man as such, are now frequently used for the opposite purpose (Spaemann 1996). The introduction of a distinction between human beings that are not persons and those who are, defends the thesis that a huge class of "deficient" unborn, mentally handicapped, or dying humans lack personal dignity.

Thus the true dignity of the human person persists even when he is unconscious, but at the same time requires that the human person, whose "whole dignity consists in thought" (Pascal), be left conscious as long as possible.[17] For a new dimension of personal dignity, which involves rights to freedom of conscience, education, religion, and so on, comes into play only when a person is awake as person. It is of this dignity, bound to consciousness and thinking, that Pascal speaks.

Pascal elucidates the intrinsic dignity of consciousness and conscious life itself as well as the fact that even the dignity of permanently unconscious human life in the "persistent vegetative state" can only be understood when one grasps the ordination and in-principle faculty of the person of conscious life. In a being endowed with intellect, freedom, spiritual emotions, morality, language, culture, and religion, we encounter an essentially higher, inviolable, and nonnegotiable value called personal dignity.

Regarding the relationship between dignity and specifically personal consciousness, there exists a marked contradiction in modern medical practice and theory: between an exaggeration of the role of consciousness and its virtual negation. On the one hand, the first recommends the killing of human persons who are persistently deprived of consciousness because it identifies their dignity with consciousness and quality of life. This fails to recognize the objective ontic status of the person as an individual and unique substantial being of rational nature and the fact that human life is ontologically deeper in human persons than its awakening and conscious actualization. Persons never owe their existence to some act of adoption or decree of society, nor do they inhere in matter. They stand in themselves in being. Without this autonomy of being, freedom and personhood would be unthinkable. A person's life therefore cannot be reduced to conscious life (think of states of unconsciousness that only an absurdly "actualistic" metaphysics, like that of Derek Parfit, can hold to end the person's identity; Parfit 1984). Consciousness is just one decisive condition of actualizing in an essential and unique way the personal being in the multiplicity of his acts and conscious relations. Reduction of the person to his consciousness constitutes a grave error.

Conversely, the role of consciousness is belittled. Its absolutely fundamental role as the condition for personal cognitive and rational life, including religious life and adequate preparation for death, is overlooked. Patients are frequently deprived of consciousness for superficial reasons, such as to spare them the trauma of imminent death, as if they were animals. The "snowing" and "quieting" of dying or suffering patients involves a lack of seeing the high value of personal consciousness as the condition of all rational, moral, and religious life and for a properly human death, dying with the dignity of a person. Recognition of this dignity of conscious human existence applies in particular to pain management in ICUs. The dignity of persons demands that we provide for persons' remaining consciousness in order to bid farewell to loved ones, and to prepare religiously for a good Christian death. Also, the personal act of dying—or, more precisely, because the *event of dying* is not within our control and hence not a personal act—of surrendering one's life freely to God, of repenting one's sins, of awakening one's faith, of accepting death freely, as well as the whole moral drama preceding a person's death, all require the consciousness of the dying. Their dignity demands that one respect conscious life as much as possible, including administering painkillers that leave their consciousness intact as long as bearable, even if they are in grave pain. The first and second sources of dignity are closely linked. An inalienable dignity is grounded in the very substance as well as in the vocation of the human person to conscious life.[18]

Acquired and Moral Dignity of Persons

Still another and more sublime root and dimension of personal dignity depends on the good use of freedom. For a morally evil person fails in his or her fundamental human vocation. One could say with more justification than Pascal about thought: the whole dignity of the person lies in the goodness of his will and his fundamental moral attitudes (1973). For the Catholic, this moral life culminates in holiness and in the perfection of the love of God and of neighbor, as well as in all other virtues of faith, hope, humility, forgiveness, and so on. This moral dignity of the person, unlike the first two dimensions of human dignity, has as opposites the unworthiness and violation of personal dignity through evil. It is extremely important to recognize the distinction of this third source of personal dignity from the other two in order to understand that a person can only reach this dimension of his dignity by fulfilling his moral vocation as a person. The ultimate dignity of the person can only be realized with his free cooperation and culminates in holiness. If we understand that conscious life is a *condition* for acquiring and actualizing this source of human dignity and that the whole value of the person culminates in it, we have to give, from a purely human but even more from a religious standpoint, attention to avoid any privation of consciousness of ICU patients that is not strictly necessary and to provide for them all occasions and opportunities to face their death in a properly personal and Christian way.

Bestowed Personal Dignity

The fourth source of human dignity, gifts bestowed upon the human person, lies at the root of many human forms of dignity: the dignity of parents, judges, kings, and others. Bestowed dignity originates in an incomparably deeper way in the restoration of human dignity through redemption and grace. The Catholic Church liturgy in the Tridentine Mass says that God restored by grace the dignity of the human person more admirably (*mirabilius*) than He had created it. The Ambrosian hymn and Preface of the Catholic Easter Liturgy proclaims more drastically that it would not have profited us anything to have been born if we had not been redeemed as well. Thus for the Christian this source of human dignity is in a certain way perfecting and integrating also the second and the third sources, it is the most profound: the divine life of grace and of God's presence in us which sanctifies us and makes us active participants in redemption through the sacraments.[19] Any Catholic ethics, but also any humanitarian ethics that respects religious freedom and the religious faith of persons, has to take into consideration this dimension of the value of the life of human persons and do everything to guarantee the right of persons to access it. This presupposes not only that patients in ICUs should not be "snowed" and deprived unnecessarily of consciousness, but also that they should be properly informed of the danger of their death, and given an opportunity to express their wish to talk to a priest and to receive the last sacraments.

Neither the source of the value of a human life in his being as a person nor its sources in conscious awakened existence and in his fulfilling his vocation can be understood without comprehending the human person's relationship to God, which can be brought to evidence even by reason.[20] To understand this includes an understanding of the greatness of man as well as of human finitude, misery, and the human limitations that follow from trying to achieve his ultimate dignity through his own strength. In the light of these insights, all hospitals, especially all Christian and all Catholic hospitals, should take all necessary care not only to accompany and to console the dying, but also to let them gain access to the means of their eternal salvation.[21]

The Irreducibly New Dignity Seen by Religious Faith

The Catholic Church insists on the irreducibly new dimensions of human dignity that become visible in the light of faith (to which we have already referred). The admirable Jewish religious vision of the dignity of each person is fully shared by Catholicism without denying the further overwhelming new elements added by Christian and Catholic faith. Christian faith adds entirely new moments of dignity in comparison with all pagan philosophies and even in comparison with Judaism. For we as Christians believe that *God Himself,* the *eternal Logos,* the Second Divine Person, *sarx egeneto,* became flesh, became man, without ceasing to remain God, and that God loved man so much that He delivered His only-begotten Son, (of Whom the Psalmist[22] has the Lord say "today have I begotten thee") for each one of us on the Cross. We understand the dignity of each human person in a far different and more profound light than by just observing human beings. Unfathomably deeper than all purely secular and humanistic concepts of a person's dignity is this vision of human dignity through the looking glass of the *Redemptor hominis.*[23] In his encyclical of this name, Pope John Paul II quotes the two Gospel sentences that summarize the Christian message: "The Word became flesh and dwelt among us," and elsewhere: "God so loved the world that He gave His only Son, that whoever believes in him should not perish but have eternal life" (John Paul II 1979).

But the fact that the Christian sees an incomparably more sublime dignity in each person than the secular humanist, à la Camus, or adherents of other religions, does not mean that there is no universal ecumenical basis for such dignity that can be reached in principle. Although the question of a broad consensus about this dignity is very different from the question of its cognitive accessibility, the dignity of the human person does command a very broad consensus; it underlies demands for rationality and peaceful dialogue.[24] Virtually all of mankind agrees that the dignity of persons, at least when they are in full possession of their conscious life, forbids genocide, rape, torture, and many other horrors. Most will also agree to the more subtle ethical requirements that proceed from the four roots of human dignity regarding the treatment of patients in ICUs. This consensus presupposes the recognition of the intrinsic dignity of persons. More important is the cognitive evidence with which this dignity is grasped. Human dignity becomes evident philosophically when we ponder those essential marks that distinguish the person from any other being. It emerges even more clearly when we contemplate the mysteries of Christian faith. There are infinite degrees of clarity and depth in the existential perception, as well as in the philosophical and theological grasp of this dignity of the person. One of the important insights into this dignity, expressed by Socrates as an argument against suicide and euthanasia, is that man is a "possession of the gods"; he owes his existence to God and *as person* is uniquely related to God, such that he has no right freely to dispose of his or any other person's life.

On the Greatness and Limits of Earthly Human Existence

It can only be in this light—against the background of a metaphysics and religious vision of the human person in relationship to the totality of being and of goods and in relationship to a living God—that we can situate our specific problem as Christians with regard to a proper ethics of limiting access to critical medical care. Reasons of many different sorts may prompt us to limit in an ethically defensible way access to medical intensive care technology: impossibilities of various kinds, excruciating pain, extreme expense, and so on. There is also a very different sort of reason to limit access and not to use unboundedly available medical treatments: the spiritual temptations that flow from an un-Christian and proud concern to extend earthly life at all costs, idolizing earthly life while forgetting the meaning of suffering and death, as well as the higher good of eternal salvation. Such reflections lead back to the ultimate vision of man that underlies any ethical stance of limiting access to medical technology: Besides the awareness of the immense preciousness of each human life, there is insight into the enormous but nevertheless limited value of earthly human life.[25]

In this essay, I wish first to show in a systematic way the ethically acceptable, and even perhaps morally obligatory, ways of limiting access to critical care. Concurrently, I will point out several illicit ways of seeking unlimited access to, and use of, medical technology, particularly in ICUs. Second, I will show that there are immoral ways and reasons for limiting access to critical care or for neglecting to exhaust the full capacities of medical technology. Third, I will argue that in the light of both reason and Catholic faith—between which I see no possible reducibility but nonetheless perfect harmony—such reflections can be understood and realized in deeper ways than through secular reason alone, and in new and content-full ways. In this latter context, I shall be pointing at the far deeper and more perfect light that Catholic faith sheds on all such ethical issues.

OVERVIEW OF ACCEPTABLE AND OBLIGATORY WAYS OF LIMITING ACCESS TO MEDICAL SERVICES AND INAPPROPRIATE WAYS OF SEEKING UNLIMITED ACCESS TO MEDICAL TECHNOLOGY

Limiting Access to Intrinsically Immoral Treatment Is Obligatory

First, one ought to limit or even entirely prevent access to medical treatments in any cases in which the respective medical service provides a disservice or violates objective, morally relevant goods, such as human life or health. Intrinsic wrongness is found when viable infant survivors of abortions are refused admission to ICUs, or when high-risk female patients are admitted for "treatment" of cardiac problems, which includes the abortion of their babies. Intrinsic wrongness is also attributable to acts of euthanasia or assisted suicide when these are put at the disposal of ICU patients in order to limit their access to medical treatment or to free machines for other incoming patients. I regard euthanasia and assisted suicide, both as a philosopher and as a Catholic, as crimes that the state should never permit and that, even if "legalized," no person ought to introduce as a means of limiting access to prolonged medical treatment in ICUs.[26] If I am correct, it is morally obligatory to limit access to any medical treatments in ICUs that involve intrinsically immoral acts. Such treatments do not deserve any access from a purely ethical point of view, and physicians or nurses ought never deliver these services.

Here we find a distinction insisted on (and in my opinion seriously exaggerated) by Engelhardt: the distinction between what a state in a pluralistic modern society should legally permit and the moral point of view. This distinction was always made. For example, Saint Augustine and Saint Thomas Aquinas held that kings should permit brothels to be established, if to forbid them would lead to assaults on decent women and because adults have a certain "freedom to sin" when they do not violate the rights of others. From a legal point of view, therefore, inasmuch as we need to respect the freedom and liberty of individual persons, as long as they do not violate the rights of other persons, freedom to commit even some noncriminal, intrinsically immoral actions should be granted in some measure, as long as these actions fall within the field of legality and outside the sphere of what gravely disturbs "public morality." The "legality" meant here is not merely the conformity of actions with positive law, because laws can be intrinsically evil and therefore what is in conformity with them ought not always be permitted, but concerns a special sphere of natural law: not its purely moral sense but natural law in the sense of that part of prepositive legal and moral values and norms that prescribe those acts that ought also to be forbidden by positive law. Other wrongs, such as envy or vicious words spoken in private, cannot or ought not be positively outlawed.

Limiting access to medical treatment by allowing or enforcing euthanasia or assisting suicide of patients who desire it, however, does not belong to the class of intrinsically evil acts that ought not to be outlawed by the state. Even when they are "allowed" by positive law, physicians and nurses ought to follow their own conscience and not that of patients or states. When actions are immoral or even criminal, according to natural law, even limited access should not be given to these services. At stake here are the essential connections between medicine and values, and between medicine, natural law, and fundamental human rights.

The fundamental ethical question of whether or not there are intrinsically immoral acts (*intrinsece malum*) has a profound impact on our problem. Consider, for example, the difficulty of defining an appropriate futility policy for ICUs (Brody and Halevy 1996, 571–74). Considering possible definitions of futility, one can understand how the fundamental ethical positions of ethicists who recognize that certain acts are wrong in all cases—versus consequentialist ethicists. who believe that any action may be justified if good consequences exceed negative ones—influence solutions to the ethical problem of limiting access to medical technology in critical care. Consider the following consequences of utilitarian reasoning:

1. Provided that a sufficient demand for critical care exists, whole groups of persons (e.g., the handicapped) might be denied access to ICUs or eliminated from access to medical technology (e.g., by starvation through terminating their tubal feeding). This happens in a great number of cases, even in Catholic hospitals.

2. Utilitarian reasoning may also justify euthanasia if current patients will profit less from treatment than newcomers to the ward. In such circumstances, euthanasia might be used as a means to free up ICU space, or to avoid prolonged suffering of the respective patients, to administer a painless and quick, and thereby "more merciful death," to the patients one disconnects from artificial life-support systems.

3. If the number of anticipated patients for ICUs is too great and one anticipates that handicapped children will use scarce ICU resources, utilitarian reasoning would justify the use of preventive eugenic abortion to prevent this conflict of interest.

4. Pregnant women treated in ICUs, for whom pregnancy complications reduce chances of successful ICU treatment, might be relieved of these problems by therapeutic abortion.

5. Physiological futility, imminent-demise futility (the patient will die before discharge), lethal-condition futility (the patient is bound to die in a short time from incurable disease), and qualitative futility (expectation of low quality of

life) will each suffice to make many kinds of life-terminating decisions regarding ICU patients, dependent only on the overall sum of expected desirable consequences.[27]

The position of the official magisterium of the Catholic Church on this is clear, as was recently reiterated by the papal address to the U.S. Catholic bishops: The church condemns any direct killing or discontinuation of feeding with the intention to kill, whether in or out of an ICU. The many dissenting Catholic theologians—who reject a "deontic ethics" and adopt a consequentialist teleological ethics—disagree.[28] Thus we see profound moral disagreements within what calls itself "Catholic moral theology" about principles that deeply affect the ethics of limiting access to medical technology in ICUs. Such disagreements, however, do not change the fact of the unity of ethical doctrine of the magisterium on all central moral issues. On this issue, there is a clear Catholic moral teaching.

To summarize, recognition that intrinsically wrong medical services should never be delivered does not depend so much on religious convictions (although Catholicism in its magisterial teachings strongly affirms this *intrinsece malum*) as on whether one understands the absolute character of the "ought" linked to moral values. Situation ethics and so-called teleological ethics object to any designation of general types of acts, such as suicide or euthanasia, as intrinsically wrong. Some believe that the insistence on acts whose *finis operis*, whose very nature and purpose, is morally wrong, is an exclusively religious or even a sectarian Catholic viewpoint and the consequence of some false rationalism in Catholic moral theology derived from scholasticism. In reality, however, it is not limited to Catholic moral theology as it is part of the magisterium,[29] but includes also the great ethical insights from Confucius, Socrates, Cicero, Kant, and many contemporary philosophers. Each concurs regarding the existence of intrinsically evil acts. Being and value are intelligible and therefore open to intellection. Things themselves teach us clearly which acts committed as a means of limiting access to medical technology, or of limiting access by limiting and reducing the number of patients in ICUs through euthanasia, are intrinsically wrong.[30]

Does the Recognition of an "Intrinsece Malum" *Entail Rationalism?*

In the light of Catholic faith, all the reasons that condemn these "services" as unjust are seen far more deeply, clearly, and convincingly. In addition, specifically religious arguments taken from Christian revelation and the Catholic magisterium solidify the knowledge of the truth about essentially wrong actions. In the light of these reflections on the relationship between faith and reason, I cannot agree with Engelhardt and others that Christians are separated from others by their understandings of knowledge, reality, morality, epistemology, and metaphysics, as well as by their understandings of history, axiology, and appreciation of the sociology of knowledge and value (Engelhardt 1996). Granted that all these elements contain important distinctions between Christians and non-Christians, they do not involve per se any "separation" of Christians from truth-seeking non-Christians. I rather think that all genuine epistemology, axiology, and so on unites Christians with non-Christians. Christians just know many more things than can be understood through secular reason alone. Indeed, they can know the things known by reason much more deeply. To believe that such a view of the relationship between reason and faith in ethics is rationalistic, which is the view the Catholic Church expresses in many of its documents, calls for some crucial distinctions.

If I understand the essays of some of my colleagues correctly, they suggest that a more or less undefined "rationalism" has crept into traditional ethics and Catholic moral theology. Although I concur with them on several bad senses of "rationalism," and also on the claim that much false rationalism has entered into Catholic manuals of moral theology, it is necessary to distinguish radically different phenomena that are intended by the terms "rationalism" or "rationalistic." It is generally unfounded and intellectually dangerous to raise the reproach of rationalism against anyone without extremely careful distinctions among entirely different senses of this term.

First, one might call "rationalism" any recognition that natural reason, prior to the life of religious faith, knows any objective ethical truth. Such rationalism is inseparable from Catholicism. I wholly agree that Catholic moral theology contains this sense of rationalism. Yet, I think to be rationalistic in this sense is not bad but, quite the contrary, beautiful and true. It is simply false that reason can in no way derive ethical foundations and criteria for public ethics. Why should the human person know mathematical laws and logical truths while not also comprehending some ethical laws? We could not even consent to our religious faith if we did not grasp in it the light of ethical truth evident already to our reason to some extent. The fact that ethical knowledge has some moral conditions, without fulfillment of which blindness instead of moral knowledge will be found in an individual, in no way contradicts the objectivity of ethical knowledge. Consensus therefore is no condition of objectivity or of the character of philosophy as a rigorous science (Husserl 1987; Seifert 1983a, 1983b, 1987). When rationalism means simply the insistence on the understanding of a natural law and of a rationally graspable moral order that can be perceived by truth-loving reason prior to any Christian faith,[31] then the mere recognition of the universal presence of ethical knowledge is falsely called rationalism in any negative sense. Saint Paul's claim that the divine law is inscribed in every man's heart, allowing each pagan to understand right from wrong, would thus mark him as a "rationalist" in this sense (Romans 2:4).

Regarding the claim inherent in Catholic moral theology that there are certain valid ethical intuitions and a moral "natural law,"[32] I do not agree that Catholic moral theology has fallen victim of false rationalism. Nor is there good reason to believe that only skepticism regarding ethical reason lacks such a rationalistic character. The sheer recognition of the existence and function of ethical human reason, characteristic of the Catholic teaching that, although sin has wounded human nature, it has not completely destroyed it, is no valid meaning of rationalism. It means simply the positive rejection of any historicism, cultural or general relativism, and skepticism that discard the capacity of human reason to recognize truth, and also ethical truth. Socrates, Plato, Aristotle, Gandhi, Confucius, Cicero, and many other men and women in history prove that there is reason as well as ethical rational knowledge of values everywhere and at all times.[33]

Catholicism is distinct from many other fideistic, antiphilosophical, or philosophically relativistic versions of Christianity because it approves of philosophy, not only in encyclicals and teachings but even on the level of dogma. Catholicism is a religion for philosophers and philosophical objectivists: first of all by recognizing that all of the most central Christian dogmas, such as those of Chalcedon, are imbued with reason and contain philosophy as an integral part.

This formula for the most central Christological dogma was greatly inspired by the work "Tome" of Pope Saint Leo the Great, which contains the core of the essence of the utter mystery of the Christian faith and simultaneously a thoroughly philosophical language. The Catholic Church even dogmatically declared content-full philosophical knowledge independent of faith to be possible in the First Vatican Council. The knowledge of God was declared possible for all. Thus Roman Catholicism, more than the Orthodox Church, and over against Protestantism, insists on the union of faith with reason. It rejects all *Averroist* and *Siger of Brabantian* concepts of double truth, considering the marriage of the greatest philosophical discoveries of the Greeks with Christianity as a great providential event and not as a hellenization of Christianity to be replaced by some *sola fides* doctrine or irrationalistic and skeptical fideism.

A different reason for calling the church's moral stands rationalistic is its rejection of any pure situationism (i.e., the thesis that only situations determine the moral quality of acts). The church affirms that there are some universal essences of human acts and actions that make these morally licit or illicit always and everywhere, regardless of circumstances. This teaching is closely related to the famous Catholic doctrine recently expounded in many documents that there is an *intrinsece malum*. Hearing this, many immediately disagree, because they just think of *Humanae Vitae* and other documents regarding specific sexual issues that many reject. In rejecting these teachings and understanding their connection with the view that there are intrinsically evil acts, one fails to see the full accordance with natural human reason of the general ethical teaching on an *intrinsece malum* implying the nonutilitarian dimension of morality. To call the insistence on rationally evident *intrinsece malum* "rationalistic" implies that only situational or consequentialist ethics—which precisely denies the morally wrong character of some human acts *under all circumstances*—would overcome this rationalism. Yet, at least the extreme examples of intrinsically evil acts such as perjury, slaughtering the innocent, or rape allow us to see clearly that this position on *intrinsically wrong acts* is simply true and also rationally knowable, being in no way negatively "rationalistic."[34]

Second, a good and important thing wrongly disqualified as mere rationalism lies in the making of basic rational moral distinctions found in classical ethics, as well as in Catholic moral theology and the magisterium, such as distinctions between ordinary and extraordinary means, between proportionate and disproportionate means, among quantitative and qualitative meanings of "futility" (Engelhardt and Khushf 1995), and the identification of the conditions under which the principle of double effect comes into play. Not more deserving of the negative qualifier "rationalistic" is the crucial distinction between the *finis operis* (i.e., the constitutive essential end of an action that makes it into the kind of action it is, such as self-defense, life saving, and assassination), and the *finis operantis* (i.e., the further subjective or accidental purpose of an action, such as the aim or motive of the action). Without this distinction, the sphere of human actions cannot be properly understood. These positive senses of rationality must not be debunked as rationalism, even if conceptual rational distinctions and principles neither *exhaust* the qualitative depth of the moral life nor solve the infinity of situations.

Third, and more negative, rationalism may mean a reduction of virtues and fundamental moral attitudes to moral actions aimed at realizing states of affairs in the world and the additional reductionist conception that this obeys a set of definable moral principles that would make them good or evil. Such a reductionism of morality to concrete actions—and the additional reduction of the morality of these external actions to their conformity to some principle or categorical imperative—would be a wrong rationalism indeed.[35] In reality, morality includes, besides actions that realize or omit realization of states of affairs in the world, free inner stances to all kinds of goods and values as well as superactual attitudes and value responses, such as love and humility, virtues and vices, and even sanctioned affective responses, which can in no way be thus reduced.[36]

Fourth, rationalism as a significant concept in ethics often refers to a reduction of specifically Christian attitudes and virtues to pagan or purely rationally founded ones, overlooking the overwhelming new qualities, motivations, and fulfillment of the moral life through the specific objects of religious faith and the specifically Christian life of holiness. Indeed a phenomenological ethics, philosophy of religion, and specifically Christian narratives can unfold the wholly new attitudes of a life in Christ, a life of holiness. It is in no way true that the tradition of Catholic moral teachings overlooked these, however.[37] Consider, for example, any great collections of sermons, such as those of Saint Augustine on the letters of Saint John and the Fourth Gospel (Reale 1994), those of John Henry Cardinal Newman, or of the tale in the *Fioretti* of Saint Francis, which reports how he treated three robbers and murderers sent away previously by the guardian with harsh words.

Fifth, a very different meaning of rationalism, brought out by Engelhardt, lies in a lack of understanding regarding the specifically connatural moral knowledge that *presupposes* virtue, an ethical knowledge that is not an isolated, merely intellectual affair, but grows from the humble, loving, holy heart. Rationalism in this sense includes the wrong opinion that the neutral attitude of the amoral man is the best foundation of objective knowledge in ethics, instead of the heart that opens itself to God and that perceives the depth of moral goodness by the mediation of humility, purity of heart, and love (Scheler 1955). More generally speaking, such rationalism overlooks the manifold influence of moral and immoral acts and attitudes on ethical knowledge and on moral value blindness (von Hildebrand 1982b).

A sixth form of rationalism lies in overlooking the new dimensions of moral knowledge that are not open to the virtues of the natural man, but only through a life of contemplation of the Scriptures, a life of grace and of Christian holiness. Such Pelagian rationalism is utterly foreign to the authentic Catholic teaching on grace and the supernatural virtues. It is foreign to the writings of the great Catholic mystics and saints, such as Saints John of the Cross, Theresa of Avila, or Bridget of Sweden, even though some of this false "naturalistic rationalism" may have crept into Catholic moral theological textbooks or sermons.

Seventh, is the rationalism of reducing prudential knowledge,[38] which alone can do justice to the infinite variety of ethically relevant facts, to a mere practical syllogism from a few abstract principles as ethical knowledge. This rationalism was often present in moral theological manuals. Certainly, ethical decision making in the face of countless cases and circumstances in ICUs cannot simply be deduced from a few general principles, but must be grasped by an infinitely differentiated knowledge of concrete cases. Here lies both the root of the indispensable usefulness of casuistry and the limits of books on it, which can never exhaust the variety and wealth of concrete reality that demand ever again new *Sachkontakt.* All such casuistry depends on universal ethical principles and should be seen as integrating in the sphere of essentially good and essentially wrong moral attitudes and acts. Rejecting radical situationism has nothing to do with false rationalism but only with authentic rationality.

Thus we reach the conclusion that the admission of rational ethical knowledge, including that of species of acts that are intrinsically wrong, does not have the negative implications of rationalism; nor does it contradict the acceptance of the superior life of faith or deny the need of moral reform or conversion as the source of more adequate and deeper ethical knowledge. Moreover, from an ethical standpoint, access to intrinsically wrong acts should never be demanded or offered by a physician. From a legal standpoint, giving access to intrinsically evil acts should never be demanded by the state or allowed by the state to be demanded by private institutions from those whose objective ethical knowledge and/or subjective conscience rejects such actions. Moreover, the perpetration of intrinsically wrong acts should be permitted solely where immoral acts do not violate natural and positive human rights or public morality.

Unlimited Universal Access Is Impossible, Practically Unrealizable, or Even Morally Objectionable

A second basic problem regarding "limiting access to medical treatment," concerns limited or unlimited access to medical services in all areas of genuine medical practice and with respect to actions that truly serve the goals of medicine (life, health, the alleviation of pain, etc.). Here universal access to medical treatment is desirable and morally justified. Nevertheless, universal access to all critical care may be economically impossible or at least practically unrealizable; it is, therefore, not obligatory. Besides, under some conditions, an otherwise legitimate and morally correct application of medical technology may even be morally objectionable, constituting an idolization and fetishism of earthly life. We can delineate, following Cronin's pertinent catalogue, the reasons under which not only normal medical services but even life-saving measures in ICUs may cease to become morally obligatory or even begin to become morally objectionable (Cronin 1989; Wildes 1995).

Some Impossibilities (*Quaedam Impossibilitas*)

It is obvious that physical impossibilities of treatment permissibly limit the use of and access to medical technology—for example, if the respective means of treatment lead to greater harm than good for the patient, as in the case of surgical interventions in consequence of which a patient would die.

There are also psychological impediments, impossibilities, and necessities that may permissibly limit access to medical interventions. These include insurmountable psychological inhibitions, repulsions, and irrational feelings of shame, under which a person may suffer and which prevent his accepting or even being capable of receiving certain kinds of medical treatment that require his consent and free cooperation.

More essentially related to the dignity of the person as free agent and to ethics is the central sphere of necessities and impossibilities situated within the objective and subjective moral duties of persons. When only the patient's life is at stake, rather than the lives of their children or unborn babies, the forced imposition of medical services, including such ordinary means as blood transfusions, might not only be imprudent but also constitute objectively an intrusion into a legitimate sphere of freedom, which ought to be respected even when patient choice is misguided. Forced imposition of medical services on individual persons, who autonomously reject such treatment, stands in violation of certain fundamental rights of persons to reject treatment for moral and religious duties, or even for reasons of psychological inhibitions. Thus a personalistic medical ethics must respect these "subjective" impossibilities that encompass an enormously wide spectrum of personal choices, reaching from irrational psychological inhibitions to objective moral and religious "necessities" based on imagined or real obligations. Hence they should not even indiscriminately be called "subjective" simply because they do not exert influence on human behavior without the mediation of knowledge and free decisions. Rather, they should be referred to as person-related, consciousness-related, or freedom-related necessities, such as moral oughts. Even when such "necessities" lack an objective rational basis in cognition, such as in cases of irrational psychological factors or mental disease or erroneous judgments of conscience, they often ought to be respected by medical staff and may limit duties to treat.

The situation is more difficult and requires a different judgment when the rights of other persons are affected. In this case, the rights of the other person take precedence, and one may save a life even against the scruples of relatives regarding blood transfusions and the like. For the second person's rights must be protected and in this case take priority.

Economic necessities also play a role under the category of necessities and impossibilities. One can consider such impossibilities both as they present themselves to individuals and to society at large. For individuals, and short of a sufficient public system of health insurance, it is clear that certain expensive treatments cannot be afforded by some persons, even when they are ready to make extreme personal sacrifices for the sake of their health. One might argue that a perfect system of public health services is an expression of social justice and a consequence of a Christian sense of universal solidarity. Notwithstanding the nobility and also in large measure realizable greatness of this vision, one must note that to demand unlimited distribution of public funds for all kinds of health services might not only neglect the above principles but likewise the demands of a hierarchy of values, within which also culture, art, education, and so on have high priorities. Health care is a good, but it is not the only good. Such a universal medical welfare program is also under many circumstances imprudent and counterproductive, inasmuch as it may lead to the economic collapse of public health care systems. This is the case not only in rich countries, where bankrupt insurance providers can be saved by state money, but also in poor countries, where no economic remedy against such bankruptcy is available. Therefore, the "perfect welfare system" might lead to greater damages for public health in a given society at large than a less perfect welfare system. Thus an unlimited quest for public health care not only proves to be open to abuse but is also self-defeating.

Forbidding Expenses (*Sumptus Extraordinarius*, *Media Pretiosa*, and *Media Exquisita*)

Even when they do not constitute an impossibility, the forbidding expenses of treatment may give us the liberty not to opt for them. Regarding forbiddingly high costs for health services, traditional Catholic moral theology always allowed for a cessation of duty to provide or aspire to such treatments, further distinguishing differences of status and wealth that may determine what is ordinary or extraordinary means of life support for a given individual. Of course, this presupposes that earthly life is neither an absolute nor the highest good. Noble as it is when a family starves half to death to save another family member's life by providing extraordinary means of his life support,[39] there is no absolute moral obligation to do so. Indeed, there may be a duty not to do so.

With regard to the absoluteness of the value of human personal life, one must introduce important metaphysical and ethical distinctions regarding the "absoluteness" of this value. Metaphysically speaking, we must distinguish between the value of the ultimate life of the person *qua person*, of the immortal life of the human person, intended also by Plato, aimed at by the Christian in striving for his own and other persons' eternal salvation, the "eternal life," and the more limited earthly life of the human being. The latter does not possess absolute or infinite value. It would be better, for example, to sacrifice this life rather than committing an injustice that is a greater evil than death, as Socrates notes. The life of the person *qua person*, however, possesses much more ultimate metaphysical value. Ethically, however, we must distinguish between actively promoting life and health and acting against health and life. In the latter form of acting, the moral relevance of human life over against destructive acts is in a certain way ethically absolute; it gives rise to a categorical imperative grounded in the value-content of human life, also earthly human life. In situations in which we are faced with the temptation to commit euthanasia, or other immoral acts, human life and health are morally speaking absolute goods. Although they are not absolute goods metaphysically speaking, and therefore it is permissible to forgo extraordinary means actively to save them, they demand the moral absoluteness that one never intentionally and directly seek to destroy them. This is what utilitarianism and consequentialism of all sorts fail to comprehend. Yet, it is a position already insisted upon by Socrates, who was ready to sacrifice his life rather than murder Leon or condemn the ten unjustly accused generals after the sea battle of Salamis. Similarly, physicians should rather die, or subject themselves to the excruciating consequences of Nazi terrorism, than surrender to political or other pressures that prompt them to commit intrinsically evil acts. With respect to actions of protecting or actively promoting the goods of earthly human life, however, the goods of life and health are to be seen in their limited rank, which does not demand all sacrifices. This is especially the case when it is not the life of a young person, who still has a whole life before him, and for whom the parents ought to choose to starve rather than to leave any means of life support unattempted. In contrast, it is permissible to allow an old person, who asks to be allowed to die in peace, his natural death.

There are other issues at stake here: *Social justice* and *liberty* are involved in the influence of economic factors that limit and extend access to medical treatment. Although aiming at universal accessibility of medical technology, regardless of financial and social status, may be in principle an ideal of social equity, to bar some persons from access to more expensive forms of medical care that they can afford, but that cannot be made accessible to everyone, would also go against legitimate freedom of choice. Regarding certain forms of risky or extremely expensive and unusual surgery, one may argue that even when nobody is *required* to choose such care, because of the risk and expense involved, and although in most countries it is too expensive to be included in public health plans, the freedom of the daring and wealthy to pay for such surgical interventions should not be suppressed. This inequality of health service has always existed, such as private room service in hospitals, and cannot permissibly be eliminated entirely by the state. Inequality of health care can also be the consequence of a reason far more beautiful than dire economic needs. Gratuitously and freely offered medical services exist and ought to exist in each society. These services are by their nature not "equally accessible to all," nor can they be bought for money. This sphere, particularly entrusted to genuine Christian charity, practiced for centuries in Christian communities and by religious orders, though often sorely absent even in some Catholic hospitals today,[40] will always exist and ought to be supported by the state and private donors as much as possible. One ought never to seek to substitute the freely and gratuitously offered services of physicians, nurses, and nuns with state medicare or health insurance. Rather, society must create space for such freely rendered services, because their value is great from a human and a Christian perspective. Allowing and furthering such free and intentionally underpaid or unpaid services, such as those offered by Mother Theresa's Sisters of Mercy, should always be a noble task of the state and of other bodies responsible for the allocation of means of medical support. Hence a surplus of medical services, whether purchasable only by the wealthy or gratuitously offered for humanistic or religious motives,[41] should never be prevented by minimal wage requirements nor by other forms of state totalitarianism or medical labor unionism.

Too great an effort such as very long trips (*summus labor et nimis dura*) also lessens the duty to prolong our or other persons' lives. Terrible pain (*quidam cruciatus et ingens dolor*) as well may end the duty to save a life. The same is true of immense feelings of horror (*vehemens horror*). This is clearly true of rationally founded horror, such as when a female patient refuses to expose her body to a male physician who is known to have sexually abused other patients, or when a person prone to vertigo would have to reach medical help by climbing a dangerous abyss. But it is true as well of irrational feelings of horror.

More difficult is the category of futility in its different quantitative or qualitative senses as a criterion for limiting access to medical treatment. Futility can lie (1) in the absence of reasonable hope for the health of a person from the respective cure (*spes salutis*), perhaps because other ailments afflict him or her; (2) in the absence of reasonable hope even for the immediate physiological efficiency of certain medical treatments; or (3) in the lack of hope for a life condition desirable for the patient, such as being confined to a persistently unconscious state after a life-saving operation.

Illegitimate versus Legitimate Forms of "Limiting Access to Medical Treatment"

In the following, I discuss both new concerns and formulate conclusions from previous arguments regarding legitimate versus illegitimate forms of limiting access to critical care, as well as regarding legitimate and illegitimate reasons for so doing.

Basic Health Care and Emergency Health Care Should Be Guaranteed

The necessary limitations of access to medical services for moral reasons should not prevent some basic health care, especially emergency health care, from being guaranteed everywhere and to everyone. In circumstances where this might be unrealizable factually, or with respect to certain treatments, the "ought" remains a necessary moral ideal. The demand for universal accessibility of basic health care is not a consequence of socialism, but of human solidarity and of a Judeo-Christian vision of the human person. No cruel capitalistic, unbounded free-market philosophy, or unrealistic trust in freely bestowed charity, should prevent society from making basic health services available to all. Determination of what constitutes "basic health services" and their legitimate extent is crucial here. Although it seems obvious that this basic health care ought to include all directly necessary life-saving technology for persons who do not choose to be "allowed to die a natural death," it is not truly so. Terminology regarding so-called extraordinary or disproportionate means often hides a refusal to make basic health care available to all. In many countries, such language includes new and special surgical or other life-saving interventions that cannot be made accessible to all because of unavailability or forbidding costs. Notwithstanding such circumstances, all legitimate and necessary life-saving medical services, as far as is possible and reasonable, belong to basic health care and hence should be made accessible to all. Basic health care should also include all forms of protection by preventive medicine, such as vaccinations against infectious diseases, which are realistically speaking dangerous for a certain population, and many other elements to be determined concretely by medical professionals in dialogue with philosophers and theologians. Any form of restricting access to basic or emergency health care because of greed, false value hierarchies in which wealth comes before health, negligence, or racist or sexist restrictions is morally evil.

Limiting Access on the Basis of Superficial Quality of Life Standards Is Wrong

Many of the arguments in favor of limiting access to critical care based on notions of "quality of life" are superficially grounded on misunderstandings of human dignity and of the value of human life in relationship to other economic factors. Such arguments ought to be rejected. As clear a hierarchy as possible of the objective order of goods and values ought to be developed, including an assessment of all the factors that legitimately influence decisions regarding access to medical services. It ought to be recognized that even the life of a suffering, poor, and sick person possesses immense moral, religious, and personal value. It constitutes a horrible reversal of the true hierarchy of values when health is placed above life, when unconscious life is regarded as worthy of termination, or when comparatively small defects of health, such as congenital or acquired deafness or blindness, are regarded as worse than death, and abortion or euthanasia are justified on these grounds.

We are faced today with incredibly shallow criteria of the quality of life, which do not do justice to the true dimensions of the value of an earthly human life. Ivan Sergeyevich Turgenev describes in the moving story from *Notes of a Hunter,* titled "The living relic," a girl, who once was a vivacious beauty but now is paralyzed, crippled, and hardly cared for by others. Under these incredibly gloomy circumstances, she experiences intense gratitude, love of nature, and love of others so as to touch profoundly the hunter who visits her. This girl succeeded in feeling intense love and gratitude in spite of her not being loved or cared for by anybody. Even she believes in a love that one cannot directly see; she does not doubt that preciousness in herself that allows for being loved. The person who believes that in him no value exists, which calls for recognition and love, lives in despair even if he is a world-famous movie star; he is poor even if he is the richest man on earth. Any limiting of access to medical services ought to be based on a proper understanding of human dignity and of the hierarchy of values.

Legitimate Forms of Limiting Access Are Imposed by Ethical Demands

Legitimate limitations of critical care can be seen in the following four cases in which such limitations follow from moral imperatives:

1. It is ethically justified and even morally obligatory not to provide access to critical care if the procedures themselves are objectively and always morally wrong. Medicine and medical practice does not always *serve* the fundamental goods for the sake of which it exists, such as human life, health, and liberation from pain. Frequently it acts against these goods in "procedures" and "services" such as euthanasia or assisted suicide. Because such acts should never be committed by physicians, it follows that there can be no duty to provide these "services" nor any rights to them.
2. Access to critical care is morally unjustified when the means to obtain these services, whether through research or medical praxis, involve immoral acts—for example, if one immorally procures organs for transplantation without the individual's prior consent.
3. Limiting access to critical care is justified when such care would violate the patient's subjective conscience. From this standpoint, intrinsically licit actions such as blood-transfusions should not be forced upon Christian Scientists who regard them as immoral; although there is good reason to assume that there are exceptions, such as forcibly transfusing a child over the objections of the parents. Full freedom of conscience, as long as reference to it is plausible and not a coverup of crime and unlawful behavior, should be guaranteed.
4. Limiting access to critical care may also be morally justified when its costs outweigh the goods obtained by their recipient. For example, it is immoral to procure kidneys from a healthy young person, if this involves serious risks for his health and life, in order to implant them in a dying old person who will foreseeably not even survive such an operation. Similarly, an expensive operation is not obligatory for a family when the saving of a grandfather's life will lead to the death of the rest of the family through famine. This is an application of the principle of proportionality insofar as it is part of the principle of double effect.

Critical Care that Is Impossible Economically, Scientifically, or Politically, or Imposes Truly Unbearable Burdens on Others

Besides the infinity of possible preventive and curative health care options, which are never in their entirety available to anyone, it is legitimate and unavoidable to restrict public and private health care where due to economic factors. It is permissible that certain medical equipment and services may not be available in certain places or certain times.

If neither individual nor society can afford certain critical care services or disease-preventive measures (at least not without inflicting proportionally greater harm on society than the value realized by the respective health service), or when society can make them available in all honesty only to a few, it is permissible to limit access to these services. In the choice to whom to grant access to these services, however, objective standards and value hierarchies ought to be used (along the lines of the preceding analyses). It is also legitimate to limit access to medical services if the respective service, such as expensive plastic surgery for purely aesthetic reasons, does not belong to basic health care and justly requires private financing, even if such financing is unavailable.

CONCLUSION

This essay has to be understood as a mere first sketch of the moral and immoral ways of and reasons for limiting access to critical care and of the principles underlying such distinctions. Much more work needs to be done to present the general relevant factors for the distinction between good and bad forms of and reasons for limiting access to critical care. This work can best be undertaken in the light of both reason and Catholic faith. Human dignity—as well as general moral attitudes of charity and all-encompassing love for the poor, old, and sick based on Catholic faith—cannot be reduced to the conception of human dignity attainable in a society of secular ethics and moral pluralism. Nevertheless, between the basic human experience of human dignity and philosophical insights into its fourfold roots and the sublime understanding of personal dignity by Catholic teaching and genuinely Christian faith, there is no division, at least not when one understands the true cognitions as opposed to the errors contained in a "secular" vision of bioethics. Between faith and reason we find perfect harmony, and we think we cannot do better than to search indefatigably for sources of understanding the bioethical aspects of our topic—recognizing as well the "canonical" contents derived from both, and trying to implement them as far as possible in private and public health care to the utmost benefit of humanity and of human life based on the truth of the exalted dignity of the human person and human limits.

NOTES

1. Regarding how the dignity of the human person is known, whether by a metaphysical intuition into the essence of the person or derived from human actions, according to an action-theoretical scheme, (1) I agree with Aristotle in general that the nature of a thing (substance) can best and primarily only be known by observing its activities. These reveal the nature and faculties of the being in question. If we never experienced any act of a kind of being, we would know little of its nature. (2) Once we experience the acts of a being, and in order to grasp the nature and lofty value of these actions and of the underlying faculties and subjects, we cannot avoid the direct and immediate form of cognition which, as Aristotle explains in *Posterior Analytics,* necessarily precedes all deductive arguments. Thus a metaphysical-axiological insight into the nature of these acts and the kind of being and substance which is their subject is unavoidable. (3) If the objection to a metaphysical foundation of personal dignity is based on some Kantian skepticism as to a knowledge of objective being of the person in itself, and in an alleged precedence of practical ethical philosophy over theoretical philosophy in Kant, I do not share such a Kantianism or the opinion that metaphysical facts such as the value of the person can only be introduced as postulates of practical human reason (Seifert 1976, 1987).
2. Although Engelhardt seeks to exempt metaethical considerations from such criticism, his reasoning forces him to abolish such a distinction between metaethics and con-

tent-full ethics for two reasons: (1) The principles of his seemingly purely formal metaethics are themselves not without reference to content and inevitably include, just as Kant's alleged "formalism," content-full values such as tolerance, freedom, and peace. (2) Although he concludes from the lack of consensus to the absence of binding ethical contents, the libertarian principles of his metaethics are even less the object of consensus than more content-full ethical values and thus would have to be rejected by him for the same reasons that compel him to reject ethical contents (Engelhardt 1996).

3. Two of these meanings of "canonical," (2) and (3), appear to be rejected entirely by Engelhardt (1996, 1997), whereas (1) seems to be upheld by him, but solely on religious grounds. Engelhardt holds that there is an objective canonical content for morality, but that it lies beyond the scope of philosophy and is neither open to rational philosophical knowledge nor to entitled to any claim of authority in secular pluralist society. Engelhardt denies any "canonical content" for secular ethics, not only rejecting the socially or politically authoritative character of an ethics based on reason that no longer finds majority consensus in our democratic society, but also denying any philosophically recognizable objective content of ethics, relegating therefore any ethical content to religion and religious communities of "moral strangers in a public world."

4. See the quotes from Luther and Calvin to this effect in Seifert (1978, 1989a, 1989b). Engelhardt's position is not purely fideistic inasmuch as it allows for some knowledge and experience of moral values mediated by a life of holiness and grace.

5. Think, e.g., of the dogma of the power of reason to know God in the Vatican I, or of the encyclicals of Popes Leo XIII and John Paul II, *Aeterni Patris* and *Fides et Ratio*.

6. Both Thomas Aquinas and Immanuel Kant, however, emphasize rightly that natural practical reason (moral knowledge) is far superior to natural theoretical knowledge. See Aquinas, *Summa Theologica* (1948), Ia, Q. 1, a. 1, resp.; see also the original text, corpus:

> ad ea etiam quae de deo ratione humana investigari possunt, necessarium fuit hominem instrui revelatione divina. quia veritas de deo, per rationem investigata, a paucis, et per longum tempus, et cum admixtione multorum errorum, homini proveniret, a cuius tamen veritatis cognitione dependet tota hominis salus, quae in deo est. ut igitur salus hominibus et convenientius et certius proveniat, necessarium fuit quod de divinis per divinam revelationem instruantur. necessarium igitur fuit, praeter philosophicas disciplinas, quae per rationem investigantur, sacram doctrinam per revelationem haberi.

See, likewise, Immanuel Kant, *Kritik der praktischen Vernunft* (1993), V, 91 ff.; V, 155 ff.

7. See the foundational work on sources of moral value blindness (*Wertblindheit*) by Dietrich von Hildebrand, *Sittlichkeit und ethische Werterkenntnis* (1982b [1922]).

8. Cicero, *De Legibus* (1970), I. xv. 42:

> Iam vero illud stultissimum, existimare omnia iusta esse, quae sita sint in populorum institutis aut legibus. etiamne si quae leges sint tyrannorum? si triginta illi Athenis leges imponere voluissent, aut si omnes Athenienses delectarentur tyrannicis legibus, num idcirco eae leges iustae haberentur? nihilo, credo, magis illa, quam interrex noster tulit, ut dictator, quem vellet civium, aut indicta causa impune posset occidere. est enim unum ius, quo devincta est hominum societas, et quod lex constituit una; quae lex est recta ratio imperandi ac prohibendi; quam qui ignorat, is est iniustus, sive est illa scripta uspiam sive nusquam.

Cicero, *De Legibus* (1970), I. vii. 22; VI. 19: "lex est ratio summa insita in natura, quae iubet ea, quae facienda sunt, prohibetque contraria"; I, XIV. 40 f.; I. viii. 24; I. xii. 33 ff.

9. *De Re Publica* (1970), III. xxii, 33:

> Est quidem vera lex recta ratio naturae congruens, diffusa in omnes, constans, sempiterna, quae vocet ad officium iubendo, vetando a fraude deterreat; quae tamen neque probos frustra iubet aut vetat nec improbos iubendo aut vetando movet. huic legi nec obrogari fas est neque derogari ex hac aliquid licet neque tota abrogari potest, nec vero aut per senatum aut per populum solvi hac lege possumus, neque est quaerendus explanator aut interpres eius alius, nec erit alia lex Romae, alia Athenis, alia nunc, alia posthac, sed et omnes gentes et omni tempore una lex et sempiterna et immutabilis continebit, unusque erit communis quasi magister et imperator omnium deus, ille legis huius inventor, disceptator, lator; cui qui non parebit, ipse se fugiet ac naturam hominis aspernatus hoc ipso luet maximas poenas, etiamsi cetera supplicia, quae putantur, effugerit. . . .

Vgl. auch Cicero, *De Re Publica* I. xl. 64 ff., bes. I.xLiv 68 ff.; *De Re Publica*, IV. viii. 8 f.

10. Regarding sexist language: I shall not bow to the unenlightened feminist and anti-sexist destruction of language (as I once did to some extent in *What Is Life?*) and will therefore continue to use the masculine pronoun for "person" in English because this belongs to the great tradition of the English language, just as it belongs to Latin and to all the Romance languages, as well as to my native German, to use the feminine pronoun for *persona* or for *person*. I would equally refuse in German to refer to the *person* as "*er*" or "*er oder sie*" because it would be ugly to the point of *impossible* linguistically and also would be stupid for a male reader not to understand that he is equally comprised under the common "gender," even when person and its pronouns take the feminine form. It would in fact mean a destruction of the German and of the Romance languages to "masculinize" persons. One can avoid all of this gender debate by referring to the person always as "he or she" and by avoiding the term "man" in the sense of human being (*Mensch*). Yet how cumbersome is it to never refer to the human being as such and to call the human person always "he or she"! And how wrong simply to throw away the fundamental concept of *Mensch*. I find it an equally silly and ugly destruction of the English language to bow to this fashion of our day and to become virtually possessed with the elimination of masculine pronouns when women are included. Such a use of language fails to understand the functions of grammar and language. Rather than throwing away the concept of *Mensch*, I might consider "Germanizing" and "romanticizing" English and using the "she" for person, an attractive idea indeed. But in due admiration for Shakespeare and all great English writers, I do not see any need to do that; most languages feminize us men when speaking of persons. Why should we not once enjoy including women under the *genus commune* in the masculine form? This is inevitable in English, because it collapses the different concepts expressed in the German *Mann* (man) and *Mensch* (human person) into the one term "man," for which one cannot choose a feminine pronoun without doing greater violence to English than by calling *Persons* in German or Italian "he."

I have to explain a bit more why I use the masculine personal pronoun for "person" here. I use a personal pronoun instead of the "it," which has now become customary for "person," because I find it unacceptable to refer to persons as "it," because they are not things but *persons.* I use the masculine pronoun for "person" because this is customary in English, whereas in German the feminine "she" is not only customary but necessary as pronoun for *die Person.* This has nothing at all to do with masculine or feminine "sexism." Thomas of Erfurt (or Duns Scotus) is right here who distinguishes in the *Grammatica speculativa* four kinds of gender: Besides the *masculinum, femininum,* and *neutrum,* there is a fourth "common" gender (*sexus commune*). There is a special *discretio sexus,* the *genus commune,* which in its linguistic *form* is either masculine or feminine (*quod nec differt a masculino nec a feminino*), but in its *meaning* comprises both sexes within itself, such as in *homo* (*man*) where this term signifies human persons as such!

11. See this theory of the fourfold root of human dignity in my article "Philosophische Grundlagen der Menschenrechte. Zur Verteidigung des Menschen" (1992b); and my "Die vierfache Quelle der Menschenwürde als Fundament der Menschenrechte" (1997b).

12. Historically speaking, and very briefly, the notions and word of dignity for the person is found already in some ancient philosophers. It appears also in the text of the Tridentine Catholic Mass, which was universally imposed by the Council of Trent but dates back to the earliest Christian centuries and to preceding Jewish prayers. There it is said of God that He founded and more admirably restored "dignitatem humanae substantiae." It later appears very clearly in one of the classical medieval definitions of the person favored by Saint Anselm the Great: that the person is a being "distinct by his dignity." In Kant, we find a beautiful further exposition of this notion, and it becomes a key notion in personalist thought.

13. This concept is also rejected by the secular ethics propounded by Engelhardt (1996, 1997).

14. Recently, decisive criticisms have been launched against identifying brain death with actual human death (Shewmon 1997; Seifert 1993a, 1993b).

15. See, e.g., Congregation for the Doctrine of the Faith (1988).

> *The human being is to be respected and treated as a person from the moment of conception;* and therefore from that same moment his rights as a person must be recognized, among which in the first place is the right of every innocent human being to life.

16. At the latest, through the solemn declarations of Pope John Paul II's encyclical *Evangelium Vitae,* this teaching has attained quasi-dogmatic binding force:

> Therefore, by the authority which Christ conferred upon Peter and his Successors, in communion with the Bishops. . . . *I declare that direct abortion, that is, abortion willed as an end or as a means, always constitutes a grave moral disorder,* since it is the deliberate killing of an innocent human being (John Paul II 1978, n. 62).

17. See Blaise Pascal, *Pensées* (*Thoughts*) (1973) 200 (347):

> Man is only a reed, the weakest in nature, but he is a thinking reed. There is no need for the whole universe to take up arms to crush him: a vapour, a drop of water is enough to kill him. But even if the universe were to crush him, man would still be nobler than his slayer, because he knows that he is dying and the advantage the universe has over him. The universe knows none of this. Thus all our dignity consists in thought. . . .

18. This dignity belongs to each living human being of whom we can know or assume that he *is* a person even if he cannot function as a person (Schwarz 1990).

19. From Plato on to Anselm, Thomas Aquinas, Leibniz, and Descartes up to the present, we find many arguments for the existence of God. I have attempted to defend these in *Essere e persona* (1989b, chaps. 10–13; arguments from temporality, contingency, and imperfection, chaps. 14–15; and *Gott als Gottesbeweis* [1996b], the ontological argument).

20. This is reflected even in the consequences of atheism. See Friedrich Nietzsche, *Die Fröhliche Wissenschaft* (1982, 125, 285, and the preceding text).

21. Of course, the atheist will regard this to be really impossible, but he is still bound to respect the beliefs of his patients and to allow them access to what they regard as the source of their eternal well-being.

22. Psalm 2, 7: "You are my son, today have I begotten thee."

23. This is the title of the second great encyclical of Pope John Paul II.

24. For this reason, the stark division between metaethics without content and content-full ethics proposed by Engelhardt cannot be maintained. Also, such a metaethics of tolerance and peaceful settlement of disputes cannot be founded without any content-full morally relevant value, e.g., human dignity or freedom, however much Engelhardt tries to do precisely that and to *substitute,* for secular ethics, any value ethics with a mere ethics of democratic consent to be as libertarian and tolerant as possible.

25. See the 1980 Vatican *Declaration on Euthanasia:*

    Life is a gift of God, and on the other hand death is unavoidable; it is necessary, therefore, that we, without in any way hastening the hour of death, should be able to accept it with full responsibility and dignity.

26. According to the Catholic Church, persons who perform or assist in abortion and similar acts even are by this very deed excommunicated (Seifert 1988; 1996a).

27. Baruch A. Brody and Amir Halevy (1996, 571) report that the task force entrusted with working toward a policy found any of these four kinds of futility per se insufficient to make ethically correct decisions. The "Houston Policy," which resulted from these discussions, is purely procedural and seeks to renounce to any content-full principles; these must, however, be assumed, as in any purely procedural or formal approach to ethical questions.

28. Following the terminology of the present debate, I use the term "deontic" not just for a Kantian formalistic ethics but for any ethics that recognizes absolute moral oughts: and "teleological" ethics, not for any ethics that recognizes ends and the influence of the object of moral actions on the moral quality of human acts, but for a purely consequentialist and utilitarian approach to ethics that precisely rejects the idea of intrinsically wrong acts and judges the moral quality of acts just by their consequences.

29. Think of the encyclicals *Veritatis Splendor* and *Humanae Vitae.*

30. These intrinsically wrong acts include the raping of women, sexually abusing and murdering children (which crimes provoked recently the unanimous outcry and shock of the whole Belgian nation), murdering the unborn, and others that are by their essence morally evil. Reason and faith teach us here the same thing, though the vision of Christian faith grasps this same truth far more deeply, which again does not exclude the fact that many Christians and Catholic moral theologians precisely deny these facts. For example, B. Schüller, J. Fuchs, F. Böckle, C. Curran, and countless others. Many other authors, e.g., Robert Spaemann, John Finnis, Joseph Boyle, Andreas Laun, Carlo Caffarra,

Elizabeth Anscombe, and Julian Nida-Rümelin, have criticized consequentialism in ethics (Seifert 1985).

31. This does not exclude the truth of Aquinas's observation that original sin weakens our mind's pure understanding of natural law, which, however, remains accessible to all.

32. This is also the position of Thomas Aquinas on the *species* of human acts that they receive from their directedness to a certain object: the *finis operis*. See also Aquinas, *Summma Theologica, Prima Secundae* (1948, Q1, A1, C):

> respondeo dicendum quod actionum quae ab homine aguntur, illae solae proprie dicuntur humanae, quae sunt propriae hominis inquantum est homo. differt autem homo ab aliis irrationalibus creaturis in hoc, quod est suorum actuum dominus. unde illae solae actiones vocantur proprie humanae, quarum homo est dominus. Est autem homo dominus suorum actuum per rationem et voluntatem, unde et liberum arbitrium esse dicitur facultas voluntatis et rationis. illae ergo actiones proprie humanae dicuntur, quae ex voluntate deliberata procedunt. si quae autem aliae actiones homini conveniant, possunt dici quidem hominis actiones; sed non proprie humanae, cum non sint hominis inquantum est homo. manifestum est autem quod omnes actiones quae procedunt ab aliqua potentia, causantur ab ea secundum rationem sui obiecti. obiectum autem voluntatis est finis et bonum. unde oportet quod omnes actiones humanae propter finem sint.

33. Think also of Edmund Husserl's *Logical Investigations, Prolegomena* (1975), in which general and historical relativism are refuted, or Dietrich von Hildebrand's *Ethics* (1978, chap. 9), as an excellent critique of ethical relativism.

34. Not only in the first, also in this second sense, Saint Paul is a "rationalist" when he speaks of a natural intuition (through the "heart" and "conscience") of the morally good and evil, and writes:

> revelation of the righteous judgment of God; who will render to every man according to his works: to them that by patience in well-doing seek for glory and honor and incorruption, eternal life: but unto them that are factious, and obey not the truth, but obey unrighteousness, *shall be* wrath and indignation, tribulation and anguish, upon every soul of man that worketh evil, of the Jew first, and also of the Greek; but glory and honor and peace to every man that worketh good, to the Jew first, and also to the Greek: for there is no respect of persons with God. For as many as have sinned without law shall also perish without the law: and as many as have sinned under the law shall be judged by the law; for not the hearers of the law are just before God, but the doers of the law shall be justified: (for when Gentiles that have not the law do by nature the things of the law, these, not having the law, are the law unto themselves; in that they show the work of the law written in their hearts, their conscience bearing witness therewith, and their thoughts one with another accusing or else excusing *them*); in the day when God shall judge the secrets of men, according to my gospel, by Jesus Christ. *Romans* 2:5–16.

See, likewise, *Romans* 1:19–20.

35. See against this, e.g., Dietrich von Hildebrand, *Sittlichkeit und ethische Werterkenntnis* (1982b).

36. On the significant relation between the affective life and morality, see Augustine, *The City of God* (1961a, Books 9, 14).

37. See Augustine's sermons or treatises on the Gospel and on the Letters of Saint John. For example: *Agostino. Amore assoluto e "terza navigazione"* (Reale 1994), Saint Bernard of Clairvaux's *Treatise on the Love of God* (1922, 1961), the world of Saint Anselm, Saint Bonaventure's *Itinerarium* (1987), Francis de Sales' *Treatise on the Love of God* (1942), Soeren Kierkegaard's *Edifying Discourses* (1962), Max Scheler's *Das Ressentiment im Aufbau der Moralen* (1955), Dietrich von Hildebrand's *Transformation in Christ* (1989), and countless others.

38. The *phronesis* of which, e.g., Aristotle speaks in *Nichomachean Ethics* (1962, VI, 6.13, 1144 b 17–1145 a6); and again in NE 10.8 1178 a 16–19, Thomas Aquinas, in his *Summa Theologica* (1948, I–II, Q 57, a 4–5; Q 61, a 2; II–II, Q. 47, a. 5); or Dietrich von Hildebrand in his *Morality and Situation Ethics* (1966).

39. This happened, e.g., in the case of Dr. Nathanson's grandfather, who unfortunately committed suicide when he heard of this fact (Nathanson 1996).

40. I still remember with horror the scene of a woman in the middle of hard labor being taken away from the labor room of a Catholic hospital in Dallas to be rushed to a public hospital because her husband did not have enough money to pay the bill in advance. This appears to be the absolute opposite of the mission of Christian charity of a Catholic hospital.

41. Consider also the possibility of atheist physicians, e.g., the one described in Albert Camus' *The Plague* (1984), offering such services for areligious or even antireligious reasons, as described in Sartre's *Le Diable et le Bon Dieu* (1951).

BIBLIOGRAPHY

Aquinas, T. 1948. *Summa Theologica*. Trans. by Fathers of the English Dominican Province. New York: Benziger Brothers.

Aristotle. 1962. *Ethica Nicomachea*. Trans. by H. Rackham. London: Oxford University Press.

———. 1976a. *Metaphysics*. Trans. by H. Tredennick. Cambridge, Mass.: Harvard University Press.

———. 1976b. *Posterior Analytics*. Trans. by H. Tredennick and E. S. Forster. Cambridge, Mass.: Harvard University Press.

Augustine. 1961a. *De civitate Dei* in *Clavis Patrum Latinorum*. Ed. by E. Dekkers. The Hague: M. Nijhoff.

———. 1961b. *Contra Academicos* in *Clavis Patrum Latinorum*. Ed. by E. Dekkers. The Hague: M. Nijhoff.

Bonaventure. 1987. *The Mind's Road to God*. Trans. by G. Boas. New York: Macmillan.

Brody, B., and A. Halevy. 1996. A multi-institutional collaborative policy on medical futility. *Journal of the American Medical Association* 276: 571–74.

Camus, A. 1984. *The Plague*. Trans. by S. Gilbert. New York: A. A. Knopf.

Cicero, M. T. 1970. *De Re Publica, De Legibus*. Trans. by C. Walker-Keyes. Cambridge, Mass.: Harvard University Press.

Clairvaux, B. 1922. *Traite de l'Amour de Dieu*. Paris: P. Lethielleu.

———. 1961. *On the Love of God*. Trans. by a religious of C.S.M.V. London: Mowbray.

Congregation for the Doctrine of the Faith. 1980. Vatican declaration on euthanasia. *Acta apostolica Sedis* 72: 547–49.

Cronin, D. A. 1989. *Conserving Human Life.* Braintree, Mass.: Pope John Center.

Declaration on Euthanasia. 1980. *AAS* 72: 547–49.

De Sales, F. 1942. *Treatise on the Love of God.* Trans. by H. B. Mackey, O.S.B. Westminster, Md.: Newman Book Shop.

Engelhardt, H. T., Jr. 1996. *The Foundation of Bioethics,* 2d ed. New York: Oxford University Press.

———. 1997. The foundations of bioethics and secular humanism: Why there is no canonical moral content. In *Reading Engelhardt,* ed. by B. Minogue, G. Palmer-Fernañdez, and J. E. Reagan. Dordrecht: Kluwer Academic Publishers.

Engelhardt, H. T., Jr., and George Khushf. 1995. Futile care for the critically ill patient. *Current Opinion in Critical Care* 1: 329–33.

Husserl, E. 1975. *Logische Untersuchungen.* Text der ersten und zweiten Auflage. Bd I: *Prolegomena zu einer reinen Logik,* ed. by v. E. Holenstein. The Hague: M. Nijhoff.

———. 1987. Philosophie als strenge Wissenschaft. In Edmund Husserl, *Aufsätze und Vorträge* (1911–21), ed. by Thomas Nenon and Hans Rainer Sepp. Dordrecht: M. Nijhoff.

John Paul II. 1979. *Redemptor Hominis.* London: Catholic Truth Society.

———. 1993. *Veritatis Splendor.* Vatican City: Libreria Editrice Vaticana.

———. 1995. *Evangelium Vitae.* New York: Times Books.

Kant, I. 1938. *Kant's Gesammelte Schriften.* Ed. by v. der Preußischen Akademie der Wissenschaften. Berlin and Leipzig: Walter de Gruyter and Co.

———. 1993. *Kritik der Praktischen Vernunft.* Hamburg: F. Meiner.

———. 1997. *Kant im Kontext.* Ed. by Karsten Worm, Werke auf CD-Rom, 2e erw. und neu durchgesehene Auflage. Berlin: InfoSoftWare.

Kierkegaard, S. 1962. *Edifying Discourses.* Trans. by D. F. Swenson and L. M. Swenson. Minneapolis: Augsburg Publishing House.

Minogue, B. P., G. Palmer-Fernañdez, and J. E. Reagan, eds. 1997. *Reading Engelhardt. Essays on the Thought of H. T. Engelhardt, Jr.* Dordrecht: Kluwer Academic Publishers.

Nathanson, B. 1996. *The Hand of God. A Journey from Death to Life by the Abortion Doctor Who Changed His Mind.* Washington, D.C.: Regnery.

Nietzsche, F. 1982. *Die fröhliche Wissenschaft.* Frankfurt: Insel.

Parfit, D. 1984. *Reasons and Persons.* Oxford: Oxford University Press.

Pascal, B. 1973. *Thoughts,* 5th edition. Trans. by A. J. Krailsheimer. London: Penguin.

Paul VI. 1978. *Humanae Vitae.* San Fransisco: Ignatius Press.

Reale, G., ed. 1994. *Agostino. Amore assoluto e "terza navigazione."* Mailand: Rusconi.

Sartre, J-P. 1951. *Le Diable et le Bon Dieu.* Paris: Gamillard.

Scheler, M. 1955. *Das Ressentiment im Aufbau der Moralen.* In Max Scheler, *Vom Umsturz der Werte.* Bern-München: Francke-Verlag.

————. 1987 [1916]. Liebe und Erkenntnis. In Max Scheler, *Schriften zur Soziologie und Weltanschauungslehre.* Gesammelte Werke, Bd.6. 3e. Aufl. Bonn: Bouvier Verlag.

Schwarz, S. 1990. *The Moral Question of Abortion.* Chicago: Loyola University Press.

Seifert, J. 1976. *Erkenntnis objektiver Wahrheit. Die Transzendenz des Menschen in der Erkenntnis,* 2d ed. Salzburg: A. Pustet.

————. 1978. Das Unsterblichkeitsproblem aus der Sicht der philosophischen Ethik und Anthropologie. *Franziskanische Studien,* H 3.

————. 1983a. Zur Begründung ethischer Normen. Einwände auf Edgar Morschers Position. Ein Diskussionsbeitrag. In *Vom Wahren und vom Guten,* Festschrift zum achtzigsten Geburtstag von Balduin Schwarz. Salzburg: St. Peter Verlag.

————. 1983b. Und dennoch: Ethik ist Episteme, nicht blosse Doxa. Über die wissenschaftliche Begründbarkeit und Überprüfbarkeit ethischer Sätze und Normen. Erwiderung auf Edgar Morscher's Antwort. In *Vom Wahren und vom Guten,* Festschrift zum achtzigsten Geburtstag von Balduin Schwarz. Salzburg: St. Peter Verlag.

————. 1985. Absolute moral obligations towards finite goods as foundation of intrinsically right and wrong actions. A critique of consequentialist teleological ethics: Destruction of ethics through moral theology? *Anthropos* 1: 57–94.

————. 1987. *Back to Things in Themselves. A Phenomenological Foundation for Classical Realism.* London: Routledge.

————. 1988. Abortion and euthanasia as legal and as moral issues: Some reflections on the relationship between morality, church and state. In *Bioethics Update,* ed. by N. Tonti-Filippini. Melbourne: St. Vincents Bioethics Centre.

————. 1989a. Gibt es ein Leben nach dem Tod? *Forum Katholische Theologie* 5, Heft 4.

————. 1989b. *Essere e persona. Verso una fondazione fenomenologica di una metafisica classica e personalistica.* Milan: Vita e Pensiero.

————. 1992a. Is "brain death" actually death? A critique of redefining man's death in terms of "brain death." In *Working Group on the Determination of Brain Death and Its Relationship to Human Death,* ed. by R. J. White, H. Angstwurm, and I. Carasco de Paola. Vatican City: Pontifical Academy of the Sciences.

————. 1992b. Philosophische Grundlagen der Menschenrechte. Zur Verteidigung des Menschen. *Prima Philosophia* 5 (4): 339–70.

————. 1993a. Is "brain death" actually death? *The Monist* 76: 175–202.

————. 1993b. *What Is Life? On the Irreducibility of Life to Chaotic and Non-Chaotic Physical Systems.* Amsterdam: Rodopi.

————. 1994. Essere Persona Come Perfezione Pura. Il Beato Duns Scoto e una nuova metafisica personalistica. *De Homine, Dialogo di Filosofia* 11: 57–75. Rome: Herder/Università Lateranense.

————. 1996a. Euthanasia: What is it? Is it right? *Social Justice Review* 87: 153–55.

————. 1996b. *Gott als Gottesbeweis.* Heidelberg: Universitätsverlag C. Winter.

————. 1996c. Philosophy as a rigorous science. Towards a foundation of the method of realist phenomenology in critical dialogue with Husserl's idea of philosophy as a rigorous science. *Filosofickù Áasopis* 6 (44): 903–22.

————. 1997a. Person und Individuum. Über Hans Urs von Balthasars Philosophie der Person und die philosophischen Implikationen seiner Dreifaltigkeitstheologie. *Forum Katholische Theologie* 13: 81–105.

————. 1997b. Die vierfache Quelle der Menschenwürde als Fundament der Menschenrechte. In *Staatsphilosophie und Rechtspolitik. Festschrift für Martin Kriele zum 65. Geburtstag*, ed. by Burkhardt Ziemske. München: Verlag C. H. Beck.

————. 1998. Phänomenologie und Philosophie als strenge Wissenschaft. Zur Grundlegung einer realistischen phänomenologischen Methode—in kritischem Dialog mit Edmund Husserls Ideen über die Philosophie als strenge Wissenschaft. In *Filosofie, Pravda, Nesmrtlenost. Tòi praúskå pòednáóky/Philosophie, Wahrheit, Unsterblichkeit. Drei Prager Vorlesungen*. Prague: Vydala Kòestanská akademie Òim, svacek, edice Studium.

Shewmon, D. A. 1997. Recovery from "brain death": A neurologist's apologia. *Linacre Quarterly* 64: 30–96.

Spaemann, R. 1996. *Personen. Versuche über den Unterschied zwischen "etwas" und "jemand."* Stuttgart: Klett-Cotta.

Turgenev, I. S. 1999. *Notes of a Hunter*. Paris: Bookkings International.

von Hildebrand, D. 1966. *Morality and Situation Ethics*. Chicago: Franciscan Herald Press.

————. 1978. *Ethics*, 2d ed. Chicago: Franciscan Herald Press.

————. 1982a [1922]. Durchgesehene Auflage. In *Jahrbuch für Philosophie und phänomenologische Forschung*. Vallendar-Schönstatt: Patris Verlag.

————. 1982b [1922]. *Sittlichkeit und ethische Werterkenntnis*. Eine Untersuchung über ethische Strukturprobleme. In *Jahrbuch für Philosophie und phänomenologische Forschung*, vol. 5. Vallendar-Schönstatt: Patris Verlag.

————. 1989 [1948]. *Transformation in Christ. On the Christian Attitude of Mind*. Manchester, N.H.: Sophia Institute Press.

Wildes, K. W., S.J. 1995. Conserving life and conserving means: Lead us not into temptation. In *Critical Choices and Critical Care. Catholic Perspectives on Allocating Resources in Intensive Care Medicine*, ed. by K. W. Wildes, S. J. Dordrecht: Kluwer Academic Publishers.

Equal Care as the Best of Care:
A Personalist Approach

Paul T. Schotsmans

Problems of macroallocation in health care have become increasingly important. Awareness and confrontation with such problems has come much later in nations with a very large social insurance system. This is certainly the case for my native country, Belgium, and may explain the strong reactions of unbelief and even severe critique on health care allocation experiments like those in Oregon in the United States. Some Belgian commentators even consider the Oregon experiment radically unethical (Hallet 1994, 24–25). There is quite a lot of misunderstanding about the social health care system of the democratic European countries by U.S. observers. The fact that some of them classify the Western European health care system as "socialist" may illustrate a strong misunderstanding of the ethical foundations of the European health care systems (McCarrick and Darragh 1997). At the same time, many Europeans refer to the American system as radically unjust for the reason that it excludes millions of people outside of a national system of solidarity. They are convinced that the American health care system places too much emphasis on individualism (McCarrick and Darragh 1997, 82). For Europeans, this observation is even more surprising in light of the so-called "promised land" myths surrounding the U.S. welfare state (Kilner 1995, 1071).

This very general introduction seeks to clarify why I seriously object to statements by Engelhardt in his introduction to this volume, such as:

> Much public policy has been framed in terms of a disingenuous commitment to providing all citizens equally with all the care from which they could benefit. Such an approach to health care policymaking is at best deceptive and at worst involves a corruptive false consciousness, which makes forthright health care policymaking impossible. It is not possible to provide all with (1) the best of care, (2) equal care, (3) physician and patient choice, while (4) still containing costs. One must compromise on one or more points. If resources are not unlimited, then one must limit choice and provide a basic package but not the best of care. And if one is not to impose intrusive governmental restraints, one must accept numerous forms of inequalities. (6)

In this essay, I want to make understandable how a Christian ethical approach—which also may be called a kind of social personalism—can be developed as a foundation for a social health care system, wherein the "best of care" is distributed on "an equal basis" for "all" members of a democratic society. In this way, I will argue against Engelhardt's statement. The crucial point of my reflections may be found in an analysis of how I propose to understand "best of care." In my understanding, "best of care" must refer to some standards or criteria for appropriate care, adapted to the unique situation of every patient. In line with this volume, I will then clarify the meaning of this position for patients in intensive care units (ICUs).

As a start, I will clarify the personalist approach, or what I would like to call the Louvain understanding (Janssens 1980–81). I will then apply this approach to the general problem of health care allocation, and finally explain how this may be translated into the care of patients in ICUs, including the prevention of some patients from having access to critical care.

SOCIAL PERSONALISM AS AN EXPRESSION OF THE CHRISTIAN TRADITION OF SOLIDARITY

My approach to the problem of health care allocation is inspired by the Louvain personalist model, which may be considered to be identical to the theology of the *Pastoral Constitution on the Church in the Modern World* of the Second Vatican Council (hereafter, Vatican II). First, I will situate the ethical debate on the notion of "person" and then present the personalist approach, which afterward will serve as a general framework for entering into the problem of limiting access to medical treatment.

Personalism between Collectivism and Individualism

The concept of a person is possibly the most important idea in any moral discussion. It is the one unavoidable, irreducible element that must always be present if one wishes to enter into moral discourse. This is quite obvious when one considers the subject of morality. The person is the moral agent. In the tradition of Roman Catholic moral theology, the concept of the person frequently indicated little more than this basically correct, but limited, notion of the moral agent. The object of morality was founded upon the moral law, rationally defended as a form of natural law, theologically sought after in biblical prescriptions, and canonically stipulated in the disciplinary rules of the church. It is difficult to determine when and how the concept of the person began to take on a more significant role in ethical reflection. More philosophical language appears appropriate here, for moral theology could hardly be said to have taken the lead in this area. Phenomenology and existentialism would almost certainly prove to be more fruitful places to look for the origins of personalistic thinking (Selling 1988).

At the same time that some theologians were taking their first, hesitant steps toward a personalist approach to conjugal morality, a much more profound evolution was taking place in the area of social thought. The relatively young "social teaching of the church" was facing a major crisis in the 1930s, as the world that it proposed to address accelerated the rate of change and forced both analysts and moralists to recognize that social reality, not only logically but also really, comes prior to any theoretical construct. The economic crisis of the early 1930s aggravated social and political tensions in Europe. The tradition of social teaching, couched in neoscholastic terminology and operating from the presumption of an idealistic abstraction of what social living might look like, was forced to deal with the reality of social life.

On the one side, there was collectivism (e.g., communism). Some early movements in Catholic social teaching, such as corporatism or solidarism, that seemed to envision the possibility of the church somehow stamping its own concept of a *societas perfecta* onto the secular world, became less tenable in light of the more radical forms of socialism and the perceived threat of communism. On the other side, there was totalitarianism (e.g., fascism and national socialism). Perhaps the stronger tradition, in official social teaching at least, was a kind of fundamental belief in individual initiative and responsibility. Apart from the voluntarism implicit in such an approach, placing too much emphasis on the individual begged the question of how to determine the assignment of responsibility. The answer that was acceptable enough to be clearly stated in *Rerum Novarum* (Leo XIII 1891), that there were natural differences between classes and between individuals, was now radically driven toward the conclusion that there must be a "natural" ruling class. Such a position was obviously contrary to the Gospel. The church was left with the problem of finding the middle way between these two extremes. The way that was found was based upon the concept of the human person.

If the central concept of justice was the common good, the evolved notion of social justice (Pius XI 1931) finally admitted the reciprocal relationship between the person and society. The common good was a goal, a task to which every responsible member of society should contribute. The classical idea had already served to establish the notion of duty or obligation. But the common good was also now understood to be a source, a storehouse of opportunity or provider of resources that enables persons to fulfill their responsibility, the human task. From this, one can appreciate the notion of rights, claims that are made by persons in service to the accomplishment of that task. First formulated by Pius XI in *Mit brennender Sorge* (1937), this scheme would mature into the more refined expressions of Vatican II (the sum of those conditions of social life that allow social groups and their individual members relatively thorough and ready access to their own fulfillment (Flannery 1986, *Gaudium et Spes*, 27). The pivotal concept, however, that allowed social teaching to evolve was that of the human person, created in the image of God and endowed with unassailable dignity.

The theology of Vatican II has frequently been described as personalist. The clearest evidence for this can be found in the two final documents the council produced in 1965, *Gaudium et Spes* and *Dignitatis Humanae*. Each text exhibits a profound sense of person, and each utilizes a concept of the person in developing its fundamental principles. It is therefore no wonder that moral theologians of most every persuasion do not hesitate to claim that their approach is personalist or that they would be satisfied with the claim that the person serves as the most fundamental norm. Such claims, however, do not always indicate a similar thought pattern or represent the same notion of person. For the concept of "person" itself is open to a wide range of interpretations.

When personalism began to develop in the first half of the twentieth century in Western Europe, in many Catholic circles it quickly became identified with the communitarian version of French personalism that had developed as an alternative to communism. The person was perceived as being essentially engaged in community living. Therefore, building a just society is founded upon the nature of the person. This parallels a corporatist notion of ecclesial life as well, so this form of personalism appealed to many Christians. However, it was the Northern European concern for epistemological and axiological questions that introduced more philosophical rigor into the discussion. The meaning of experience and the absolutely essential demand for interpretation of experience inevitably led into more metaphysical and sociological considerations.

An Ethic of Responsibility

This preference leans toward an ethics of responsibility, built upon a personalist foundation in the spirit of Vatican II. In the "Pastoral Constitution on the Church in the Modern World" (*Gaudium et Spes*), the groundwork for such an approach was outlined (especially in Part I). It explains the fundamental and constant aspects or dimensions of persons: a subject, not an object; a subject in corporeality (*Gaudium et Spes,* section 14); a part of the material world (33–39, 53–62); essentially directed toward each other (12); created in the image of God (12, 34); a historical being (36) and also a social being (23–32) (Janssens 1980–81).

Human persons are not only essentially social beings because they are open to each other in the I–Thou relationship (Buber 1923), but also because they need to live in social groups and thus in appropriate structures and institutions. Every human being lives in a concrete societal context. We need structures and institutions worthy of people, e.g., political structures and international cooperation. Therefore, the council reacted against an individualistic morality: Ethics demands that we respect laws and other institutions in social living, insofar as they are in service to the common good (*Gaudium et Spes*, 26, 74). But social structures and institutions are made by humans and thus are necessarily limited, imperfect, and changeable (historicity). It is therefore also a social and moral demand regularly to revise them, to accommodate them to changing circumstances, and to renew them through dynamic development, according to the growing possibilities of human dignity (*Gaudium et Spes*, 26, 39, 30).

By virtue of the historicity of the human person, which affects all the essential aspects of the human person, an ethics of responsibility on a personalist foundation must necessarily be a dynamic ethic. It is the specific task of ethics to inquire as to how the growing possibilities can be realized to serve human dignity and how the developing experience of values must enrich our activity. The promotion of the *humanum,* that which promotes the human person, adequately considered, becomes a moral obligation insofar as it becomes possible (*le souhaitable humain possible*) (Ricoeur 1975). Ethics is fundamentally a way of living, and in its own growth must keep step with human life itself as it unfolds throughout history. That is precisely what we mean when we say that it must be dynamic as human life itself, which it directs and leads.

All human persons also are fundamentally equal, but at the same time each is an original human being. We are fundamentally equal (*Gaudium et Spes,* 29), which explains why moral demands are universalizeable; that is, that the same moral obligations apply to all. But in this framework and on the basis of fundamental equality, each person is simultaneously original, a unique subject. The unfolding of each and every originality is also a requirement for a rich, fruitful social life. In society as a community-living (coexistence), for instance, I–Thou relationships are very important in order to promote the originality of each person involved in an unsurpassable way. Society as a community working (cooperation) toward the realization of culture obviously presupposes our fundamental equality, which permits us to have an interest in the same cultural values. In society as a community-sharing (coparticipation), the fruits of working together must be attuned to the needs of each and every person according to the demands of his or her originality (to each according to their needs). These orientations are equally valid for the development of an ethically adequate health care system in every democratic society.

These considerations imply that we must build a health care system that serves human dignity, that is, if it in truth, according to reason enlightened by revelation, is beneficial to the human person adequately considered with regard to both oneself and one's relations. In virtue of the historicity of the human person, this criterion requires that we again and again reconsider which possibilities we have at our disposal at this point in history to serve the promotion of the human person. In conjunction with this we must, in our acts and institutions—and thus also in the health care system—respect the originality of all as much as possible.

The Personalist Interpretation of Solidarity and Subsidiarity in Magisterial Documents

These lines of thought are very similar to the magisterial teaching on solidarity and subsidiarity in the Catholic Church. Theologians traditionally make a distinction between three periods: before John XXIII, the period between John XXIII and John Paul II, and the theologization of the social teachings of the church by John Paul II (Verstraeten 1998). Before John XXIII, the solidarity concept was a secular concept of the eighteenth century. The concept indicated the solidarity created by the process of the division of labor and the complementary competencies and capacities of those who are involved in the common labor process of a society. Durkheim made a distinction between "mechanic solidarity" (or the unity on the basis of equality, typical for primitive communities) and "organic solidarity" (or the unity in complementary divergencies). As a consequence of this sociological approach, the concept of solidarity was given more and more an ethical meaning, namely the duty to cooperate and to collaborate in such a way that the society can become "socialized." Later on, this led to an ontological meaning of solidarity, whereby every human being is considered to be ontologically oriented to society and community as an anthropological characteristic (Pesch and Lechtape 1922; Gundlach 1927). The encyclical *Quadragesimo Anno* (Pius XI 1931), strongly influenced by the "solidaristic" approach of Pesch and Gundlach, takes as a starting point the notions of "social justice" and "the common good."

This encyclical, however, made more history through its explicit clarification of the subsidiarity principle, which is understood by Von Nell-Breuning (1986) as the duty of the community to give all individuals the opportunities to develop as persons. The negative interpretation of the subsidiarity concept is prevalent in the encyclical (as much as possible, the state must give individuals the opportunity to develop their own initiatives, and only in-tervene when individuals endanger the common good).

John XXIII further developed the positive meaning of subsidiarity, stressing the need for a positive intervention of the state that has to support, stimulate, and complete. He clearly developed a plea for state intervention in the context of social security: the Western social security system functioned here as a model for his teachings. He presented a much more personalistic than ontological interpretation of solidarity; his inspiring vision of advancing the common good is based on the equality of all humankind by virtue of their human dignity. The human person is for John XXIII the foundation, rationale, and purpose of all social institutions. Every human being is a person, which implies that his or her rights and duties are absolute and inalienable: "every man has the right to life, to bodily integrity, and to the means which are necessary and suitable for proper development of life; these are primarily food, clothing, shelter, rest, medical care, and finally the necessary social services" (John XXIII 1963, 11).

There is also a shift to a more sociological foundation of the commonality of the human being: by virtue of the analytic instrument "seeing, judging and acting" (reference, e.g., Joseph Cardinal Cardijn of Belgium, the spiritual leader of social action in the Roman Catholic Church), it became very important to be open for the input of the social sciences in the promotion of human society. John XXIII is radically critical of political systems that are based only on freedom rights and are linked to a "liberal" (in the sense of individualistic, e.g., the liberal economic strategies of Prime Minister Margaret Thatcher in the United Kingdom and President Ronald Reagan in the United States) tradition. It may also be stressed that Vatican II documents further explained this personalistic interpretation of the foundational value of solidarity (*Gaudium et Spes*, 25, 26, and 27). A next shift, inspired by John XXIII, is that from national economic interest to a worldwide concept of "world-solidarity" (wereldsolidariteit) (John XXIII 1963, 157). He makes it clear that solidarity cannot be understood fully by the universal realization of individual human rights. This is also very strongly present in *Gaudium et Spes* (78). The problem of international solidarity finds, however, its brilliant completion in the encyclical *Populorum Progressio* from Paul VI (1967).

All this makes clear that the personalist approach to the creation of a just health care system is almost identical with the Catholic teaching of John XXIII and Vatican II. I will further elaborate this personalist model in relation to the problem of limiting access to medical treatment and, in particular, to critical care. To be complete, however, I cannot avoid mentioning that John Paul II has given a much more theological interpretation to the concept of solidarity in his social teachings (*Redemptor Hominis*). This shift in understanding has very important practical implications. John Paul II is essentially interested in an engaged practice (an evangelical praxis) (crucially important in the encyclical *Dives in Misericordia*). It even functions in the fundamental teachings on moral theology, where "martyrdom" becomes a task for all Christians (John Paul II 1993, 93). The most important document remains, however, *Sollicitudo Rei Socialis*, wherein he extends the concept of solidarity also to "ecological care" (John Paul II 1988, 26). The negative meaning of the concept of "subsidiarity" is for John Paul II the most important one: He is very critical about the so-called "State of Care," in which he discerns essentially negative bureaucratic forces. As an alternative, he proposes a revival of subjectivity and volunteering engagement, which has surprised many observers because they cannot accept that he would favor a radically individualistic social health care system.

LIMITING ACCESS TO MEDICAL TREATMENT: A PERSONALIST APPROACH

Christian Personalism and Health Care

We have now the necessary elements at our disposal to deal with a concrete problem in light of an ethics of responsibility on a personalist basis, namely, the problem of limiting access to medical treatment in order to reach a better balance of the health care system in our societies. To do so adequately, I must first clarify some basic concepts.

It may be clear that the problem of scarcity is strongly influenced by the culture and the values of a society. Medicalization, consumerism, and defensive medicine are key factors in the discussion of problems of choice concerning health care priorities (*Choices in Health Care* 1992). Scarcity may, therefore, be classified as a relative notion, linked with the problem of choice in health care. It will also depend on social choices concerning other priorities in a welfare state. Political and social policy concerning the ways in which we value "health" relative to other goals in our value system are hereby certainly decisive.

Central to this discussion will be how we value "health." In the recent debate on the ethics of health care, this concept has been strongly overvalued. Due to secularization and pluralistic nihilism, the only remaining target value seems to have become an idolatrous ideology of health. This has many negative consequences; for example, dependence on health care providers, who become the new moral "heroes" of the Western world. Christianity has always criticized this overvaluation of health; it refers to "human finitude" as one of the essentials of our existence. Of course, it remains a strong obligation in health care to promote the health of all people as much as possible. As the Dutch Dunning committee describes it, health is an instrumental value necessary in order to function socially. But instead of serving the sick and being devoted to the weakest, the economic and financial constraints in some Western health care systems have become extremely powerful, leaving aside the concern for real solidarity. In order to be consistent with the Christian tradition, we need, therefore, to add to the concept of health care the very concrete, daily caring for sick, dependent, handicapped, and dying patients. The structures and organizations of the health care system stand indeed primarily under the critical evaluation of the ways in which this concrete caring takes place and gets priority in the system.

This implies finally also a critique on the dominant role being given in ethical discourse to self-determination and autonomy. Notions of self-determination and respect for autonomy are important as dimensions of the human person adequately considered, but have become almost ideological instruments in self-defensive reactions to discussions about priorities and choices in health care. The classical Christian idea of health care as a service, devotion, vocation, and even a duty suffers strongly under this evolution.

In light of all these considerations, it is astonishing that Christian reaction is so poorly present in the debate on macroallocation. One of the most remarkable contributions I have seen was the reaction of the spokesman of the Roman Catholic community in Holland on the national Dunning Report (Jeurissen 1993). First, he judged that Christian social ethics must be totally personalistic for it refers to the complementary function of the individual and the society. Social justice must, therefore, be a key notion at the crossroads of individual and collective interests. Second, crucially important for every Christian approach on health care is the preferential option for the poor; every solution for eventual problems of scarcity starts with solidarity with the most vulnerable groups in the society. Finally, Christianity has its own view on health: It is a fundamental but not absolute good. Health care may be finite for the reason that we human beings are finite. This may even be the most fundamental input of Christianity in the debate on health care allocation.

Humanitarian Solidarity: A Personalist Approach to Limiting Access to Medical Treatment

So far it is clear that the basic inspiration of Christian personalism may help us to design a general outline of a just health care system. I will now turn to more concrete considerations and translate the personalist approach into a structural answer to the problem of limiting access to medical treatment. My first observation is that the recent debates on "access to medical treatment" concentrate essentially on the conditional right to health care and do not seem to be interested in health care itself. In light of the personalist approach, the promotion of the best of care in an equal way must, however, remain the target of the system. The best of care means that every individual in society has at least equal access to the highest standard of medical treatment. I understand the "highest standard" to mean that all services must be made ready so that appropriate medical care may be provided. It does not mean that medical obsession must take the lead; on the contrary, every individual patient demands an individual approach. What is appropriate for one patient may not be appropriate for other patients. In any case, solidarity implies that the social network is developed in such a way that not only the rich and privileged, but also the poor and the unemployed, may enter the health care establishment with equal access to standard medical treatment. Even more, a really Christian organization of health care implies a preferential option for "the poor, the widow, the orphan," such as chronically ill elderly patients, psychiatric patients, and severely handicapped newborns, in order to fulfill the basic requirements of a just distributive health care system.

Ter Meulen (1994) refers in this context to the notion of "humanitarian solidarity." This kind of solidarity, which is based on the dignity of the human person, seeks to protect those human persons whose existence is threatened by circumstances beyond their own control, particularly natural fate or unfair social structures. Humanitarian solidarity should be the starting point for defining necessary care. Services for persons unable to care for themselves because of psychological handicaps (e.g., Alzheimer's disease, psychiatric disorders, and mental retardation) should have priority in the basic package of health care. Defined in this way, the basic package should be equally accessible to all, without financial constraints, such as copayments or obligatory risks. A two-tier system based on the principle of humanitarian solidarity puts care, not cure, at the center of its efforts to provide an adequate level of health care for all (Ter Meulen 1994).

The implicit aspects of societal debate, such as those in Oregon and Holland, must be situated in an effort to become more open and more critical about the "hidden" priorities that guide final decision makers. The value of the Oregon plan was exactly the promotion of public concern for these decision-making procedures and the realization of wide participation by the general public in the debate. It is necessary that health care data become public—an effort many Western European countries are starting to realize. We must engage in epidemiological studies on medical treatments and provide the necessary empirical data. Transparency and information are basic instruments for keeping the social values of the system intact. The publication of these figures and eventual controls will make people alert and help them to discuss on a more open level the priorities of various health care systems. I am convinced that such a system, with all possible techniques of evidence-based medicine, revision of protocols, and so on, will provide better insights for the necessary cost containment.

But all this is only secondary to a more fundamental debate about solidarity and justice in the organization of the health care system. The goal of realizing the best of care, understood as what may be appropriate for every unique patient, on an equal basis, may not be an illusion of someone living in the thirteenth century, but a realistic challenge for all those who are concerned about the neediest. This will even be made more realistic by translating these incentives into hospital protocols, medical guidelines, and decision-making procedures. These guidelines and orientations may help hospital managers, physicians, and the public to realize necessary restrictions on investment in medical treatments that do not really adequately serve the goals of a well-functioning health care system.

In line with such a project, special attention is needed for the development of critical care. Although no one can imagine a health care system without adequate critical care units, it has become a very expensive and, at times, disproportionate service. In that way, it may be the place where cure is overvalued and care is neglected. The personalist approach must, therefore, clarify how cost containment can also be realized in the context of critical care. The following may illustrate how equal access to the best of critical care may be realized, without creating unacceptable expectations and even with the result of adequate financial balance in the totality of the health care system. Here we must shift attention from social ethics to more specific medical ethics; the subject indeed demands careful balancing between macro- and microethical considerations.

CRITICAL CARE: MEDICAL DECISION MAKING IN A CONTEXT OF SOLIDARITY AND JUSTICE

In a personalist approach, the promotion of the patient, in all his or her dimensions and relationships, adequately considered, is the central dynamic orientation. In the context of critical care, this can be translated into very precise guidelines. The suggestion is fundamentally that decisions on appropriate cure and care must be situated in the context of the physician–patient relationship and must lead to better application of medical technology in a more human approach. Personalism, however, is directed to promote the person in all his or her dimensions and relationships, which implies the need for significant value dialogue among the patient, family members or representatives, physicians, nursing teams, and the hospital administration. Decisions regarding the ethical justifiability of withholding or withdrawing medical treatment—and eventually also treatment-limiting orders (e.g., refusal to provide access to the ICU)—involves not simply an evaluation of the physical condition of the patient but that of the whole person. Therefore, it is good to be aware of an entire complex of values and norms with regard to life, quality of life, and other values. Ethical guidelines seem, however, to be essentially needed for dealing with the problems of the application of excessive medical technology.

A Proportional Evaluation as Ethical Method

Traditionally, moral theology applied in this context the concepts of "ordinary" and "extraordinary" means. Although many moral theologians still refer to these concepts, it is very difficult to make an adequate distinction between ordinary and extraordinary care. This distinction may be adequate for static and poor medical environments, but it is no longer apt to cope with the rapid evolutions of medical technology at the moment. From a more methodological point of view, we may say that these concepts functioned indeed very well in the context of the ethical model of so-called act-deontology, but they lack sufficient dynamic integration of new evolutions and changing perspectives. Treating the question of the value of life, the theme of euthanasia, and the meaning of suffering, the *Vatican Declaration on Euthanasia* introduced another terminology by referring to the proportionate use of therapeutic agents (Congregation for the Doctrine of the Faith 1980). Although treating the validity of the principle that guides the concepts of "ordinary" and "extraordinary," the document points out that, due to the rapid advances of medical treatment and because of its vagueness, today the language of "ordinary" and "extraordinary" appears ambiguous. Therefore, the declaration refers to the more recent proposals of some theologians on "proportionate and disproportionate means:"

> In any case, it will be possible to make a correct judgment as to the means by studying the type of treatment to be used, its degree of complexity or risk, its cost and the possibilities of using it, and comparing these elements with the result that can be expected, taking into account the state of the sick person and his or her physical and moral resources. (Part IV, Due Proportion in the Use of Remedies)

Also important is the opinion that proportionality is to be decided not only at the beginning of the treatment but also in the course of its application; because during the course of its application the treatment can become disproportionate due to the factors like disproportionate strain or suffering, or by being against the wishes of the patient, or due to actual results.

All this makes clear that speaking in terms of "proportionate and disproportionate means" is preferable. The general dissatisfaction with the concepts of "ordinary" and "extraordinary means" (e.g., in situations where good and evil coexist) led many eminent moral theologians, including Janssens, Knauer, Fuchs, Schüller, Van de Poel, Van der Marck, and McCormick, to explore a way of reasoning that is now well known as the "theory of proportionality." But as noted by Selling, "proportionality" is neither a "system" nor a "determinative methodology," but is only a way of "looking at things proportionally" (Selling 1986). According to Janssens (1980–81), proportionality is a question of the relation between end and good. There must not be any intrinsic contradiction between the basic or ontic good that we want to preserve and the means we use for that end. As Knauer says, this postulate of noncontradiction between the means and end is a central norm for determining the proportionate reason of any human act (Knauer 1965).

Crucially important for us, this approach makes clear that every time we must realize the most humanly possible care (Ricoeur 1975). This implies that the best of care must be understood in terms of appropriate care: What may be here and now for this patient the most humanly possible to realize? It may imply that limiting orders are decided, or that the patient is removed to a palliative care unit, or also that all possible medical technology is implemented in order to rescue the patient's life. Such decisions are of course very delicate and therefore require careful analysis of the medical condition of the patient, comprehensive clarification of personal and relational values, and extensive justification for the investment of societal resources.

Proportional Decision Making in Critical Care

Decisions in critical care must be made from the perspective of the well-being of the patient. One is only obliged to use the available medical means for the prolongation of life if the well-being of the patient (individually or socially) is genuinely being served. The point of departure here is respect for the patient as person and the process of care as an interhuman event. When a decision must be made concerning critical care, the physician—in communication with the patient, his or her eventual representative, and the family—must weigh the various values and disvalues that are at stake, including all the important elements (personal and familial as well as medical), as well as the extent to which particular treatments promote human fulfillment. This "proportionate" judgment needs to be made in each particular case: *one must evaluate the possibilities by considering the type of treatments available, their degree of complexity, the costs, and their possibilities of application along with the result that can be expected, taking into account the condition of the sick person and his or her bodily and moral strength.* In collaboration with nurses, colleagues and other health care professionals, physicians should dialogue with the patient, his or her representative, and the family to justify proposals for concrete decisions.

This creates an open atmosphere, avoids excessive application of medical technology, and helps lead to sincere cost containment. Indeed, the use of excessive medical technology is meaningless when it functions only to preserve physiological life. The best of care for a patient in the ICU may be the decision to forgo all medical treatment and to give priority to basic care by transferring the patient to patient-caring departments.

At the same time, this approach makes a trustful encounter with patients (and their families) possible. The responsibility for the final decision, which is at the end also a fully clinical decision, lies, in my view, best in the hands of the physician, functioning as the medical gatekeeper of the system. The physician indeed is the only one who has the skill, experience, and responsibility to bear the load of such decisions. This is not medical paternalism, but an expression of full respect for the relational structure of the medical profession. The physician can only come to a conclusion when taking the caring and curing relationship with the patient seriously. The profession of physicians is a relational profession, because medicine is one of the best illustrations of the relational structure of the human person. When physicians finally make decisions, they are not acting on their own, but as agents of the relational structure and of devotion to the patient (Pellegrino and Thomasma 1993).

On the practical level, this concern for cost containment and adequate medical decision making has led to proposals for several treatment-limitation policies (Bone 1994; O'Toole et al. 1994; see Appendix A). It also has made possible the transition from critical care to palliative care, because there may come a moment where the medical data clearly indicate that further acute care will become disproportionate. Care is always present, in every medical activity, but will take now the lead to help a patient, who is no longer critically but terminally ill, peacefully to die (Delooz 1995).

Is this microethical approach sufficiently taken into account in the macroethical restraints on health care systems? I am convinced this may be very convergent, really starting where one has to start: in the concrete and daily patient-physician relationship. Three conditions need to be fulfilled to bridge the eventual gap between the individual and society (Society of Critical Care Medicine Ethics Committee 1997).

First, decision procedures must be developed in an open and communicative atmosphere. This may be promoted by wide participation of hospital ethics committees in the process of information and education. Second, physicians and staff members functioning in ICUs must be prepared to cooperate in evidenced-based medical strategies. This openness is growing and will facilitate in the future an adequate evaluation of eventual outcomes of medical technologies. Finally, the societal evaluation of investments, costs, and outcomes must be totally transparent. This is crucially important for making societal decisions about priorities in health care allocations.

TENTATIVE CONCLUSIONS

Cost containment is essential to keep health care systems properly functioning. I am convinced that this may be possible, while at the same time providing all with the best of care and with equal care, under the conditions that we understand by "best" of care the appropriate care for every unique patient. This implies that the medical profession in dialogue with the representatives of the patients (e.g., mutual insurance funds) must define adequate health care in general and adequate critical care in particular. Concerning the former, the value of "health" must be balanced against other values in current value systems. Concerning the latter, adequate critical care can best be defined by setting general standards of care, many times expressed in intensive and critical care units by "codes of treatment."

This system seems to be perfectly realistic in a context of free physician and patient choice. It remains, therefore, crucial to develop the physician–patient relationship as fully relational and to give the medical responsibility to the health professional. Excesses of patient autonomy must be made impossible by favoring more important values as authentic responsibility and solidarity. Excesses of medical paternalism must be made impossible by controlling bodies with adequate representation of all those involved. Here the value of solidarity and the promotion of equal care are the guiding principles. Those who want to purchase care that would not be provided in these standards can do so freely, but it will be totally left to their own expense. The preservation of a just and equal society may not be threatened by these excessive demands. Crucially important, however, remain consensus agreements about a basic and equal amount of care that should be provided to all.

Christian social personalism has helped to create as much as possible the best of care on an equal basis for all citizens in many Western European countries. It is of course a permanent challenge: Again and again, we must inquire how the growing possibilities of medicine can be integrated in order to promote human dignity. But the challenge is at the same time also an exercise in a continuous conscientious effort to realize the Kingdom of God in the world.

APPENDIX A: LEUVEN CODING

Consider, for example, the "Leuven Coding" regarding critically ill patients (Department of Intensive Care Medicine, University Hospitals, K. U. Leuven, Belgium) (Peter Lauwers, M.D., professor, director of the Department of Intensive Care Medicine, University Hospital, Leuven).

Note: Each coding can, by specific orders, be defined with greater accuracy, not in a way though that a different code would be the result.

Code 1   Maximum care (unrestricted)

Code 2   All care except for a number of (prescribed) restrictions (e.g., hemofiltration, circulatory-assist, re-operation, transplantation)

Code 3   Therapeutical options (unaltered) continued as prescribed, without however increasing care or initiating a new therapy. In case of progressive deterioration or circulatory arrest: no initiation of CPR (= DNR [do not resuscitate]), except when arrest is due to an accident (e.g., disconnection of the ventilator, . . .)

Code 4   The therapy is reduced to comfort care, as decided and prescribed on the written order. Only this comfort therapy can be modified or increased. In case of circulatory arrest: DNR

Code 5   Stop ALL therapy, including respiration and feeding (e.g., in case of cerebral death)

Guidelines with Regard to the Coding of Critical Patients in Intensive Care

The determination of the code is always done by the responsible medical supervisor(s).

- The medical supervisor of the patient decides for Code 1 and 2.
- For the transition to Code 3, 4, and 5, the decision making must be done by a group of three supervisors (the supervisor responsible for the patient and two other supervisors), of whom at least one is a Senior (>5 years of experience in intensive care medicine). The decision making is always formal and carried out with the utmost care, after joint discussion between the three supervisors, the registrar, the nurse in charge for the patient, and a senior nursing officer. The responsible supervisor determines whether the referring physician is drawn into the discussion.
- From Code 2, the decision made will be explicitly written down in the medical file.
- The family of the patient will always be informed about the decision and the further evolution in all objectivity and with all the discretion and tact necessary.

- The referring physician(s) is (are) also immediately informed about any change of code.
- By CPR (cardiopulmonary resuscitation) is meant: the restoration of cardiac activity in case of circulatory arrest, through cardiac massage and/or defibrilation, and all activity necessary for reaching this goal (e.g., increasing $FiO2$, artificial ventilation, cardiac drugs).
- DNR (do not resuscitate) means: no actions will be taken to reverse a cardiocirculatory arrest.
- Codes 3, 4, and 5 always presuppose DNR. Therefore this statement (DNR) is not written down on the order page.
- In case of codes 2, 3, 4, and 5, the code-statement will be signed by the supervisor.

"Comfort care" is not a confined concept, it is defined by the supervisor. Comfort care is generally related to: thirst, hunger (feeding: enteral or parenteral); pain, and discomfort (analgetics, sedation, anti-emetic drugs…). Comfort care can, however, also stand for respiration and oxygen therapy (in connection with asphyxia) or a change of position (in connection with decubitus), etc.

BIBLIOGRAPHY

Bone, R. C. 1994. Concepts in emergency and critical care. *Journal of the American Medical Association* 271: 1200–03.

Buber, M. 1923. *Ich und du.* Leipzig: Insel-Verlag.

Choices in Health Care. A Report by the Government Committee on Choices in Health Care. The Netherlands. 1992. Rijswijk: Netherlands Ministry of Welfare, Health and Cultural Affairs.

Congregation for the Doctrine of the Faith. 1980. Vatican declaration on euthanasia. *Acta Apostolica Sedis* 72: 547–49.

Delooz, H. 1995. Ethical issues in critical care: Criteria for treatment. In *Critical Choices and Critical Care. Catholic Perspectives on Allocating Resources in Intensive Care Medicine,* ed. by K. W. Wildes, S.J. Dordrecht: Kluwer Academic Publishers.

Flannery, A. 1986. *Vatican Council (2nd: 1962–1965).* Northport, N.Y.: Costello Publishing.

Gundlach, G. 1927. *Zur Soziologie des katholischen Ideenwelt und der Jesuitenordens,* Freiburg: Herder.

Hallet, J. 1994. Y a-t-il une limite à la prise en charge des soins de santé par la solidarité? In *Solidarité. Santé. Ethique,* ed. by J. Hallet, J. Hermesse, and D. Sauer. Louvain: Garant.

Janssens, L. 1980–81. Artifical insemination: Ethical considerations. *Louvain Studies* 8: 3–29.

Jeurissen, R. J. M. 1993. De gemeenschapsgerichte benadering in het christelijk-sociaal denken. In *Solidariteit volgens Dunning: Gemeenschap of Gemeenplaats?* ed. by M. A. M. Pijnenburg. Utrecht: Katholieke Vereniging van Zorginstellingen.

John XXIII, Pope. 1961. *Mater et Magistra.* Vatican City: Vatican.

———. 1963. *Pacem in Terris.* Vatican City: Vatican.

John Paul II, Pope. 1979. *Redemptor Hominis.* Vatican City: Vatican.

———. 1980. *Dives in Misericordia.* Vatican City: Vatican.

———. 1988. *Sollicitudo Rei Socialis.* Vatican City: Vatican.

———. 1993. *Veritatis Splendor.* Vatican City: Vatican.

Kelly, D. F. 1991. *Critical Care Ethics. Treatment Decisions in American Hospitals.* Kansas City: Sheed and Ward.

Kilner, J. F. 1995. Health care resources, allocation of. I. Macroallocation. In *Encyclopaedia of Bioethics,* 2d ed., ed. by Leroy Walters. New York: Macmillan.

Knauer, P. 1965. La détermination du bien et du mal moral par le principe du double effet. *Nouvelle Revue Théologique* 87: 356–76.

Leo XIII, Pope. 1891. *Rerum Novarum.* Boston: Daughters of Saint Paul.

McCarrick, P., and M. Darragh. 1997. A just share: Justice and fairness in resource allocation. *Kennedy Institute of Ethics Journal* 7: 81–102.

O'Toole, E. E., S. Yougner, B. Juknialis, B. Daly, E. Bartlett, and C. Landefeld. 1994. Evaluation of a treatment limitation policy with a specific treatment-limiting order page. *Archives of Internal Medicine* 154: 425–33.

Paul VI, Pope. 1967. *Populorum Progressio.* Vatican City: Vatican.

Pellegrino, E. D., and D. C. Thomasma. 1993. *The Virtues in Medical Practice.* New York: Oxford University Press.

Pesch, H., and H. Lechtape. 1922. *Der christliche Solidarismus.* Freiburg: Herder.

Pius XI, Pope. 1931. *Quadragesimo Anno.* Vatican City: Vatican.

———. 1937. *Mit brennender Sorge.* Vatican City: Vatican.

Ricoeur, P. 1975. Le problème du fondement de la morale. *Sapienza* 28: 313–37.

Selling, J. 1986. The development of proportionalist thinking. *Chicago Studies* 25: 167–75.

———, ed. 1988. *Personalist Morals. Essays in Honor of Professor Louis Janssens.* Leuven: University Press.

Society of Critical Care Medicine Ethics Committee. 1997. Consensus statement of the Society of Critical Care Medicine's Ethics Committee regarding futile and other possibly inadvisable treatments. *Critical Care Medicine* 25 (5): 887–91.

Ter Meulen, R. 1994. Are there limits to solidarity with the elderly? *Hastings Center Report* 24 (5): 36–38.

Verstraeten, J. 1998. De betekenis van solidariteit en subsidiariteit in kerkelijke documenten. *Ethische Perspectieven* 8: 210–20.

Von Nell-Breuning, O. 1986. The drafting of *Quadragesimo Anno.* In *Official Catholic Social Teaching* (*Readings in Moral Theology,* 5), ed. by C. E. Curran and R. McCormick. New York: Paulist Press.

Wildes, K. W., ed. 1995. *Critical Choices and Critical Care. Catholic Perspectives on Allocating Resources in Intensive Care Medicine.* Dordrecht: Kluwer Academic Publishers.

Quality of Life and Human Dignity: Meaning and Limits of Prolongation of Life

Ludger Honnefelder

Within only a few decades, the development of contemporary biomedicine has enlarged the possibilities of medical diagnostics and therapy to a hitherto unknown extent. That in turn has led to questions, which until now we have hardly had to address with the same scope and urgency. The most fundamental of these asks: Is everything that is technically possible also medically mandated? Moreover: Does the patient desire what is technically possible and medically mandated? This leads to the further question: Can what is technically possible, medically mandated, and desired by the patient be made available to everyone within the resources of a public health care system? Those questions then yield several restricting perspectives: individual restrictions, from the perspective of the patient; medical restrictions, from the perspective of the physician; and economic restrictions, from the perspective of the health care system.

Within each of those perspectives, what restrictions are both required and responsible? Because ethics demands that restricting possible courses of action through omission must be justified as much as actually following a particular practice, we are obliged to furnish a moral justification for the restrictions within each of those perspectives.

What are the criteria for such a justification? Because the problem of restricting possible courses of action arises within each of the three perspectives, and because all are necessary conditions of contemporary medical practice, we can address that question only according to the criteria that are regarded as morally relevant within each perspective. That approach yields the following proposition: We can only find an adequate justification for restricting medical practice, especially in the area of contemporary intensive care medicine, if we succeed in relating the relevant moral criteria of the different perspectives to one another in a convincing way.

In its approach, this proposition is identical to the position developed within the Catholic tradition of Christian theology, at least if one accepts as the fundamental assumption of that tradition that the moral criteria for our actions emerge from an insight of reason into the law-like structure of the type of actions in question. However, this by no means exhausts that position. For it holds that all of human life, from beginning to end, including all its manifestations, evolves within an order to which the concepts of faith, hope, and love give meaning. This order does not replace the, albeit limited, insights of reason, but rather transcends them. What then are the roles of faith, hope, and love over and above the moral norms that reason can grasp when it comes to managing those limits that apply to humans as finite beings, especially with respect to illness and death?

In what follows, I will therefore first look at the different dimensions of medical practice as well as the moral criteria that are relevant to restricting access. I will then inquire into the role that the tradition ascribes to the premises of the Christian faith for this issue. Following that, I will attempt to demonstrate how the different perspectives influence the decision to restrict medical treatment and how the moral criteria from those perspectives relate to one another. Finally, I will address the need for and the difficulties of relating the different sets of criteria to one another, if we want to justify restrictions of practice in intensive care medicine. For reasons that will become clear below, the problem of limiting treatment will be discussed with respect to patients in a persistent vegetative state as a limiting-case example of individuals in critical care.

RELEVANT MORAL CRITERIA

In contemporary industrial societies, medical interventions and their limits must be understood as a multidimensional network of practices. (1) As interventions in the psycho-physical identity of humans, they affect their basic rights. (2) As actions of medical and paramedical practitioners, they are governed by the rules of medical practice. (3) As practices that occur within certain institutionalized individual and social conditions, they are governed by those institutions. (4) As far as they require certain resources, they are governed by the rules that apply to the distribution of those resources under conditions of scarcity, especially the conditions of a market-based economy, albeit that the influence of the market varies according to the health care system in question. Whereas the first two dimensions have a more or less universal character, the last two vary greatly from health care system to health care system, according to social, cultural, and other factors.

What then are the relevant moral criteria for each of the dimensions in question? As far as (1) is concerned, we can refer to individual and social basic rights as contained in the globally accepted ethics of human rights. As for (2), we can refer to medical ethics as it results from the goals of medical practice and the associated doctor–patient relationship as presented in professional codes. However, there are no universal criteria of an institutional nature covering (3); here we have to take into account the ethos that is linked to the social and cultural manifestation of the institutions we encounter and to which the individual and society are committed. As far as (4) is concerned, we must refer to the rules of economic morality, particularly those of the market, which in turn are determined by the social and economic order in which the market is embedded.

Human Rights

Under the title human rights, we recognize certain dimensions of humanity that are so fundamental that everyone must respect them (Honnefelder 1996, 139–60). Underlying this claim is the assumption that human beings are creatures who are to be respected as such and have, to use Kant's terminology, not just a price (i.e., a substitutable value), but also dignity (i.e., inherent worth). The basis for that dignity is the capacity of human beings to act as moral subjects, that is, to set their own goals. Because the creature (natural being) has that capacity to act as a moral subject, a human being has dignity *qua human being* (as a member of the species). For the same reason, basic rights protect the natural and social conditions without which a human being could not realize the capacity to act as a moral subject. This is most evident in the basic right to integrity of body and life, which directly entails the prohibition of killing innocent human beings.

As the term "human" or "basic" right indicates, such rights arise from moral claims, which precede all others and which as such cannot be compared or traded with other entitlements. This also applies vis-à-vis the demands of medical ethics. Contemporary medical ethics acknowledges this in the principle: that no medical intervention can be regarded as legitimate without the explicit or at least implicit consent of the patient in question.

The precedence of moral claims that ground human or basic rights is easily recognized in cases of defensive rights against third parties; that is, in cases of negative rights, such as the general prohibition against killing. The argument becomes more complex when positive rights come into play. First, it only makes sense to grant such rights if real entitlements are available. Second, it is notoriously difficult to delineate which of these rights must be explicitly granted to everyone and which ones can be left to the free play of other forces.

As regards medical interventions and their limits, that problem appears as the question of whether everyone has a right to health care (Bole and Bondenson 1996). I cannot here discuss the extent or the arguments in favor of such a right in detail. Only this much must be said: If it can be argued that such a right is entailed by rights to integrity of body and life, to self-determination, and to the free development of one's personality, then it has the same rank as a human or basic right.

With respect to restricting medical practice, negative human or basic rights function to set certain limits, such as the one set by the prohibition of killing. Inasmuch as we can formulate and argue as binding positive human or basic rights, such as the right to health care, we are facing consequences that result from economic limits. Health care may then no longer be regarded as a service that is distributed according to market forces. There would have to be at least a basic level of care available to everyone. That, however, entails the difficult question of what constitutes a basic level of care.

The Goals of Medical Practice

Medical Ethics lists, in the form of professional codes, the moral criteria that have emerged from the goals of medical and paramedical practice, the *lex artis*, and the structure of the doctor–patient relationship. The triad of diagnosis, therapy, and prevention determines the goals of medical practice; the *lex artis* determines the choice of the right means. The structure of the doctor–patient relationship demands that any intervention is subject to the patient's informed consent and the specific circumstances of the case. What is morally required, therefore, is only what falls within those parameters of medical teleology; that is, what serves the goals of diagnosis, therapy, and prevention; follows best-practice guidelines; acknowledges the patient's specific circumstances; and has the patient's informed consent.

The concrete decision by which the physician determines the therapeutic goal—and thereby which interventions to carry out and which ones to omit—must therefore always be regarded as the result of a practical deliberation, in which the means are determined with respect to the required goal, according to best practice, with respect to the individual patient and his or her circumstances, and recognizing the patient's informed consent. Thus, such deliberation takes into account moral, functional (scientific as well as pragmatic-technical), and circumstantial criteria. The physician's decision, inasmuch as it is a determination of the therapeutic goals, is therefore about interventions on an individual patient and thus practical and subject to the principle of proportionality. To be distinguished from it is such *basic care* as is required even when therapy is no longer possible or sensible. (I will address the problems that ensue from this distinction below.)

Medical Social Contexts

Contemporary medical practice is dependent on a wide range of conditions. Among them are research, the production of pharmaceutics and other medical products, laboratories, surgeries and clinics of various kinds, a mixture of different professional roles and their respective training regimes, emergency and permanent care services, and rehabilitation facilities, as well as public and private insurance schemes. In short, it requires a complex social system, which differs from country to country. This means that medical practice must follow the rules that are constitutive of the local social system of health care, including its balance of demand and supply, as well as the criteria discussed above.

At its core, every social order is constituted by certain value judgments. This holds especially for those goods that, like health, are considered "basic." As a good that is both basic and contingent, however, health cannot be left to the prudent provision by the individual alone. That is the reason why it makes sense to speak of a basic right to health care. Conversely, assuming such a right exists does not in itself determine in which way and by what means it is to be granted. Even the demand for justice with respect to the distribution of limited resources does not determine which form of distributive justice is to be considered adequate.

Rather, a society's preferences with respect to basic goods and its sense of justice regarding their distribution are the result of a sociocultural development, which is linked to the respective socially relevant manifestation of an ethos. Accordingly, there will be different moral rules for the distribution of basic goods, particularly the good of health care, subject to the social system and its fundamental ethos. That is not to deny, however, that any system to be considered as morally sufficient must have regard for the claims inherent in the basic rights as well as for the overall goal of justice. Nor is it implied that those claims can be met only in one particular way.

The Limited Role of the Market

The structure of a health care system is made more complex by the larger or smaller role played by the market as an instrument of distribution within it. The market gains its moral dignity from the fact that it can manage the efficient allocation of scarce resources demanded by the principle of justice better than any other distributive mechanism. Efficient use of resources occurs only where agents in a market environment are interested in the best cost-benefit ratio. To be sure, the market delivers the desired allocation outcome only if it is left undistorted and if access to it remains open. Over and above that, however, the claims guaranteed under basic rights require that those who are unable to act as agents in the market are protected. For well-known reasons of social morality, a free market economy, therefore, needs certain restrictions; for example, Germany utilizes a social market economy.

The role of the market is particularly important with respect to the good of health care. For if health care were left entirely to market forces, there would be a danger that it could not meet the demands arising from basic social rights, as well as the twin goals of justice and solidarity. A health care system without any market elements, however, is in danger of missing the most efficient allocation of scarce resources, which results only in a functioning market.

Besides the moral criteria governing actions and omissions in medical practice, there are then also demands for the efficient use of scarce resources. We are thus faced with the following question: How far can the distribution of health care be left to the market, and which criteria need to be applied for it to function without distortions? Figure 1 summarizes the relationships among these considerations.

THE LIMITS OF MEDICAL INTERVENTIONS

If the dimensions of medical practice shown in Figure 1 are correct, then the criteria for restricting access to a health system characterized by scarcity of resources can only be the

FIGURE 1. *Ethics and the Distribution of Health Care*

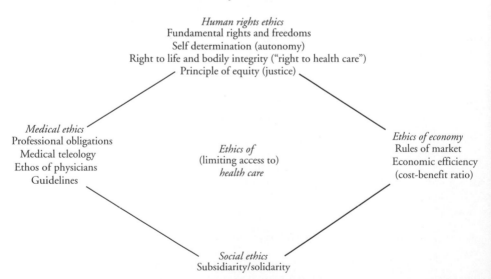

ones I listed for each of the dimensions above. But how are they related to one another? To be sure, basic human rights criteria and medical-moral criteria must be regarded as necessary, though not sufficient, conditions for morally responsible restrictions of access to the health care. That does not imply, however, that the four groups of criteria form a foundational system. Rather, they are to be seen as a matrix of mutually dependent norms.

This means, however, that the concrete moral norms applicable to the management of scarce resources in a health care system and especially in the area of intensive care medicine and its consequences cannot simply be deduced from the framework criteria but must be won in a process of practical deliberation. Thus we are dealing with judgments in a form that has long been central in moral philosophy: for example, *phronesis* in Aristotle, *modus determinationis* in Aquinas, *practical judgment* in Kant, and *reflective equilibrium* in Rawls.

What role, then, do religious beliefs and prescriptions play in restricting access to the health system? How do they relate to the above-mentioned norms? As far as the Catholic tradition of the Christian faith is concerned, the beliefs and norms developed in it do not constitute an additional fifth complex of norms. Inasmuch as there is a Catholic Church–developed doctrine regarding this area, it presents a certain approach with regard to each of the four dimensions; this approach is characterized by specific assumptions of the Christian faith, as well as experiences that have emerged from the life of the church.

Behind this understanding lies the view that revelation and the faith based on it do not contain any immediate norms for human action; instead, they form the horizon within which reason has to search for those norms. On the basis of Romans 1:20 (and following) and the philosophical ethics of antiquity, reason is seen as participating in God's law in such a way that reason *as reason* can grasp what is morally required: That grasp of the natural law (*lex naturalis*) is restricted to first principles, that is, metanorms, which are both nonarbitrary and open to active interpretation and thus require concrete elaboration through human law (*lex humana*) (Honnefelder 1989, 81–98). Here, practical deliberation in the sense of *prudentia* mentioned above means that the norms cannot simply be deduced from the principle but must be the result of a determination (*modus determinationis*), that is, of active interpretation. Thus, the contribution of the Christian faith to the formation of norms in the area with which we are concerned can be differentiated on the following four levels (Böckle 1977).

Human Moral Autonomy

First is the *deeper grounding* of human moral autonomy in a comprehensive theonomy. *Deeper* grounding means that the plausibility and binding force that human moral autonomy has by virtue of reason is seen to rest on that theonomy as on a *second* layer. For example, the belief in a creator God deepens the reasons to respect the dignity and moral autonomy that other people have as human beings. In Aquinas's language, this means that the human law (*lex humana*) proves to be the determination of the natural law (*lex naturalis*), which within the horizon of faith can itself be interpreted as participation in God's eternal law (*lex eterna*). Within the horizon of a belief in a God, Who is Creator of the world, the mutual acknowledgment of the moral autonomy that belongs to us as humans and of the dignity that results from it proves to be the will of God.

Individual Motivation

Second is the motivating, stimulating, critically selecting role that the Christian faith has with respect to the ethos and norm-building function of reason. For example, we can point to the influence of the Christian faith in achieving recognition that human beings as human beings have equal dignity and that certain demands of justice and solidarity must be met.

Paradigmatic Influence

Third is the paradigmatic influence that models of the Christian life have on the formation of the ethos and the norms of other groups in society or of society as a whole. As the ethos that commands discipleship of Jesus, the Christian ethos goes beyond the moral norms demanded of everyone and includes commands such as those from the Sermon on the Mount (the Beatitudes), which within the horizon of faith, hope, and love yield specifically Christian virtues and obligations. During the history of the church, these imperatives of discipleship have produced various models and visions of the imitation of Christ, which in turn have had a broader social influence. Thus, from very early on there have been models of church-based care for the sick, which have had and continue to have significant influence on the development of modern health care.

Providing Meaning

Fourth is the function of giving meaning to the experiences of suffering and death, as well as the limits of human care for the sick. This allows us to find sense in suffering, futility, and death, which goes beyond a merely human perspective. Such a horizon of meaning is important for patients themselves; it is the horizon within which they decide and accept the limits of their lives. It is also relevant to those who treat and care for patients, especially when that happens under conditions of futility. Such a horizon becomes action guiding through specific virtues and rules of behavior, such as guides to a Christian death (*ars moriendi*) or codifications of a Christian professional ethos for physicians and paramedics.

LIMITING ACCESS TO CRITICAL CARE

Using an example, I will now further explicate the criteria that are relevant in applying restrictions on access to health care. This example focuses on the limiting case of the therapy and care of patients whose state is often the result of intensive care medicine; that is, those patients who have survived injuries to the skull and brain, yet have not regained consciousness and (using current medical indicators) are not expected to. The ethical problems of restricting therapy appear even more pronounced with respect to this group of patients than in the general area of intensive care medicine.[1] There, the basis for making medical decisions is even more problematic than here. For because the state of those patients is as yet unfamiliar to medical practice—because research only delivers limited answers, and even an appropriate definition of that state is subject to debate—diagnosis and prognosis carry the burden of high uncertainty. In addition, the estimation of how much quality of life remains for such patients, which is an integral part of determining therapeutic goals, is nowhere more the subject of debate than for patients in a persistent vegetative state. This is accentuated by the fact that most of those patients have not left their doctor or their relatives with a living will, which means that decisions more often than not have to be made and justified by doctors or relatives. Further, relative to the determination of therapeutic goals, we are faced with stark questions about therapeutic measures: which ones may or must be stopped, when may or must they be stopped, and which ones must always continue to be employed?

Thus, the example of patients in a persistent vegetative state should serve exceptionally well to clarify the moral criteria for settling conflicts over decisions about restricting medical care. This applies to three questions in particular. (1) What does it mean that humans have an inviolable dignity and, therefore, enjoy the right to integrity of their bodies and lives? (2) What does it mean that we have both a right to life and a right to a natural death, and what role does quality of life play as a criterion in this context? (3) How much does the professional teleology that guides physicians' decisions determine the limits of what has to be done?

Human Dignity

The concept of human rights expresses the view that every human has an inviolable dignity and enjoys the protective rights that follow from it, independent of any characteristics or achievements (i.e., independent of one's health or state of consciousness).

It is the living being which has that capacity; its identity through time is both that of a living individual and that of a subject, of nature and person. But if the I and the body are an inseparable unity, then it is enough to be a living being of that species to determine what is a human being. Thus, if the basis of human dignity is the subject and if creature and subject are an integral unity, then the criterion for ascribing that dignity can be nothing other than being human. The notion of human rights, therefore, not only expresses the inviolability of that dignity but prohibits making the ascription of that dignity depend on anything other than being human.

Further, if the I and the body are an inseparable unity such that life is the condition for the possibility of being a subject, then the right to have one's dignity respected directly entails the right to have the integrity of one's body and life protected. The right to life of a human being is something that is acknowledged, not something that is ascribed. Thus it must be regarded as a right that precedes all legislation. Consequently, the prohibition of killing another human being is of a general kind.

In view of these deliberations, the patient in a persistent vegetative state must at the core be considered as a living human being who is deprived of some functions. This yields a first claim: The patient in a persistent vegetative state is a human being like any other, and therefore has the same dignity and right to life.

This claim is sometimes disputed on the basis of a distinction between being human and being a person, combined with the ascription of human dignity only to persons. However, that distinction contradicts the identity of human beings through time, which we ascribe to one another in all theoretical and practical contexts. Further, the moral implications of such a distinction run counter to the consensus, which is contained in the notion of human rights, that the ascription of human dignity must not depend on anything other than being human. At least those who dispute that point have the onus of proof (Honnefelder 1996). In practical terms, this means that patients in a persistent vegetative state have the same rights to therapy and care necessitated by their illnesses as any other patients. What is more, if the notion of human rights is regarded as the basis not only of fairness between the equally strong but also of solidarity with the weak, then the demands of the extremely needy gain special weight.

Human Nature

The demands and limits identified thus far must be further specified by a detailed explication of human nature. For although I am identical with my physical and physiological nature, I also experience myself as one who transcends that nature; as a person who speaks and acts and suffers, I find fulfillment in a life of communicating with others. Because the human being *is* a corporeal individual that *has* a body, that body can become the object of diagnosis and therapeutic intervention; at the same time, any intervention must take into account the individual as a whole. If the individual and the body form a unity of "mediated immediacy" (Plessner 1981, 396–419), then it is clear why mere life or survival is a necessary condition of the possibility of a fulfilled life but not yet identical to it.

Humans have always struggled with the question of how the good of life (survival) is related to those goods that make a fulfilled life. An initial though unsatisfactory answer interprets that relationship as functional. Life (survival) has value only inasmuch as it is an instrument for achieving the life of a person. Such an interpretation is based on a dualistic anthropology in which life (survival) remains external and merely functional with respect to a fulfilled life. However, any interpretation of personal identity as a continuity of consciousness without the dimension of life faces problems with respect to its consistency, forcing John Locke to resort to a theological argument for the prohibition of killing; it also contradicts our practical experience of identity through time. Another, similarly unsatisfactory answer assumes that life is so integral to the person that it must have absolute value. Yet that interpretation, too, cannot accommodate our practical moral experience. If life were an absolute value, it would have to be extended at any cost, even the cost of great pain and suffering. Any omission would amount to killing. Risking one's life for others or martyrdom would be a violation of life. Even one's own free decision against life-prolonging measures would be illegitimate.

If we accept the legitimacy of such actions, then it appears that only a third approach is consistent. Moral philosophers have long distinguished between basic and higher-order goods (Schockenhoff 1993, 365–69); within that structure, life is an inherent human good, which, as the condition of all human activity, has fundamental value, yet does not represent the highest of all goods. Because it is a fundamental good, it yields the right to integrity of body and life, though that does not exclude the right to a natural death. Because nobody may hold someone else's life at his or her disposal, any intervention by a physician must seek the consent of the patient. This implies the patient's right to set limits for that intervention.

The position sketched above does not, however, entail that the fundamental good of life is at anyone's disposal where the link to higher goods, such as independence, communication, or a fulfilled life, can no longer be made out. Why not? If life is the human task that grounds the dignity of a person's moral existence, then human freedom, which must be protected, includes the freedom to decide what counts as a fulfilled life. The protection of human dignity, therefore, demands the inviolability of one's freedom of conscience. This does not establish one particular way of life as the only one compatible with human dignity; but a line is drawn that guarantees the conditions for such a life, opens up the space in which humans can make their own decisions about a fulfilled life, and provides protection from unwanted outside intervention.

Any judgment by a third person, which "from the outside" regards certain states of life as no longer worth living, would be a judgment about the quality of life and its relation to a fulfilled life, which only the patient himself can make. This is true especially of any calculus that, from a lack of certain aspects of the quality of life, draws an inference to a restriction on the right to life. Conversely, patients must have the space to exercise their freedom to reject a particular intervention as diminishing their quality of life, because the intervention is experienced not as meaningful but as painful and senseless.

If a judgment about the quality of life can be made only from the perspective of the person who leads that life, then that person's will must be decisive. As regards persons in a persistent vegetative state, who are unable to express their will, the legitimacy of any intervention from outside must depend on their will, either previously expressed or presumed, and must be based on the beliefs and preferences that can be gleaned from their biographies.

This yields a second claim: Life is a human good, which—as the necessary condition for the possibility of higher-ranking goods—has a fundamental value. What quality a particular state of life has with respect to those higher-order goods can only be decided by the individual. This includes the right to reject an intervention judged to be meaningless and prolonging a state experienced as painful and distressing. Any decision not based on the (presumed) will of the patient, but rather on external criteria, would be a violation of the right to self-determination.

The Teleology of Medical Practice

How can we accommodate patients' rights to appropriate treatment if, on the one hand, an "objective," "external" judgment about the quality of their lives is problematic but, on the other hand, the physician has to make decisions and justify both actions and omissions? The only answer that preserves the limits that have been drawn appears to be one that grounds the decisions on the teleology of medical practice. To be sure, even the physician has to make a judgment about the actual or expected quality of his or her patient's life; otherwise, it would not be possible to determine any therapeutic measures. However, those judgments are limited by the structure of medical practice and, unlike external ones, appear to be morally justified.

Medical practice is related to the individual patient and determined by the twin goals of cure and relief. It must be the result of a diagnosis and prognosis that are essentially related to the individual case. Interventions must be in accordance with or at least not contrary to the patient's will and, in a kind of shared action, supported by the patient's relatives or attorney. Even judgments about the actual or expected quality of life, which are implied in the prognosis as well as the subsequent therapeutic actions, are limited to the individual case and its context.

The difference between an "objective" judgment and one made within an individual patient–physician relationship is akin to that between the subsumption under rules or under practical deliberation. Whereas in the first case the concrete treatment of a patient appears only as an instance of following an overarching obligatory rule, in the case of practical deliberation it is the individual case itself from which the inquiry into the appropriate rules and the development of criteria for action begins. Those criteria will be no less strict, but they do not constitute a simple calculus, unlike those used in the application of a rule.

The second aspect of medical practice relevant here are the twin goals of cure and relief. According to the traditional notion of a physician's work, curing comprises the preservation and restoration of the conditions of a fulfilled or at least tolerable life. As a goal of therapeutic action, it is neither identical with a fulfilled life nor conceivable without reference to it. Thus the determination of the therapeutic goal hinges on the question of whether and how it can help patients attain a position in which they can pursue the aims and purposes of human life. If in the eyes of the physician the therapy can no longer achieve such a position, it has reached its limits, and all medical action must be restricted to appropriate comfort care and pain relief.

If the process of dying has commenced, a restriction of life-prolonging measures can be justified. At any rate, the second goal, that of relief, excludes any life-prolonging therapy that involves unreasonable pain for patients; conversely, pain relief appears to be legitimate, even if it has life-shortening side effects.

However, the treatment of a patient in a persistent vegetative state is usually not the treatment of a dying patient. It happens under an uncertain prognosis and without the possibility to refer directly to the patient's will. Thus the physician will have to act according to a careful diagnosis and a presumed prognosis; he or she will have to evaluate the patient's circumstances as well as balance the "intensity and gravity of the interventions and strain to which the patient is subjected" with the "expected therapeutic success and the life expectancy of the patient" (Schweizerische Akademie der Medizinischen Wissenschaften 1995). Here the entire responsibility rests with the physician. Acting under someone else's instructions would be contrary to the medical ethos. At the same time, the remaining uncertainty of the prognosis demands appropriate consideration of the patient's presumed will. This includes any expression of the will to live, previous instructions of the patient, and his or her moral and religious beliefs, including the value preferences entailed by them. If the restoration of a state in which the patient can return to a "life of interhuman communication" is possible, his or her consent to the necessary measures must as a rule be presumed. If the patient cannot consent, the treatment must be supported by the patient's relatives.

This implies a *third claim*: The treatment of a patient in a persistent vegetative state results from the teleology of medical practice and the circumstances of the individual patient. The necessary judgment about the patient's expected future life, which is the result of careful diagnosis and prognosis and determines the therapy, must be based on the individual circumstances and the (presumed) will of the patient. The therapeutic measures, for which the physician must take sole responsibility, should be supported by the patient's relatives. It seems almost obvious that one also should consult with a third, independent party.

The three claims together entail the following consequences: As long as there is no clear indication that the patient's state is irreversible, the physician must employ all diagnostic, therapeutic, and rehabilitative measures that are suitable for the restoration of the patient's health. As long as the prognosis is uncertain, the principle *in dubio pro vita* applies. The deliberate omission of what is obligated by the goal of medical practice would be a case of killing.

Rationing Scarce Resources

What about the problem of restricting the therapy or treatment of patients in a persistent vegetative state because the health care system as a whole has limited resources? On the basis of the moral criteria developed above, there can be no restriction of the treatment because of a preferential order determined by the allocation of resources. Where basic rights are at stake, restrictions can only be justified as triage; that is, as not doing what is due in the face of competing, yet simultaneously unachievable, claims and rights, which must be accepted as the lesser evil. This applies to patients in a persistent vegetative state at least as far as their basic care is concerned. Whether restrictions of therapy contrary to the therapeutic goal can be justified depends on whether one accepts a basic right to health care or not. If one does not accept such a right, the problem becomes a test case for the moral standards that characterize the health care system in question.

PERSISTENT VEGETATIVE STATE: LICIT LIMITS

We can now return to our initial question. How does the proposition outlined in the first part of this essay hold up in our sample case; and how do we assess the result with respect to the Catholic tradition and the relevant church teaching outlined in the second part above?

Moral Justifications for Restricting Care

The difficult area of the treatment of patients in a persistent vegetative state has highlighted the need to employ a combination of mutually dependent and supporting criteria in deciding actions or omissions in contemporary medical practice. Among the criteria are those based on human rights, which highlight that even the patient in a persistent vegetative state can claim basic rights that must be observed. However, only the criteria of medical teleology allow the determination of a therapeutic goal compatible with those basic rights. This observation demands that any restrictions that may result from the determination of the therapeutic goal must apply only to the therapy itself and not to the basic care of the patient.

This shows that the moral justification for restrictions depends on certain distinctions. One of these is the distinction between decisions that are covered by the declared or deemed will of the patient and those for which reference to such a will is impossible. Then there is also the distinction between a lack of intervention (even if that has life-shortening consequences) and actively life-ending measures, where the declared or deemed will of the patient can only relate to the former. Also important is the further distinction between therapy and basic care; as regards the latter, we must distinguish natural feeding from feeding by way of medical intervention, the latter requiring at least the deemed consent of the patient. In such situations, we are facing the problem of delineating what we regard as artificial.

There are analogies to the Catholic tradition's distinction between ordinary and extraordinary measures, as well as to its development under the title of proportionality.[2] I will discuss this shortly.

If my sketch of the moral criteria is correct, then the answer regarding restrictions of treatment based on the scarcity of resources must be a differentiated one. Where basic rights are at stake, restrictions can be justified only as the result of triage—that is, a decision about the lesser evil as well as about the distinction between therapy and basic care. Furthermore, triage decisions are always a criticism of the supply and demand structure of the health care system in question.

The Role of Church Doctrine

In seeking to relate the above-mentioned moral criteria to the Catholic tradition and the church teachings associated with it, we discover briefly the following aspects. As regards the criteria that are based on human or basic rights, such as the inviolability of human dignity and the entailed right to life, we can undoubtedly speak of a deeper grounding through the church doctrine discussed above (Hilpert 1998, 670–79).

As regards the extension of the notion of basic rights to health care, we can assume a motivating, stimulating, critically selecting role for church doctrine. Such an extension can be seen as covered by the social teachings of the church and its comprehensive concept of solidarity, even if the argument for a basic right to health care does not depend exclusively on assumptions based on faith.

With respect to the distinction between ordinary and extraordinary measures in the area of medical and paramedical practice and the wider notion of proportionality, church doctrine has a paradigmatic role. This brings into focus the concept of appropriateness with respect to means and achievable goals, which is part of the determination of the therapeutic goal made by the physician, as well as the distinction between due care and broader therapy, the latter of which depends on whether the therapeutic goal is achievable. Paradigmatic is also Pope Pius XII's 1954 evaluation of restrictions based on the availability of resources. Assuming a scarcity of resources, he regards a lack of intervention for the sake of equal- or higher-ranking goods (i.e., a choice of unavoidable evil) as justified. As concerns a right to a natural death, too, that doctrine can be regarded as having a paradigmatic role. For such a right ensues where the irreversible progress of a disease means that patients, having met their obligations to others as well as to themselves, are no longer morally obliged to make use of all life-prolonging measures. What that older doctrine did not take into account in the same way as we would today is the reference to a patient's declared or deemed will. In that respect, it displays the vestiges of a paternalism characteristic of the medical ethics of the day. What justifies the doctrine's paradigmatic role is the position traditionally assigned to the criterion of appropriateness or benefit and the evaluation associated with it; that position is based on the doctrine's reception of Aristotelian ethics.

We can generally speak of the doctrine's role in giving meaning to our dealing with sickness, suffering, and death in the face of finality and contingence. More important, it appears to play that role specifically where our human limitations force us to make decisions about what is appropriate and beneficial.

NOTES

1. Cf. PVS '9: An International Conference on the Implications, Progress, and Opportunities in the Management of Persistent Vegetative and Low Awareness States; March 6, 1995, organized on behalf of the EC BIOMED I Programme by the Centre of Medical Law and Ethics, King's College, London; and March 7, 1995, organized by the Royal Hospital of Neuro-disability, Putney, London.
2. See, e.g., the essay by Taboada in this volume.

BIBLIOGRAPHY

Böckle, F. 1977. *Fundamentalmoral.* München: Kösel.

Bole, T. J., and W. B. Bondeson. 1996. *Rights to Health Care.* Dordrecht: Kluwer Academic Publishers.

Hilpert, K. 1998. Menschenrechte. In *Lexikon der Bioethik*, vol. 2. Gütersloh: Gütersloher Verlagshaus.

Honnefelder, L. 1989. Güterabwägung und Folgenabschätzung. Zur Bestimmung des sittlich Guten bei Thomas von Aquin. In *Staat, Kirche, Wissenschaft in einer pluralistischen Gesellschaft*, ed. by Dieter Schwab and Paul Mikat. Berlin: Duncker and Humblot.

———. 1996. The concept of a person in moral philosophy. In *Sanctity of Life and Human Dignity*, ed. by Kurt Bayertz. Dordrecht: Kluwer Academic Publishers.

Plessner, H. 1981. *Die Stufen des Organischen und der Mensch. Gesammelte Schriften IV.* Frankfurt: Suhrkamp.

Schockenhoff, E. 1993. *Ethik des Lebens: Ein theologischer Grundriß.* Mainz: Matthias-Grunewald-Verlag.

Schweizerische Akademie der Medizinischen Wissenschaften. 1995. Medizinisch-ethische Richtlinien für die ärztliche Betreuung sterbender und zerebral schwerst geschädigter Personen. In *Schweizerische Ärztezeitung*, Band 76, Heft 29/30.

PART V

Moral and Public Policy Challenges

Beyond the Question of Limits: Institutional Guidelines for the Appropriate Use of Critical Care

George Khushf

Concerns about cost and the use of health care for individuals that have a very poor quality of life have led to increased reflection on the need to limit treatment. However, such reflection usually involves implicit assumptions about the nature of medicine that need to be questioned. It is assumed that medicine is grounded in value-neutral science, and that any intrusion of socioeconomic values into medical decision making involves violation of its integrity and of the ethical norms of the medical profession. When institutions and other health care providers come to exercise authority over matters that are thought to be physicians' prerogative, the language of externally imposed limits on medicine is used. I challenge these assumptions and call for a more radical reflection on the relations among medical science, economics, and ethics. I argue that we should move beyond the question of limits, and directly consider how the values and available resources of health care institutions direct the way the norms of medicine are constructed. I thus seek to shift the focus of discussion from the microethical issues of the physician-patient relation and the macroethical issues of broad social and political policy, in order to bring into view the interethics of health care institutions.

WHY ARE PEOPLE TALKING ABOUT LIMITS?

From the 1950s through most of the 1970s, it was assumed that one should not ask about limits on health care (Rodwin 1993; Morreim 1995). In the United States, most people obtained treatment in a fee-for-service, indemnity-based system that insulated them and their physicians from costs. Insurance reimbursed on a "cost-plus" basis, and then passed on costs in the form of increased premiums (Goodman and Musgrave 1992). Additionally, physicians worked with an understanding of professional ethics, and of the fiduciary relation in particular, which called for doing whatever was in the patient's interest, no matter how marginal the benefit. As a result of the economic structure and the conceptualization of ethical norms, costs rose exponentially.

Generally, if something could be done, it was thought that it should be done (Amundsen 1978). A technological imperative motivated increasingly aggressive medical intervention. Further, it was thought that any limits on treatment, especially if they were based on cost, involved placing a value on human life. Quality of life was not even considered, and many even thought that the withdrawal of treatment amounted to euthanasia.

The economic structure and ethical norms worked in tandem with a particular conceptualization of modern medicine (Khushf 1997b, 1998a, 1999). It was assumed that medical practice was grounded in the basic sciences. Medicine was understood as a value-free, scientific endeavor, where decisions about treatment were independent of any outside, distorting influences. Ethical codes were developed to insulate physicians from economic and societal considerations that could distort clinical judgment. It was assumed that physicians, thus insulated and directed by their professional ethical norms, would only provide interventions that were called for by science. Reimbursement should then follow, covering whatever costs were incurred.

This traditional approach to the science, ethics, and economics of medicine led to major problems in cost control, access, and quality of health care. Because physicians did not recognize the role that economic incentives unavoidably play, they did not sufficiently respond to the rapid increase in utilization and cost of services that attended the incentives in fee-for-service, indemnity-based health care. Double-digit inflation in the health care sector continued until it consumed about 14 percent of the U.S. yearly gross domestic product. This, by itself, would not have been bad, if people valued the services. However, many felt that the cost escalation was due to inefficiency in the system, and they questioned the types of services offered. As costs rose, so did premiums for health insurance, making it more difficult for employers and individuals to purchase coverage. Cost escalation thus led to reduced access, with the demand curve for insurance providing a measure of the proportionality between increased cost and reduced access.

Further, in addition to the high cost of care, it was felt that some types of care were inappropriate, driven by a skewed understanding of the role of medical science and technology. This is especially the case at the end of life or when there is very poor quality of life: for example, when patients in a persistent vegetative state are put on life support in critical care units, when expensive care is used on persons who are almost certain to die in a few days in the intensive care unit (ICU), or when anencephalic children are aggressively treated in neonatal intensive care units. In each case, it seems as if something has gone wrong; that the services are being used in an inappropriate way.

These concerns led many people to challenge the economic structures and ethical norms that had led to the overuse of health care. An extensive literature mounted on the need for health care reform, especially on the rationing of services that were only marginally beneficial. A separate literature also developed on "futility," attempting to identify care that is not "medically indicated," and thus care that cannot be demanded by patients. In both cases, the central focus is on limits, constraining what a patient could demand of the insurer or physician.

Driven by cases of inappropriate care and framed by problems of rising health care costs, it seems natural to raise questions about the utilization of health care in terms of limits. However, when the problem is raised in this way, one takes for granted the traditional conceptualization of medicine; namely, medicine is viewed as a scientifically based, value-neutral practice, determinable independent of economic and ethical structures or norms. Ethics is thought to come in as a second step, considering the use and abuse of independently formulated, scientific medicine. Similarly, economic factors are thought to influence the over- or underuse of medical services, but they are thought to be independent and separable, playing no role in the implicit norms of that practice. They do not play a role in the determination of the meaning of "appropriate" utilization, which presumably is a function of science, not economics.[1]

It is time to move beyond the question of limits and consider the way economic and ethical considerations work together with scientific considerations in the construction of medical reality. It is not simply a question of limits, but of how medicine should be conceptualized and its practice directed. As outcome information is used to develop practice protocols, and as quality-of-life considerations as well as assessments of well-being are integrated into ICU guidelines, one must ask what roles ethical and economic factors should play in clinical practice. It is no longer a question of whether values play a role, but which values and what role.

MACRO-, MICRO-, AND INTERETHICS

The question of limits has been asked in different ways, depending on whether one asks from the perspective of an individual, a governmental or policymaking body, or an institution. In each case, different considerations are emphasized.

Microethics

There are two ways to consider the questions of limits from an individual perspective, depending on whether one asks from the perspective of the physician or patient. For the patient, individual values may lead to the rejection of health care that physicians consider appropriate. Refusal directives are rooted in a broadly recognized right of patients (or their surrogates) to determine what will be done with their own bodies; they are tied to the logic of informed consent, and the concrete limits that result cannot be easily generalized, because the values involved are not necessarily generalizable. The question of limits is thus framed in terms of a process that assures that patient values are given due weight in treatment decisions.[2] Patients can also make requests (and sometimes refusal involves an implicit request), which involve a demand on those who provide the health care services. If that request is regarded as inappropriate by the physician, it may be declined (limits may be drawn). If the limit on request depends on values inherent in medical practice (the "integrity of the profession," what is "not medically indicated," etc.) then one can generalize from those limits.[3] If the limit depends on a physician's individual values (religious or secular), and the refusal becomes an issue of conscience, then the case is more complex; it may or may not be appropriate for the physician to decline offering the care, depending on the values involved and the way one understands the physician's obligation to provide care.

There is a broad consensus that patients have the right to decline unwanted medical treatment. The debate surrounding this issue took place at an earlier stage and is now largely resolved. However, much of current reflection on limits focuses on the ability of the physician to decline a requested treatment, when that treatment is deemed "futile." The argument is made that certain types of interventions violate the goals or instrumentalities of medicine, and thus can be unilaterally rejected by the physician. The attempt is thus made to set such issues outside the realm of societal or individual choice and make them a function of the scientific, professional judgment of the physician. In the name of the "integrity of medicine," the physician is to be able to prescribe limits on patient demand.

Nevertheless, behind this debate, there are broader disputes, which require that deliberations move beyond the microethical domain. There are many different types of futility, including a narrowly physiological futility (i.e., the means in question cannot realize its end, as understood within the domain of medicine's scientific instrumentalities), probabilistic futility (i.e., the chance of realizing the end is too small for the intervention to be worthwhile), quantitative futility (i.e., the prolonging of life obtained is too small), and qualitative futility (i.e., the quality of life obtained is insufficient). Physiological futility is so narrow, it encompasses virtually none of the cases at issue and cannot provide a basis for a realistic discussion of limits (Brody and Halevy 1995; Halevy, Neal, and Brody 1996). All other discussions of futility involve values associated with reasonable risk, quality of life, quantity of life, or cost-benefit analysis, and such values vary, depending on the cultural and religious commitments in question. They cannot be seen as simply a question of some value-neutral medical science, separable from broader reflection on social and economic context.

This does not imply, however, that medicine is indeed value neutral, and the futility debate depends on nonmedical values. Schneiderman and Jecker (1995), along with other advocates of the use of futility assessment, are correct to note that medicine does indeed involve implicit commitments regarding values associated with risk, costs and benefits, and the appropriate ends of medicine. But they incorrectly assume that because in the past medical professionals have unilaterally determined those values inherent in medicine, this means they should be allowed to do that in the current debate. The previous authority was tied to an older medical paternalism, and to the hidden character of value judgments. In the futility debate, these implicit commitments are made explicit and require more open deliberation about the way social values can and should play a role in the construction of medical reality.

In sum, although the issues may initially be framed in microethical terms, questions of futility cannot be fully resolved in those terms. In addition to moving beyond the microethical domain, one must also move beyond the question of limits, and consider the values that play a role in the construction of medical reality.

When it is recognized that the futility debate cannot be resolved with a neat line between treatments that are effective and not effective, it becomes clear that there is *continuity* between discussions about futility and broader discussions about the use of quality-of-life assessments and outcome studies in health care generally (Knaus, Wagner, and Lynn 1991, 392). Medicine regularly makes assessments of trade-offs involved in various treatment decisions. This may be in the form of a direct trade-off between morbidity and mortality, as in the case of treatment immediately after a stroke, where the chances of permanent loss of function can be greatly reduced by treatment that involves a small, but clearly identifiable increase in the risk of mortality. One thus has a clear value decision about the appropriateness of increasing risk of death in order to avoid diminished quality of life. There are also a host of more subtle tradeoffs between alternative assessments of quality of life: for example, how one weighs different kinds of risks and losses of function against one another.

Such questions about cost-benefit analysis and values do not just come in as a second step, where ethics can provide procedures for navigating the value differences, and medicine can step back, having done its foundational, scientific work. These value issues go to the heart of medicine. As Murphy (1997) notes, they are even involved in something as basic as drawing the line between the normal and the pathological. Often, such a line is seen as a simple question of minimizing the error rate for false positives and false negatives. However, Murphy shows how a bias of ascertainment that is a reflection of social configurations of the way people seek care plays a direct role in the relative population sizes of healthy and diseased (1997, 292), a factor that will determine where the two distributions intersect, and thus where one draws the line. Further, Murphy even challenges the assumption that false positives and false negatives should have equal weight, since in some cases (e.g., tuberculosis), there may be a greater potential harm from a false negative (1997, 293). He thus suggests a weighting of relative harm in the determinations of the line between the normal and pathological (1997, 294). Financial cost is simply one additional factor included with other values in the cost-benefit assessments that are at the heart of medicine.

Because futility assessments are not of a different kind from other judgments of appropriate care in medicine, they should not be singled out as if they provided the key to limiting treatments. Problems surrounding futility are simply a subset of the broader problem of determining what is "medically necessary," and that question is not best addressed by just asking about limits (Khushf 1998a). To ask in that way assumes that "what is not medically indicated" has a certain epistemological priority, so that one can get at the medically necessary by excluding that which is its opposite. Many wish to address futility in this way, because it enables them to avoid the impression that they are importing value judgments into medicine or rationing care. They claim that what they are excluding as not medically indicated is something of a completely different kind, something that can be recognized as inappropriate simply by looking at it. Instead, one should consider in a more nuanced way the complex interaction among scientific, ethical, and economic factors that makes for an appropriate medical intervention, and recognize that sometimes there will not be an in-kind distinction between what is included as medically indicated and what is excluded as futile (i.e., not sufficiently useful).

In the case of critical care, the need for such a nuanced account of the determination of medically necessary treatment is outlined by Knaus, Wagner, and Lynn (1991). Although their essay still sets up the issues as if they are simply about the "empiric basis for difficult but increasingly common decisions to forgo treatment" (i.e., they frame the discussion as if it is primarily about limits), they also note that their analysis could equally be used "as the basis of more informed decisions by clinicians and patients about the desirability of alternative plans of care" (1991, 389). They also acknowledge the continuity between futility determinations and other kinds of clinical reasoning (392) and continually emphasize the need for collaborative decision making between physicians and patients about end-of-life care. Unfortunately, the essay stops short of bringing into view some of the extremely difficult questions that their analysis raises. By citing an essay by Schneiderman, Jecker, and Jonsen (1990), they give the impression that the kinds of professional judgments found in futility assessment and other clinical decisions are something separate from the kinds of judgments about forgoing treatment that are made jointly by physician and patient (392). However, everything they argue in their essay leads to the opposite conclusion; namely, that these "professional judgments" are continuous with the kinds of "collaborative judgments" found near the end of life, because all involve values associated with the setting of a threshold, weighing of quality-of-life factors, the use of subjective and objective probability assessments, and so on.

It is likely that Knaus, Wagner, and Lynn stop short of explicitly acknowledging and developing this continuity thesis because it has disturbing implications for traditional assumptions in both medicine and bioethics. It is generally assumed that where values are present, physicians should no longer be unilateral and paternalistic in their decision making, but rather should involve patients in the process. If medicine involves such values at its core, however, the standard bioethical recommendation immediately becomes unrealistic. Patients cannot be involved in the subtle and intricate biomedical assessments of trade-offs involved in all clinical judgments. How then does one draw the line between those situations when patients are to be involved as co-decision makers, and those when unilateral professional decision making is appropriate?

Veatch (1995) has addressed this issue in his discussion of informed consent, arguing that patients, especially when ill, are not able to participate in the full range of reflection on values needed for making important clinical decisions. He suggests that the value judgments, which go to the heart of the construction of medical reality, should rest with institutions that espouse values that patients share. Patients can then exercise autonomy in the medical decision-making process by opting into institutions whose values are similar to those that the patient espouses. Veatch thus shifts from the microethical domain to that of middle-level institutions, and finds in institutional ethics the capacity to resolve issues that were irresolvable in more traditional categories of medicine and medical ethics. It is also not coincidental that a multi-institutional working group on futility ended up turning to *institutional* procedures—rather than to a particular account of medical professional ends or immanent medical norms—when it arrived at its consensus statement (Halevy and Brody 1996).

Macroethics

Where there is a presumed social obligation to provide health services (whether understood in terms of justice or charity), some limit must be placed on the services that will be guaranteed. Resources available will necessarily play a role in determining the limits; some marginally beneficial services will not be provided. This may be done implicitly, as in the United Kingdom (through the use of global budgeting) or in managed care (through financial incentives to decrease utilization). Or it may be done explicitly, as in the case of the prioritization scheme developed as a part of the Oregon Plan. Macroethically, one can also consider the limits that can be placed on limits: for example, the nature and appropriateness of contractual agreements between an insurer and policyholder, or regulations that constrain possible agreements; for example, the recent U.S. policy that does not allow insurance to require that a woman leave the hospital within twenty-four hours after childbirth.[4]

At the macroethical level, it is important to ask how health care services should be prioritized relative to other social goods such as education, and to consider the obligation it is reasonable to impose on a population for the funding of those services. One can consider the procedures needed for determining limits, as well as the range of substantive limits that are appropriate. However, it is also important to recognize that there are limits to rationalizing any health care system. If we focus on health outcomes rather than inputs, and consider the full range of factors that influence such outcomes (including education, environment, employment, religious affiliation, etc.), then it becomes very difficult to even approximate cost-benefit assessments needed to weigh alternative configurations. Further, some things are much easier to quantify than others, and one must also make decisions about the importance given to the more intangible considerations. In the end, much will depend on aesthetic and ethical intuitions on the relative merits of alternative weightings of diverse factors that contribute to communal well-being.

Intrinsic limits on the rationalization process, and the need to consider alternative configurations as a whole, raise important questions about the way in which quality improvement or quality decrement can be measured. Consider, for example, a Montefiore Hospital policy to have respiratory therapists intubate patients in respiratory arrest or receiving cardiopulmonary resuscitation, rather than require that this be done by a physician. Rie (1997) suggests that it is inappropriate to implement such a policy without assessing the loss in quality that results, and he uses this case as an instance of the type of "quality decrement" that is introduced by current transformations in health care; in this case, by the trends toward de-skilling. Although his recommendations have much merit—especially his emphasis on the need to incorporate outcome assessments into clinical practice (something that has been too often lacking in medicine)—there are also problems.

Rie's analysis implies that one can single out particular policies such as that of intubation by respiratory therapists and assess the cost-benefit of such a policy (i.e., its "quality decrement") independent of a broader account of institutional policy and the relative merits of medical care relative to other types of health care. This assumption is only valid in certain contexts of analysis. Consider, for example, the broad movement toward de-skilling, which encompasses not just the particular policy Rie discusses, but also the use of general practitioners as gatekeepers, an increased role for nurse practitioners, and a shift of responsibilities from registered nurses to nurse technicians. All of these developments are part of the transformations that accompany the vertical and horizontal integration of health services, and they tend to be correlated with the development of institutional quality-review mechanisms that incorporate some of the outcome assessments that Rie seeks to advance. Further, along with some of these shifts, there is an increased emphasis upon educational and wellness efforts that seek to keep people out of institutions and minimize the need for more aggressive medical services. Often, one cannot assess these changes by focusing on an isolated policy, because one change may be intertwined with a host of others. A constellation resulting from all the combined changes may, for the health of a given population, be preferable, even though any one change may be considered deficient when compared with its alternative.[5]

Although it is important to consider issues of resource use at a global level, the macroethical issues cannot be fully separated from the microethical concerns associated with the physician-patient relation. Many seek to distinguish macro- and microethical domains in order to insulate a patient's physician from the need to make triage decisions with respect to that particular patient. Thus, for example, Boyle argues (in his essay in this volume):

> Physicians seem duty bound by virtue of their professional obligations toward their patients to act only in their interests, and certainly not to refuse to offer treatments because of the impact on other people. At the very least, therefore, it seems to me that physicians should not, as the helpers of the patients they serve, function as gatekeepers to medical treatment or as triage officers. If those functions must be fulfilled, then others, or physicians at arms' length, or with significant procedural caution and oversight, should carry them out. (93)

The fiduciary relation as understood within professional codes of ethics involves the obligation of the physician to act as the agent of the patient. If a physician balanced the interest of a particular patient against the interests of the patient population, or if a patient's interest came into tension with a physician's own economic incentives (as it may in managed care incentive structures), then a conflict of interest is introduced. Boyle and others assume that the economic structures of medicine must be configured so that such conflicts are avoided.

Morreim has provided some reasons for thinking that a neat line between rationing and clinical decision making cannot be fully sustained. She distinguishes between commodity scarcity, where one can sustain a distinction between macro- and microethical domains, and fiscal scarcity, where such a distinction cannot be sustained. The limited number of organs for transplantation is used as an example of commodity scarcity. In this case, one can separate the decision about who gets the organ from the multiple decisions about individual patient management. The former decision can be vested in others than the particular patient's physician. However,

> Fiscal scarcity is profoundly different from this. Because every medical decision has its economic cost, literally every medical decision is now subject to scrutiny for its economic as well as its medical wisdom. Suddenly, not this or that special item, but all of medicine is an allocation issue. Every lab test. Every x-ray. (1995, 49)

The only way to avoid this is to come up with practice guidelines or clinical protocols that would be used in a cookbook manner. However, this would take away decision-making authority from physicians, and medicine cannot be practiced that way. "In fiscal scarcity virtually all allocation decisions are ultimately micro" (Morreim 1995, 50). The problem is that there is not a neat line indicating when an x-ray should be ordered or a lab test performed. In many patients there will be a gray area, where one could go either way. Any economic system will provide economic incentives that unavoidably play a role in configuring those gray areas and determining how medicine manages uncertainty.

Summarizing, cost-control considerations do not simply lead to the limitation of treatment. Different economic structures lead to different configurations of medicine. When one does not have a test that could be of marginal benefit, one must manage the uncertainty differently. When there are long waiting periods for certain services (as there are in, e.g., Canada and the United Kingdom), one must manage patients in different ways. Macroethical resolutions thus play an indirect role in the construction of medical reality.

Interethics

We have seen how futility and quality-of-life considerations cannot be simply re-solved at the micro level; and they call for a move beyond limits to an account of the role that values play in the construction of medical reality. Similarly, questions of cost and health policy cannot be resolved simply at the macro level. They also call for a move beyond limits to an account of the role economic structures and incentives have in the construction of medical reality. These issues intersect to form the problems of interethics, where mid-dle-level institutions and their values configure the norms of medical practice.

Many of the most important decisions about limits on care are framed by the poli-cies and culture of the institutions where the treatment is being offered. Increasingly, issues of payment and provision merge at the institutional level, and administrative and organiza-tional policy plays a central role in the coordination of medical care. This circumstance is seen most clearly in managed care, where the key issues are not hidden, but it is present in any system. However, with few exceptions, deliberations about limiting access have taken place at micro- or macroethical levels, and the particular characteristics of institutions have not been considered. Guidelines on the use of health care resources are developed in a way that assumes the institutional context does not matter. This is unfortunate. As with individ-uals, institutions have values that (ideally) influence the way they approach treatment (Khushf 1997a). These values are embodied in mission statements and in the religious and cultural life of that institution.

The increasingly important role of institutions can be seen in the "Consensus State-ment on the Triage of Critically Ill Patients." When the Society of Critical Care Medicine (SCCM) addressed the issue of limiting treatment, it focused on institutions. It suggested that each hospital should develop its own policy, and thus refrained from providing the de-tails of a global policy in macroethical terms. Further, although it made concrete sugges-tions about individuals who *should* be excluded from ICUs (e.g., "those in a persistent vege-tative or permanently unconscious state") and those that *may* be excluded (e.g., "those with severe, irreversible brain damage or irreversible multi-organ failure"), it also recognized that "religious or moral convictions may legitimately be the basis for the provision of treatment to such patients" (1994, 1202). Thus, the SCCM acknowledged the role that institutional values may play in configuring the care provided.

Perhaps of greatest interest for our purposes is the mechanism that the SCCM rec-ommended for addressing triage decisions at the institutional level. They argued that policy should be set and implemented by a "critical care unit (ICU) committee":

> The ICU committee should include a broad range of health professionals and other appropriate individuals. When appropriate, the ICU committee should seek the ad-vice of members of the medical and nursing staffs, hospital administration, hospital ethics committee, patient advocacy representatives, and/or legal advisors. (SCCM 1994, 1202)

This interdisciplinary committee "should have *medical* oversight and responsibility for tri-age decisions" (my emphasis). Its activities include postponing elective operations, review-ing outcome information, evaluating backup capacity, and educating (among other things).

Although the committee stopped short of directly acknowledging it, these activities amount to the practice of health care, at least in one restricted but important area. By making the ICU committee interdisciplinary, the SCCM implicitly acknowledged that health care decisions are no longer simply made by individual physicians. They are also made by institutions and involve nurses, administrators, and a host of other professionals and paraprofessionals. That is why the questions of triage cannot be resolved in traditional microethical terms, which focus just on physicians and their interaction with patients.

It is not coincidental that when the SCCM sought to "develop a moral framework for distributing the available resources efficiently and equitably," it struggled in interethical terms (despite the relatively undeveloped state of such ethical reflection), rather than respond to the needs for allocating critical care in traditional micro- or macroethical terms. The practical wisdom of the committee members led them to advance guidelines, which were responsive to the current realities of health care. In the end, the SCCM did stop short of fully acknowledging the role that institutions play. They still present their conclusions as limits on medical care, and speak as if one could separate the practice of health care from decisions about resource use. But their analysis brings us to the threshold of more explicitly acknowledging the central role institutions now play in both resource use and health care practice.

In important ways, health care is no longer practiced just by individual physicians; it is now practiced by institutions. They integrate payment and provision, coordinate various professionals, paraprofessionals, and other health care workers, and integrate the outcome information with incentives for cost control, thus structuring the way medicine manages uncertainty. Institutional guidelines on treatment involve considerations that bridge individual and governmental or policy considerations (thus the term "interethic," because deliberations take place between micro- and macroethics).

To clarify how an organizational ethic frames the provision of health care, I will address the relevant considerations of a Christian health care institution in determining appropriate (i.e., proportionate) health care, with a focus on critical care. Although the results of such deliberations are relevant to micro- and macroethical deliberations, they do not provide the whole solution. I will thus only address a subset of the broader discussion about limits.

ETHICAL PROBLEMS WITH FRAMING QUESTIONS OF HEALTH CARE IN TERMS OF LIMITS: THE NEW ROLE OF INSTITUTIONS IN CONFIGURING CLINICAL PRACTICE

When the questions about the use of health care are framed in terms of limits, the focus today is almost always on some consideration that constrains the claim a person or population makes upon services.[6] The two considerations most often addressed are those associated with finite resources (with the need for cost-benefit assessment) and quality of life. These considerations lead to triage or futility judgments, which determine when health care providers are no longer obligated to patients. Limits are thus aligned with the stage at which countervailing considerations (e.g., the common good, integrity of medicine) relieve one from the claim generated by patient need or demand; the stage when one can legitimately abandon the patient, either because the costs of attendant care are too high or the patient's life is not of sufficient value (a life not worth living).

To avoid a digression into a crude utilitarianism or a "quality-of-life ethic" it is important to keep in view the positive obligations that lead to the provision of health care in the first place. This means appreciating not just why physicians practice, but also why institutions are involved in health care. Some institutions and individuals may simply provide services in order to obtain financial profit. However, for most institutions (especially Catholic ones), the primary motive is not profit. These institutions do not simply limit care to save costs. Further, a limit on a certain kind of care (e.g., critical care) does not necessarily mean that no other care will be offered. Catholic institutions do not simply abandon patients who have a poor quality of life. Thus, instead of asking about limits, it is better to ask about the appropriate type of care; namely, care that involves an appropriate response to the need of the patient. One must ask this question from an institutional perspective.

To ask about proportionate care in interethical terms that do justice to the current realities of health care, it is important to move beyond two common assumptions. First, one must move beyond the assumption that the nature of medical services (e.g., critical care services) is fully determined independent of the decisions about their utilization, as if one could neatly distinguish the clinical "research" in which the standards of care are formulated from the socioeconomic factors that constrain the use of those standards in "practice." On this assumption, ethical reflection about the use and abuse of health care comes in as a second step and plays no role in the construction of medical reality (presumably a value-free, purely scientific enterprise). Thus, (1) one has critical care, and (2) it is utilized. The key question in this account is how one limits such care; that is, how one controls utilization. However, if we ask in a more radical way, challenging the neat distinction between substance and use, then we must move beyond the question of limits and ask about the way institutional values frame the nature of the critical care provided.

The second important assumption that needs to be challenged is related to the first, but considers the issue from another side. It is clear that we are in the midst of major structural transformations in health care. Often these changes are simply understood as the outcome of market forces, which are altering medicine from a profession to a business venture. On this account, the sole reason why institutions have emerged as active agents of health care, influencing clinical decisions, is because they have an interest in managing financial resources (Rodwin 1993; Morreim 1995; Hall 1996). Organizations are thus aligned with economic considerations, whereas physicians and other professionals are aligned with clinical practice. The reason why administrators of institutions "interfere" with clinical decision making, the argument concludes, is because they want to reduce utilization.

Although this emphasis on the economic reasons for transformation captures an important part of the story, it does not give the whole picture. In addition to economic factors, there are considerations related to quality and to the altered nature of health care services that are equally important in understanding the new, more active role that institutions play. In *Clinical Decision Making*, Eddy (1996) provides an outstanding review of some of these quality-driven developments. They include the use of outcome information, physician profiling, and other more informal mechanisms to provide feedback on practice and thus influence the standard of care, the development of guidelines, and the shift from an individual-based to a population-based orientation. The important thing to see in each of these developments is that new skills related to health services research and administration do not just involve medical professionals, but draw on the broader skills of others and the resources of the institution to influence the standards of clinical practice (Khushf 1998b). Further, by coordinating diverse professionals to address the needs of a particular population, institutions provide health services that are broader than those provided by the physician. The types of institutional coordination and decision making in the SCCM's "Consensus Statement on the Triage of Critically Ill Patients" are thus characteristic of much more than end-of-life care.

Finally, it is important to note that different institutions may have different missions, leading to very different conclusions about how health care should be provided. Because health care is broader than medicine, and important balancing questions need to be addressed in any account of health care, there may be a concrete trade-off between medical care provided by physicians and other types of care; for example, preventive or wellness care provided by nurses or pastoral care. If one just focuses on the trade-offs from the perspective of the physician, these trade-offs will be put in terms of limits. However, from a broader institutional perspective, the balance may reflect care that is thought to be more appropriate for the needs in question. This may be especially important at the end of life, when spiritual values may need to be given overriding consideration, and when it may be more important to focus on responding to the disruptive life-world of the patient, rather than on some underlying disease process. Moving beyond medicine enables us to move beyond framing the question of proportionate care in terms of limits.

In fact, moving beyond medicine need not necessarily lead to limits on medical care. It may actually lead to a use of critical care that goes beyond that which is recommended by medical professionals, a point made by the SCCM statement on triage (1994, 1202). Consider the following, admittedly stark example. In speaking about patients in a persistent vegetative state (PVS), Edward Hughes notes:

> The time spent quietly in a coma, for all we know, may be a period of internal reflection and recollection, of sorting things out and coming to peace with God and self. . . . If we actively "liberate" them prematurely, before their internal spiritual work is done, we may deprive them of what God may have given them as the means of their salvation. (Hughes 1995, 344)

In this context, Hughes is attempting to counter arguments for assisted suicide or euthanasia, and thus is not discussing limits on treatment. But one can, on the basis of this argument, imagine a health care institution formed for the sole purpose of providing critical care for permanently obtunded patients, the equivalent of a monastery for those wealthy enough to afford the expensive care, founded to promote and sustain such internal contemplation. One could even form such an institution with the express purpose of countering quality-of-life judgments about what lives are worth living. Such an institution could be taken as a public affirmation about the value of the afterlife, and the need properly to prepare for it.

My point here is not to argue for such PVS care (I generally consider it to be inappropriate). Rather, I seek to make clear that the appropriate scope and limits for medicine are determined by institutional values that may actually construct the norms and use of medicine in a counterintuitive, countercultural way. An institution with critical care for permanently obtunded patients would nevertheless be fully compatible in principle with another Orthodox institution that sought to provide care for the poor and, because of resource limits, failed to provide any critical care at all. The type and nature of care would thus depend on the mission of the institution. Again, instead of framing questions in terms of limits, it would thus be better to frame them in terms of the appropriate or proportionate response, given the institutional vision, values, and available resources.

AT THE INTERSECTION OF TWO DOMAINS OF DISCOURSE: OPERATIONALIZING INSTITUTIONAL VALUES

To determine the appropriate (i.e., proportionate) provision of care, one must operationalize the values and mission of the institution, working out their implications for concrete treatment decisions. It is through reflection on institutional ends that the criteria for determining what is proportionate will be formulated. However, this operationalization of values may be difficult, because the ends are often expressed in a language that is not easily translatable into terms that can concretely direct clinical decision making. For example, Christian health care institutions may seek "a corporate life-climate designed to foster and deepen belief in and insight into the basic structure of our lives as this is revealed in God's self-disclosure in Jesus" (McCormick 1995, 111). And the Christian is to "take great care to employ this medical art . . . not as making it wholly accountable for our state of health or illness, but as redounding to the glory of God and as a parallel to the care given the soul" (Basil 1962, 332). How do such ends, formulated in the language of faith, translate into decisions about critical care?

The challenge for an institution is to develop the bridge work needed between its broader ends and the concrete areas where decisions must be made, so that the broader values and mission of the organization can provide guidance for the complex, new situations associated with modern health care. Here the task for a Christian health care institution is similar to that addressed by the *Catechism of the Catholic Church* (1994); namely, "to illumine with the light of faith the new situations and problems which had not yet emerged in the past" in order to initiate all in the health care arena into the realities of Christian life (1994, 4 and 8; sec. 5). This must involve an appreciation of the rules and integrity of both domains of discourse, so that guidelines are simultaneously faithful to both the institutional mission and the realities that guide norms of clinical practice.

Of course, even before this is done, there must be clarity regarding the ends of the institution. Why, for example, are Catholic institutions directly involved in the provision of health care? This question becomes especially pressing in contexts where services are readily available through other institutions, and where indigent care is provided by a community hospital. In this context, is a religiously affiliated institution needed? What makes the Catholic hospital different from a non-Catholic one? Is it analogous to a Catholic grocery store? Is health care provided in a unique way, seen in the norms and content of practice, or is the only difference found in the motivation of the health care providers?[7]

Among Catholic health care institutions, there are two competing tendencies. On one hand, there is a tendency to sharply separate the secular and scientific from the spiritual elements of care. On the other hand, there is a tendency to integrate diverse elements of care and order all toward the deeper mission and end of the church.

The tendency to separate the secular and religious elements of care aligns with assumptions that medicine does not depend on the faith for its norms and practices, and thus there will be no difference between Catholic and non-Catholic health care. McCormick, for example, argues that the only difference between the Catholic and secular physician can be found in the motivation for practice. If this is the case, then one can sharply divide regular health care from religious practices such as anointing the sick and pastoral care. When indigent care is provided by other means (e.g., state or community hospitals), then there is no loss, according to this view. The key concern is whether people have the health care, and it does not matter who provides it any more than it matters who grows or sells the food people eat. Because the nature of health care is in no way dependent on the faith, the trajectory of such care moves in a secular direction, and the analogy to the Catholic grocery store is quite apt. Thus, for example, the Sisters of Mercy Providence Hospital in Columbia, South Carolina, recently merged with the for-profit chain, Columbia/HCA, in order to establish a Conversion Foundation whose assets could be used to address various social issues. This action is not untypical for Catholic institutions in the United States, and it follows from a conceptualization of organizational mission that allows for a strong division between secular and spiritual elements of care.

For some Catholic thinkers, this separation is justified by a distinction between matters of natural reason and revelation, with the determination of proportionate care relegated to the former. The question of "limits" is addressed by philosophical means, and the appropriate use of treatments at institutions is made on the basis of independent medical professional codes or guidelines such as those developed by the SCCM (1994) on the use of critical care.

An alternative approach is reflected in the "Health Care Guide" of the Catholic Health Association of Canada:

> Catholic health care institutions are both communities of service and communities of work. Their raison d'être and the basic orientation of all their personnel are respect for the dignity of every person and concern for the total well-being of their patients/ residents. They affirm the centrality of the resident/patient and recognize the importance of family, friends, and the wider community in the health care endeavour. Underlying the care given is a comprehensive understanding of the health that includes attention to the need for a balance of the biological, psychological, social and spiritual forces that interact within the person, the society and the ecosystem. . . .
>
> The healing ministry of the Catholic health care facility is an expression of the ministry of Christ and the church. Since we are creatures of body and spirit, we need visible, tangible, human institutions to assist us to work as a believing community bearing witness to the Good News. Physical, emotional, social and spiritual healing is to be a clear sign of the presence and compassion of Christ the Healer.
>
> In order for this to happen, the total atmosphere of our institutions needs to be permeated with the love of Christ and with the visible signs of faith that characterizes the authentic Catholic tradition. (1991, 2694)

Regarding moral reflection and decision making, this same document notes that:

> Our moral decisions should be based on an understanding of human life per-
> ceived by human reason and in conformity with the best medical information
> available, enlightened by what is revealed in the life, death and resurrection of Je-
> sus Christ. . . . The Catholic moral tradition is the fruit of an on-going dialogue
> between our understanding of human nature and our experience of God as re-
> vealed in Jesus Christ. (1991, 2695)

In contrast to the separating tendency, which is associated with the secularization of health
care, this tendency to integrate leads to a sacralizing of health care. The function of health
care is united with the ministry of Jesus generally, and with the sacrament of the anointing
of the sick in particular.

> "Heal the sick!" The Church has received this charge from the Lord and strives to
> carry it out by taking care of the sick as well as by accompanying them with her
> prayer of intercession. She believes in the life-giving presence of Christ, the physi-
> cian of souls and bodies. (*Catechism of the Catholic Church* 1994, sec. 1509)

These words, developed in the *Catechism of the Catholic Church* as a justification for the sacrament of the anointing of the sick, also provide the warrant for health care generally. As in
the case of the sacrament, health care can have four functions:

1. It can provide encouragement to those afflicted with illness, leading them to
   the "healing of soul," but also restoring health to the body, when possible
   (*Catechism,* sec. 1520).
2. It can unite one to the passion of Christ. "Suffering, a consequence of original
   sin, acquires a new meaning; it becomes a participation in the saving work of
   Jesus" (sec. 1521).
3. It enables the sick to contribute to the good of those at the health care institution, by providing them with the opportunity to participate in Christian service and community (sec. 1522).
4. It brings to view the ultimate end of humanity and gives "a preparation for the
   final journey," when the person is fully conformed to the death and resurrection of Jesus Christ (sec. 1523).

When properly developed at a Christian institution, such comprehensive care can
manifest the integrated response to the whole person that is provided by the church. Health
care becomes a part of the broader witness of the church, showing the form of Christian life
to the world. When viewed in this way, there would be a great loss when secular institutions
or state health care systems take over Catholic institutions.

The way health care institutions approach the "question of limits" depends on
whether they take a secularizing or sacralizing approach to health care. The tendency to separate secular and spiritual aspects of care is associated with attempts to articulate through
philosophical means alone the norms for limits. As in the secular arena generally, the ques-

tion of limits is associated with economic constraints that lead to rationing of "medically indicated" service. The tendency to integrate secular and spiritual care situates the question of limits in the context of the broader question about the proper, integrated response of the church to illness and suffering. Before there can be any discussion of limits on care at Catholic institutions, there should thus be more foundational reflection and reassessment of the central mission and ends of such institutions. Only then can one move toward operationalizing those ends.

CURE VERSUS CARE: DETERMINING WHAT IS UNIQUE TO THE CATHOLIC MISSION

There are deficiencies associated with critical care that do not first arise when services are provided to a certain subset of the patient population, such as those in a PVS. They are deficiencies related to health care generally, as it is often practiced, and to all of critical care in particular. Here I have in mind criticisms associated with the objectivizing, depersonalizing, reductionist orientation at the heart of modern medicine; a broad cultural and ethical iatrogenesis that comes with medicalization (Illich 1976; Leder 1992). When considering appropriate use of medical care (including limits), it is important to ask questions in a more radical, comprehensive way, placing health care in the context of other responses to the suffering and assault on personal identity associated with illness. The question of limits on care should not be separated from other questions and problems associated with modern medicine, especially problems of reductionism and medicalization.

When considering the mission of a Catholic health care institution, it is important to include a broad spiritual response to the needs of patient and family. There should be a culture and practice of care that includes religious values unique to the institution. These values will play a direct role in framing the proportionate response to needs. I thus argue for an approach that resists the secularizing tendencies that have characterized health care at many Christian institutions.

To appreciate the limits on critical care, it will be helpful more generally to consider the nature and limits of medicine, as well as the way medicine can "redound to the glory of God" and serve as a "parallel to the care given to the soul" (Basil 1962). This will involve philosophical and theological reflection on the nature of medicine and the way it may be ordered to personal and spiritual life. With such reflection, there should also be an appraisal of the hubris of medicine and its inappropriate use, including the medicalization of death.

In this brief sketch, I cannot provide the needed appraisal of medicine and its place within the economy of life, as conceived within the Christian church.[8] However, a more detailed account would involve the recognition of three realities:

First, illness and death are to be understood within the context of the Christian account of human purpose, sin and death, and the life that has been manifest in Christ and the church, as the Body of Christ. In the illness experience, a patient's life-world is disrupted. There is an experienced alienation from self, others (community), and those frameworks of meaning and purpose that orient life among the well. Experienced time and space shrink, as hope is constricted and reoriented. In that illness experience, the Church has always seen an analogy of the broader and deeper brokenness of the human condition (*Cate-*

chism, sec. 1500–01). Similarly, the medical response to suffering associated with illness has been taken as an analogy for the Gospel about God's response to a broken humanity. Health care can thus serve the same function as the healings that Jesus performed. "His healings were signs of the coming of the Kingdom of God. They announced a more radical healing: the victory over sin and death through his Passover" (*Catechism*, sec. 1505). The analogy is rooted in an analogical relation between health and salvation (Mordacci 1995). It is the parallel between healing of body and healing of soul that has given medicine a special place, and provides unique opportunities for that discipline to "redound to the glory of God."

Second, apart from medicine and any natural knowledge about the healing arts, the church has had an ethic of care for the sick. This is "palliative" in the deepest sense, and it involves a communal response to the disrupted life-world that attends the illness experience. In the response of faith, where suffering and need are understood within the economy of salvation, and where a new community is made possible for the alienated other, the church has its primary concern (Khushf 1995). For this ethic of care, illness and death are not medicalized. They are grasped within a theological context that, for the Church, is truer to the reality of the phenomena.

Third, to the degree that medicine is effective—either as a means to restore health or as a vehicle for conveying that deeper spiritual healing—it has been positively appropriated by the church. To the degree it clouds the deeper ethic of care and leads to a medicalization of the important events in life, medicine should be rejected. Although a proper discernment of the appropriate role of medicine must involve more detailed reflection on the ends and means of medicine, we can minimally note that (1) when the end of medicine (health) is put forth as the summum bonum, or (2) when the objectivizing, depersonalizing means of medicine cannot realize their end, then medicine becomes inappropriate. The first involves idolatry of health, the second involves disrespect for the person (Khushf 1995).

Measured response to illness and death will involve an appreciation of the full mission of the church and the natural and spiritual reality of the phenomena in question. For a religious institution, proportionate care should entail an integration of the spiritual ethic of care and medical care. De facto limits on medicine generally will indicate where the medical response is no longer appropriate. De facto limits on a certain kind of medicine (e.g., critical care) may indicate where another medicine is more appropriate (e.g., palliative care). Such de facto limits are simply the one-sided articulation, from the perspective of medicine, of the proportionate response to need. They do not show when it is appropriate to abandon a patient, but how best to respond at every stage to the patient and family implicated in the suffering and death to which the church responds. The question of limits should thus move beyond a simple account of when a patient's request may be declined and capture the full rationality and mission of health care for the institution in question.

Finally, it should be noted that such an approach does not mean that one can avoid the more traditional concerns involved in determining limits on critical care. The question of proportionate care is raised from within the health care sector, driven by concerns with the integrity of medicine, finite resources, and so on. To resolve these questions, values and ends are required that are not fully specified within medicine. When the debate about limits is abstracted from the institutions where concrete decisions are made, the question must remain unresolved. The resolution of the debate is thus open apart from the institution's mission and values. By deemphasizing the traditional deliberations about futility, financial incentives, and the like, I do not mean to downplay their importance. I assume that they will be an important part of any deliberations, as they should be. My intention has been to highlight additional concerns that should be important for institutions, and which are largely absent from the broader debate on the utilization of health care. Only when these additional organizational issues are addressed can we develop the norms for the appropriate use of critical care.

NOTES

1. On the problems with this assumption, see Khushf (1998a, 1998b).
2. In the Roman Catholic tradition, similar concerns are addressed by the distinction between ordinary and extraordinary care (Wildes 1995).
3. This is the approach found in much of the debate about futility (Engelhardt and Khushf 1995).
4. For a good critical assessment of these kinds of regulation, see DeVille (1999).
5. This discussion could be fruitfully situated within the context of the debate about underdetermination and incommensurability in the philosophy of science. Rie's approach assumes that particular components can be treated as isolatable units that can be evaluated independently, much as advocates of the Received View thought particular components of a theory could be isolated and tested. I am suggesting that elements such as de-skilling must be seen as part of a broader constellation, which provides a comprehensive alternative to the traditional, Flexnerian paradigm of medicine (Khushf 1998a). As in semantic conceptions of theory, I suggest that elements are not in a simple way isolatable, although I do think limited intertheoretic comparison is possible.
6. The other way the question of limits is framed involves a focus on the obligation a patient has to submit to a treatment regimen that others consider appropriate or even obligatory. This way of framing the problem characterized the earlier stage of the debate, and it focused on the ability of the patient to say "no" (Amundsen 1978). The more recent stage focuses on the ability of society, physicians, etc., to say "no" (Meilaender 1993).
7. On this question, see the dispute between McCormick (1995) and Khushf (1995).
8. For a more detailed account of these issues, see Khushf (1995).

BIBLIOGRAPHY

Amundsen, D. 1978. The physician's obligation to prolong life: A medical duty without classical roots. *Hastings Center Report* 8 (4): 23–30.

Basil, Saint. 1962. *Ascetical Works*, trans. by Sister Monica Wagner. Washington, D.C.: Catholic University of America Press.

Brody, B., and A. Halevy. 1995. Is futility a futile concept? *Journal of Medicine and Philosophy* 20 (2): 123–44.

Catechism of the Catholic Church. 1994. Ligouri, Mo.: Ligouri Publications.

Catholic Health Association of Canada. 1991. *Health Care Guide*. Ottawa.

DeVille, K. 1999. Managed care and the ethics of regulation. *Journal of Medicine and Philosophy* 24 (5): 492–517.

Eddy, D. 1996. *Clinical Decision Making: From Theory to Practice.* Sudbury, Mass.: Jones and Bartlett Publishers.

Engelhardt, H. T., and G. Khushf. 1995. Futile care for the critically ill patient. *Current Opinion in Critical Care* 1: 329–33.

Goodman, J. C., and G. L. Musgrave. 1992. *Patient Power: Solving America's Health Care Crisis.* Washington, D.C.: Cato Institute.

Halevy, A., and B. Brody. 1996. A multi-institutional collaborative policy on medical futility. *Journal of the American Medical Association* 276 (7): 571–74.

Halevy, A., R. Neal, and B. Brody. 1996. The low frequency of futility in an adult intensive care unit setting. *Archives of Internal Medicine* 156: 100–104.

Hall, M. 1996. Physician Rationing and Agency Cost Theory. In *Conflicts of Interest in Clinical Practice and Research*, ed. by R. Spece, D. Shimm, and A. Buchanan. New York: Oxford University Press.

Hughes, E. 1995. The act of death and the gift of suffering: A response to Breck, Amundsen, and Breshnahan. *Christian Bioethics* 1 (3): 338–45.

Illich, I. 1976. *Medical Nemesis: The Exploration of Health.* New York: Pantheon Books.

Khushf, G. 1995. Illness, the problem of evil, and the analogical structure of healing: On the difference Christianity makes in bioethics. *Christian Bioethics* 1 (1): 102–20.

———. 1997a. Administrative and organizational ethics. *HEC Forum* 9 (4): 298–309.

———. 1997b. Why bioethics needs the philosophy of medicine: Some implications of reflection on concepts of health and disease. *Theoretical Medicine* 18: 145–63.

———. 1998a. A radical rupture in the paradigm of modern medicine: Conflicts of interest, fiduciary obligations, and the scientific ideal. *Journal of Medicine and Philosophy* 23 (1): 98–122.

———. 1998b. The scope of organizational ethics. *HEC Forum* 10 (2): 127–35.

———. 1999. The aesthetics of clinical judgment: Exploring the link between diagnostic elegance and effective resource utilization. *Medicine, Health Care and Philosophy,* 2 (2): 141–59.

Knaus, W., D. Wagner, and J. Lynn. 1991. Short-term mortality predictions for critically ill hospitalized adults: Science and ethics. *Science* 254: 389–94.

Leder, D., ed. 1992. *The Body in Medical Thought and Practice.* Dordrecht: Kluwer Academic Publishers.

McCormick, R. 1995. Does Christianity make a difference? *Christian Bioethics* 1 (1): 97–101.

Meilaender, G. 1993. *Terra es animata.* On having a life. *Hastings Center Report* (July–August): 25–32.

Mordacci, R. 1995. Health as an analogical concept. *Journal of Medicine and Philosophy* 20 (5): 475–97.

Morreim, E. H. 1995. *Balancing Act: The New Medical Ethics of Medicine's New Economics.* Washington, D.C.: Georgetown University Press.

Murphy, E. 1997. *The Logic of Medicine*, 2d ed. Baltimore: Johns Hopkins University Press.

Rie, M. 1997. Rationing critical care services in the United States. *Current Opinion in Critical Care* 3: 329–33.

Rodwin, M. 1993. *Medicine, Money and Morals.* New York: Oxford University Press.

Schneiderman, L. J., and N. S. Jecker. 1995. *Wrong Medicine: Doctors, Patients, and Futile Treatment.* Baltimore: Johns Hopkins University Press.

Schneiderman, L. J., N. Jecker, and A. Jonsen. 1990. *Annals of Internal Medicine* 112: 949.

Society of Critical Care Medicine Ethics Committee. 1994. Consensus statement on the triage of critically ill patients. *Journal of the American Medical Association* 271 (15): 1200–03.

Veatch, R. 1995. Abandoning informed consent. *Hastings Center Report* 25 (2): 5–12.

Wildes, K. W. 1995. Conserving life and conserving means: Lead us not into temptation. In *Critical Choices and Critical Care*, ed. by K. W. Wildes. Dordrecht: Kluwer Academic Publishers.

Developing the Doctrine of Distributive Justice: Methods of Distribution, Redistribution, and the Role of Time in Allocating Intensive Care Resources

M. Cathleen Kaveny

In the United States, the proportion of the gross domestic product that is consumed by health care currently hovers around 14 percent. Although the United States conceivably could provide every person living within its borders with the full range of potentially beneficial health care, we seem to have reached a consensus not to exceed current levels of spending in this area. Consequently, the health care financing and delivery system has increasingly focused upon reducing costs and providing cost-efficient care. Many hospitals have closed; those that remain in operation have downsized in order to enter into affiliations with other facilities that reduce duplication of services in a given area and achieve economies of scale. Managed care has placed increased emphasis on the need to provide medical services in the least intense setting possible, including, if possible, discharge to home care.

A particularly attractive target for cost-cutting measures is the intensive care unit (ICU). First, the ICU is extremely expensive. Second, it is not self-evidently cost-effective, at least in some cases. Third, it has come to symbolize the excesses of late-twentieth-century industrial-world medicine, as well as its more dehumanizing elements. Intensive care will provide many patients with the life support that enables them to survive an acute illness or injury and return to a relatively acceptable level of functioning. To them, it doubtless appears nothing short of a miracle. But for other patients, intensive care will not even enable them to survive long past discharge from the hospital, if even that long. For them, intensive care arguably counts as a harm. Not only does it fail to save their lives, but it also imposes intrusions, distractions, and isolation that prevent them and their families from coming to terms with the waning of their earthly lives.

Assuming that the number of available intensive care beds continues to shrink as health care restructuring continues, how should we allocate those that are available in cases

177

of scarcity?[1] Before addressing this question, it is important to distinguish and set aside the superficially similar problem of determining when patients continue to benefit from intensive care. It may be that many patients will choose to forgo intensive care, when sufficiently informed about its nature, risks, and potential benefits. But reducing the number of willing patients will not eliminate all competition for intensive care resources. Hard decisions will still need to be made. What criteria should be used to compare and resolve the claims of patients competing for scarce ICU beds?

In the world of managed care, it is entirely possible that the question will be answered in the following manner. A patient would be admitted or denied admission to the ICU on the basis of her score on a specified particular instrument, such as Acute Physiology and Chronic Health Evaluation (APACHE) III, which predicts a patient's likelihood of survival to discharge (Knaus et al. 1991). The physician would need to obtain authorization for each additional day of her ICU stay, which would be granted or denied by the managed care organization (MCO) on the basis of practice guidelines specifying the "appropriate" length of stay for each illness. It is also possible that MCOs would impose a yearly or a lifetime limit upon the number of days a particular patient may receive intensive care, as they already customarily do with inpatient mental health services. The "predictive score" required to gain admission to an ICU could be set in a number of ways. It could take into account solely the potential benefit to the patient (however "benefit" is defined), or it could be broadened to take into account the costs and benefits to the managed care plan itself. More specifically, the requisite score could be set high enough to justify substantially downsized ICU units, while minimizing the appearance of conflicts among qualified patients.

But what happens if there *is* a conflict? Suppose one patient receives a bed in the ICU on Tuesday, and on Wednesday another patient comes along with a better score on the predictive measure in use. Assuming there is no other bed, should we discharge the first patient in order to admit the second, thereby maximizing the possibility of achieving the best outcome for the unit? In its "Consensus Statement on the Triage of Critically Ill Patients," the Society for Critical Care Medicine Ethics Committee stated that as a "general rule, obligations to patients already hospitalized in an ICU who continue to warrant ICU care outweigh obligations to accept new patients." Why? The Consensus Statement goes on to assert that "there may be circumstances, however, when it is justified to discharge a patient from the ICU to admit another patient" (Society for Critical Care Medicine Ethics Committee 1994, 1201). How are these circumstances identified?

The purpose of this volume is to see what wisdom can be gleaned from the Roman Catholic moral tradition regarding how a society can justly limit access to medical treatment, particularly intensive care. In this essay, I assume that the Roman Catholic tradition's perspective on justice and health care can indeed shed some light on the vexing moral issues involved in the just distribution of intensive care resources. I will argue, however, that the tradition needs to be developed in specific ways if it is to have the necessary subtlety to tackle the problem and to provide adequate answers to the questions identified in the previous paragraph.

More specifically, I will suggest that the tradition's strong emphasis on choosing the right *principle* of distribution needs to be supplemented by two additional concerns. First, we must pay attention to the *way* we carve up the good of intensive care medicine for distribution, and in particular to the nature and size of the units in which we choose to parcel it out. More specifically, we need to ask whether it is appropriate to distribute access to intensive care beds in temporally based units, such as days (or hours), as managed care plans might be inclined to do? Second, we must consider whether it is appropriate to *redistribute* the good of intensive care. More specifically, is it ever appropriate to discharge one patient from intensive care in order to admit another? I do not claim, of course, that these two points exhaust the respects in which Roman Catholic thought will need to expand to grapple with contemporary problems of distributive justice and health care. But at least they are a beginning.

A ROMAN CATHOLIC PERSPECTIVE ON DISTRIBUTIVE JUSTICE AND HEALTH CARE

The Roman Catholic tradition recognizes that all human persons have a claim in justice to basic health care. This claim is grounded in two essential features of Catholic anthropology. First, each human person, embodied and ensouled as a psychosomatic unity, possesses an essential dignity as a being created in the image and likeness of God. Respect for that dignity calls not only for nonmaleficence, but also for beneficence, for positive acts of care and protection, particularly on behalf of the weakest and most needy.[2] Because all human beings are at their most vulnerable when afflicted with physical or mental illness, caring for them at this time honors and respects their innate dignity. Second, human persons are essentially social, called not to live in splendid isolation, but to contribute their God-given gifts and talents to the community, even as they draw strength from the gifts and talents of others. From a Catholic perspective, individuals have a right to those basic goods that will enable them to *participate* in communal life with others.[3] As the U.S. Catholic bishops noted in their pastoral letter on the economy, "human rights are the minimum conditions for life in community" (U.S. Conference of Catholic Bishops 1986, §§78–79).[4] The provision of basic health care is an indispensable precondition for communal participation; it enables persons to overcome injuries or illnesses that would otherwise prevent them from functioning as active, contributing members of their families and societies.[5]

But the right to basic health care, even in industrial countries, does not mean that every person has a moral claim on the community to provide any form of medical treatment that could conceivably ameliorate her medical problems, even severe or life-threatening problems.[6] After ensuring that each person living within its borders has access to a basic level of care, a community can decide to devote its money to projects that will benefit the common good in other ways.[7] It is arguable that, even in wealthy countries such as the United States, unrestricted access to state-of-the-art ICUs does not constitute part of the basic package of health care to which the Catholic tradition contends each person is entitled.

However, if an advanced type of health care *is* made available within a certain society, the method of its allocation must be subjected to ethical constraints. Health care is a public good, which means that it is "not created by any individual person acting alone or even through the activities of persons banding together through contract, consent, or some other form of strictly autonomous choice." Consequently, its distribution is subject to the norms of distributive justice (Hollenbach 1979, 147–48). What, concretely, counts as distributing a complex good such as health care in a just manner?[8]

The Catholic Christian tradition already offers a good deal of wisdom that bears on this question. More specifically, contemporary Catholic and Christian thinkers have recognized that there are different principles of distribution that are morally appropriate for different types of goods. For example, although it is suitable to distribute advanced academic scholarships according to the principle "to each according to merit," and civic awards according to the principle "to each according to his past contribution to the community," it is not appropriate to distribute health care according to either principle. As recent Christian ethicists have persuasively argued, health care should be distributed according to the principle "to each according to medical need" (Outka 1987, 632–43; Boyle 1987, 643–49).

Why does choosing the correct principle of distribution matter so much? As Michael Walzer explains so eloquently in *Spheres of Justice* (1983), distributing a good according to a principle not suited to it distorts the very nature of the good and corrupts the relationship of the people who interact with one another with respect to that good. For example, if the prize committee distributes the award for best first book according to the principle "to the contestant who gives the biggest bribe" or "to the contestant with the most personal charm," it may very well hold up the wrong essay as the best, thereby corrupting the criteria that people apply in writing and judging such compositions. Contestants "in the know" will focus on impressing the judges not with the quality of their writing, but with the size of their checks or the sparkle of their smiles. If the situation disintegrates far enough, the very idea that there can be defensible criteria for identifying some pieces of writing as superior to others will be substantially eroded.

So it is with choosing a principle to govern the distribution of health care. For example, one function of health care is to enable individuals to draw upon the physical and mental strength they need to fulfill their vocations as family members, members of voluntary associations, and members of the larger political community. No matter what our role in life, illness and injury prevent us from fulfilling it as we experience ourselves as called to do. Physical suffering renders us all vulnerable, in essentially the same manner. By distributing health care according to medical need, we recognize our common lot as mortals subject to the frailties of the flesh and the vicissitudes of chance accidents. If, conversely, we chose to distribute health care according to the principle "to each according to ability to make a political contribution," we would undermine the equal dignity of all human beings. The brouhaha precipitated almost thirty years ago when it was revealed that the Seattle "God Committee" was distributing scarce and life-saving access to kidney dialysis according to their own criteria of social contribution and worth (which consistently favored middle-aged, middle-class white males) is one sign of broad support for the general principle that medically necessary health care should be distributed according to need.[9]

Thus the Catholic tradition of social ethics has rightly recognized that choosing the correct principle of distribution is crucial to the just allocation of health care.[10] Yet in its current state, it is insufficiently well-developed to grapple with the moral challenges posed by the need to distribute scarce medical resources, particularly intensive care services. One task is to specify what the principle "to each according to need" means in the context of medical care. For example, who "needs" intensive care more: the person who is going to die sooner without it or the person who has a potential for a longer life of higher quality with it? Although this set of questions is extremely important, it is not the focus of this essay.

Instead, I would like to concentrate my efforts on identifying moral considerations we need to articulate and apply in addition to developing our understanding of the principle "to each according to need." More specifically, that principle does not help us decide whether MCOs can justly distribute scarce health care dollars by allocating to each enrollee a certain number of days in an ICU, per year and per lifetime. Nor does the principle tell us what to do when we are confronted with two patients competing for scarce intensive care beds. Can, for example, a unit refuse to admit a patient with an APACHE score above a certain cutoff, despite the fact that her chances for survival would be increased with intensive care, in order to save that bed for a possible future patient who might or might not appear to claim it? Could it justify that refusal to save money for the managed care plan, which could eventually be devoted to other patients? Can a unit "evict" a patient benefiting from intensive care to make room for a patient who also needs such care and whose lower APACHE score suggests that she is more likely to benefit from it?

In order to begin addressing these questions, Catholic reflection on distributive justice needs to develop in two distinct steps. First, Catholic moralists must recognize that it is necessary but not sufficient to adopt the correct principle of distribution in order to ensure a just distributive scheme. We must expand the tradition's critical scope to consider two additional aspects of distribution schemes that are morally salient: (1) the method and unit of distribution and (2) the constraints, if any, placed on redistribution.[11]

These questions are moral questions, not merely pragmatic questions. By choosing the wrong principle of distribution, we distort the meaning of the good to be distributed and erode the character of the relationships mediated through that good. In choosing the wrong method and unit of distribution, or giving the wrong answer to the question of redistribution, we do precisely the same thing. For example, recognizing the essential connection between the appropriate distributive unit and the good to be distributed allows us to take a fresh look at the biblical story of King Solomon and the two women fighting over a baby. Solomon's proposal to solve the dispute by cutting the baby in half involves a method of distribution that would literally destroy the good in question. By agreeing to this proposal, one woman demonstrated that she truly did not understand the meaning of that infant's life; consequently, the King concluded, she could not have been its mother. However, think of how much more difficult the question would have been to resolve if Solomon had proposed joint custody and equal visitation (i.e., temporal division of the good rather than spatial division). In short, I will argue that the Catholic moral tradition must be developed to recognize explicitly that in deciding how we will "divide up" a good for distribution, as well as whether and according to what criteria we will redistribute a nonperishable good, we can honor or distort the nature of the good being distributed, and support or undermine the relationship between persons as equal in fundamental dignity and made in the image and likeness of God.

Second, Catholic moralists must grapple with the application of these new insights to the problem of the just distribution of health care, intensive care in particular. So doing requires us to understand the moral meaning of the good of health care and the aspects of health care that are embodied in ICUs. Just as choosing the correct principle of distribution requires us to understand the purpose for which the good is distributed, and the nature of the interpersonal relationships that are affected by the distribution, so too does choosing the correct way to divide the good and measure distribution. More specifically, we must ask whether it is consistent with the meaning and purpose of intensive health care to distribute the good it embodies in time-based units. The nature and purpose of the good distributed also should be considered in deciding whether or not it is subject to redistribution. Is it consistent with the nature and purpose of intensive health care to institute policies that allow a bed in an ICU to be taken away from a patient who desires to remain and for whom such care is not futile, in order to give that bed to another patient who has a higher likelihood of surviving to discharge from the hospital? Needless to say, I cannot complete these twin tasks within the confines of this essay. But I do hope to make some progress in its remaining pages.

HEALTH CARE AS A POLYVALENT GOOD

Before we consider the appropriateness of using units of time to divide and distribute health care, or the legitimacy of redistributing it, we need to understand its nature and purpose. As practiced and provided in contemporary industrial countries, health care is a complex, polyvalent good. We can identify three basic purposes: (1) improving public health, (2) curing individual patients, and (3) providing comfort care to individual patients.[12] At times, two or three of these goals may be pursued simultaneously; on other occasions, they may find themselves in substantial tension with one another. All three aspects of the good of health care reflect the twin fundamental anthropological presuppositions on which Roman Catholic thought bases its recognition of a right to health care, although perhaps to different degrees. More specifically, each aspect assumes that human beings are psychosomatic unities whose well-being is constantly threatened by illness, injury, and ultimately, death. Second, each aspect recognizes that human beings are not isolated monads, but essentially social creatures, whose identity and well-being are partially constituted by relationships with other human beings and directly affected by the general good of the community to which they belong. Let me briefly consider each of the three aspects of the good of health care in turn.

First, some aspects of health care are designed to improve the health of whole populations, rather than the individuals receiving the intervention in question. Population-wide vaccination programs, screening programs, and public health and safety programs are examples. Many, perhaps most, of the individuals who participate in such programs do not "need" them; as it turns out, they were not destined to suffer from the disease corresponding to the intervention. Nonetheless, the implementation of such programs results in an appreciable improvement in the health status of the population as a whole. From a theological perspective, this type of health care contributes directly to the common good. By fortifying the level of health of the whole community, it enables more members to pursue their vocations unimpeded by the challenges of ill health. Because the community's general level of health is enhanced, fewer communal resources will be consumed by the effort to cure those members who fall and the responsibility to care for those who cannot be cured. Less directly, it contributes to the good of particular individuals, whose own particular health status might be improved by particular public health interventions.

Second, some aspects of health care are directed toward curing or ameliorating a particular health problem suffered by an individual, in order to enable her to resume as normal a life as possible. Obviously, some types of treatment are more successful in achieving this purpose than others. With the tremendous strides that medicine has made in the past fifty years or so, this curative purpose of health care has dominated public imagination and expectations. This aspect of health care can contribute directly to the good of the individual and indirectly to the common good by enabling individuals to remain active participants in society. Yet at a certain point, the pursuit of cure for individuals may find itself impeding rather than advancing the common good. The prohibitive financial cost involved in discovering and implementing new interventions designed to cure or ameliorate specific problems bears significant responsibility for the skyrocketing costs of health care in the United States (and to a lesser degree, in other industrial countries). Some of this money could be dedicated to medical programs designed to improve the health of targeted populations, such as childhood immunization programs, as well as to nonmedical interventions that improve public health, such as food subsidies.

Third, there is an aspect of health care centered on its role as a corporal work of mercy. It finds its purpose in offering comfort, care, and a pledge against final loneliness to those whom medicine can no longer cure. In the end, that will be each and every one of us. For much of human history, this third aspect of health care was its dominant one, given the very limited ability of medicine to cure disease or repair injury. In the contemporary era, it can draw upon advanced techniques in the management of pain, depression, and other symptoms of a serious illness, as we see in the hospice movement. Yet at its core remains the call to solidarity, as witnessed in the work of Mother Theresa.

The virtue of solidarity is at once personal and social. On the personal level, it expresses and motivates recognition on the part of one person of her fundamental relationship with another person, particularly one in need. As the work of Mother Theresa demonstrates, it directly honors the transcendent dignity of the individuals toward whom it is directed. On the social level, solidarity expresses the conviction that no human being made in the image and likeness of God can be allowed to remain isolated and alienated from her fellow human beings. As Pope John Paul II so eloquently argues in *Evangelium Vitae*, it also contributes directly to the common good, because the character of a community and a culture is revealed and shaped by its attitude toward its weakest members.[13]

I believe the virtue of solidarity has three general components. First, it calls upon us to relieve the suffering of another, to overcome our initial desire of avoiding any confrontation with our own impending mortality in order to come to the aid of someone who confronts this facet of human existence here and now. In the context of health care, the core focus is on stopping physical and emotional pain and suffering; it calls for an immediate response to an immediate need. Second, it asks us to resist the temptation to isolate the weak and the vulnerable, to incorporate them into our community in the recognition that what we have in common (including vulnerability) is more important than what distinguishes us from one another. In the context of health care, the prohibition against abandonment of patients becomes an absolutely central requirement of solidarity. Third, it challenges us to recognize what even the most weak and vulnerable have to give to us. (In the case of the very ill and the dying, that may simply be the awe-full privilege of accompanying them in the transition from this life to the next.) Needless to say, medical practice in general has not placed great emphasis on the virtue of solidarity. In my view, the greatest challenge that Christian bioethics poses to contemporary health care is to recover that virtue as it has historically been embodied in the emphasis that many religious orders have placed on corporal works of mercy.

The third aspect of health care may at times be in tension with the first two aspects. Most efforts to improve the health of populations involve some form of preventive medicine; by definition, they do not focus their efforts on those who already suffer from a disease. Indeed, the broadly gauged focus of public health workers may not be conducive to the more finely grained attention to individual need that is at the heart of corporal works of mercy. Moreover, although the second and third aspects of health care are compatible in that they both focus on the well-being of an individual patient, the means they require are frequently incompatible: Chemotherapy can be painful, the aggressive monitoring involved in attempting to save a victim of an automobile accident can interfere with the dynamics of a caring relationship, and the isolation of a burn victim or a recipient of a bone marrow transplant can impede solidarity.[14] There is, I believe, no way entirely to reconcile the competing aspects of the good of health care; minimizing their conflicts calls for practical wisdom on the part of both policy experts and decision makers for individual patients.

What aspects of the polyvalent good of health are most involved in intensive care medicine? In my opinion, that specialty incorporates significant aspects of the second and third aspects of the good of health care. Clearly, it is directed toward bringing a particular individual through a specific, life-threatening medical crisis. This is the aspect of intensive care medicine that most dominates our experience. We judge its success or failure by its ability to allow a patient to survive to discharge from the unit, or to live outside the hospital for a designated period of time. Yet, precisely because the fate of some of those who enter ICUs is so uncertain, it is essential to recognize that such patients stand in need of the third aspect of health care, which is care: the support and company of fellow human beings as they prepare to confront their own deaths.

This understanding of the aspects of the good of health care involved in intensive care medicine allows us to focus our questions more precisely. First, in deciding whether it is appropriate to "carve up" the good of intensive care in terms of days spent in the unit or "bed-days," we must consider whether choosing units of time to divide this good preserves or warps its meaning, either as a curative intervention or as a corporal work of mercy.[15] Second, we must ponder whether allowing redistribution of the good of intensive care (i.e., by taking a bed away from a current patient to give it to a newcomer with a better APACHE score) supports or undermines the relationship of the persons that is mediated by the good.

USING TIME AS A METHOD OF DISTRIBUTING INTENSIVE CARE

General Considerations

To distribute a good, we need to know a number of things: the principle of distribution, the method we will use to divide the good, the size of the units of division, the time frame over which the distribution is expected to operate, and whether there can be redistribution. As noted above, much philosophical attention has been devoted to identifying the correct principle of distribution with respect to specific goods. But a moment's reflection shows that the method chosen to distribute a good will affect how well we meet the objective lying behind the principle of distribution we have chosen. So will the size of the units of distribution. For example, assuming that we are distributing food according to the principle of "to each according to biological need," our ability to meet the nutritional requirements of persons contending for the food will depend upon whether our unit of distribution is whole cows, or cuts of meat. In fact, one can "hide" normative decisions about which principle of distribution is actually being used "behind" choices about how a good is to be carved up for distribution. Consider someone who says that the principle of distribution of food is "first come, first served" and distributes that food in shopping carts rather than in meal-size portions. If members of her clan happened to be at the head of the line, we would have reason to suspect that the real principle of distribution was "me and mine first, last, and always." Consequently, the method of distribution and size of the unit of distribution deserves far more attention from moralists than it has heretofore received.

There are various methods of carving up a good for distribution. Two of the most common are physical division and temporal division. With respect to some goods (e.g., birthday cake), we employ physical division. Again, we have decisions to make with respect to the precise unit of physical division. We can give everyone pieces of the whole (e.g., slices of cake) or component parts (e.g., layers of cake); the selection of a specific unit of physical distribution involves many of the same questions as choosing to employ physical division in the first place. One can also divide goods temporally, in many different ways. For example, we commonly divide a desirable toy between two toddlers by giving each of them a certain period of exclusive use. Just as choosing a method of cutting into the corpus of the good is important in the case of goods subject to physical division, so choosing a span of time to cut into the recipient's enjoyment of the good is also a crucial decision. Quite obviously, it does no good to divide a stuffed Barney dinosaur between the toddlers in ten-year increments.[16]

How should we go about choosing a distributive method and unit? First, it is necessary to recognize that there are both direct and indirect methods of distribution. Direct methods attempt to measure and divide the good itself, whereas indirect methods aim to measure and divide a proxy for the good, usually because it is too costly or difficult to divide the good directly. In choosing a direct method of distribution, the key is making a selection that will somehow preserve the identity of the good, as defined in terms of the purpose of the distribution. We do not use time as a method to distribute birthday cake, because the prospect of each guest sequentially consuming all she can eat in five minutes does not foster the common joy required at such a feast.

Once one has chosen a method, similar care has to be exercised in choosing a unit of distribution. For example, in distributing a seven-layer cake to seven birthday party guests, we do not give a layer to each guest; we cut the cake as a whole into seven pieces. However, there may be situations in which the layer-apiece approach would work equally well in light of the purposes of the distribution, such as when allocating the only remaining food to seven explorers trapped in a cave to enable them to survive until the rescue party arrives. Furthermore, there is often a convenience factor involved in choosing a unit of distribution. Sometimes, we choose a unit to divide the good that will be carried out more easily, although it will not necessarily preserve the identity of the good to the same degree that another unit would. For example, two persons dividing two boxes of Girl Scout cookies may each take one box (mystic mint and peanut butter), rather than half the cookies in each box.

This convenience factor can sometimes lead us not only to choose a less appropriate direct method of distribution, but also to rely instead on an indirect method of distribution. For example, particularly in the case of complex or abstract goods, it can be difficult or expensive to find a way of dividing and parceling up the good in order to allocate it. In such cases, we often commonly rely on indirect methods of distribution, most commonly using time or money as proxies for the primary good that we are trying to distribute.[17] Instead of dividing up the primary good, we divide up the good used as a proxy for the primary good. For example, consider the work of lawyers. Their common practice of billing by the hour suggests that we are dividing their time. Yet their time is not the primary good at issue, it is a proxy used indirectly to divide and distribute their work, which is a complex and uncertain mixture of the effort they expend and the results they produce. Increments of money can also be used as an indirect distributive unit, such as when governmental agencies allocate social services to persons on the basis of the per capita cost of such services.

Despite its convenience, there are several dangers in using an indirect method of distribution. First, at best, the good used as a proxy can function only as an imperfect stand-in for the good that we want to distribute. Consequently, using an indirect method of distribution can skew the final distribution of the good in a way that is in tension with both the principle of distribution and the nature of the good itself. For example, consider state food stamp programs, where people falling below a certain income level receive "food stamps" that work like cash to buy anything that is edible. People can buy candy, soda, too much of one staple, not enough of another. It is less expensive to distribute and administer a food stamp program of this type; it also does not fulfill the purpose as well as a program that delivers nutritious food directly to people in need.

Second, there is a constant temptation to view an indirect method of distribution as a direct method of distribution and thereby to change the meaning of the good itself. To continue the above example, cost or price is not a natural way to distribute food; in and of itself, it bears no relation to the purpose for which we are distributing food (to nourish people). We might, however, find ourselves mistakenly thinking that cost is directly related to the good that we are distributing. More radically, we might also lose sight of what is being distributed, confusing the good distributed as a proxy with the primary good itself. In other words, we might come to understand ourselves as distributing "food stamps" rather than food.

Using Time as a Method of Distribution

Generally speaking, when is it appropriate to use time as a direct method of distribution? It is clearly and intuitively appropriate to use time as a direct method of distribution in some cases (e.g., two toddlers sharing a toy) and just as clearly inappropriate in others (e.g., two adolescents sharing a piece of cake). But what are the factors that converge to yield these judgments? I believe that at least some of the considerations that need to be taken into account are as follows.

1. Will the value of the good remain stable as time passes, or will the passing of time in and of itself diminish or increase the value of the good to be distributed?
2. Is the good something that admits of sequential control or use, or will the very use that one makes of the good be something that destroys its utility for someone else? (This, of course, is the problem with the cake and the adolescents.)[18]

3. Will the fact that one's share of a good is limited by a finite time span interfere with one's ability to benefit from (or enjoy) that good? For example, if we could distribute one two-week vacation among twenty-eight stressed-out workaholics, it might be better to give each of them 1:28 odds of getting the whole vacation, rather than giving each of them half a day off. A half day of rest does no one any good; it might just make the workaholics more stressed out.

4. Will the span of time chosen to be the unit of distribution preserve the value of the good for all the persons to whom the good will be distributed? For example, having the right to sit in a seat in Notre Dame football stadium for the spring and summer, while someone else gets the seat for the fall and winter, does not spread the good equitably across the units of distribution.

As the discussion of the special dangers of using indirect units of distribution indicates, additional questions merit consideration when we are considering using time as an indirect distributive unit:

1. What is the availability (and the cost) of a direct method of dividing and measuring the good for distribution? For example, consider the purchase of legal services. It is better for lawyers to bundle their services by the project, rather than by the hour. It is the project that means something to the client; one hour of research, in and of itself, is not valuable.

2. How greatly does the indirect unit distort the meaning of the good being distributed through it? For example, consider the purchase of legal services billed by the hour. The first client who comes to a lawyer with a specific problem that needs a good deal of research will pay far more than the second client who presents it. Yet they both received the same thing, an answer to the very same problem.

3. How great is the possibility either that people will mistake the indirect unit of distribution for the direct unit, thereby distorting their perception of the good at stake, or the possibility that people will entirely lose sight of that good by believing that what they are distributing is in fact the indirect unit (time or money)? Lawyers who bill by the hour do become accustomed to seeing themselves as selling their *time*, rather than the power to change a client's situation through their services and expertise.

4. How important a good is at stake? Clearly, the good of professional legal or medical services is far more important than the good provided by a tanning salon. We may, therefore, be more willing to allow a tanning salon than a law firm to distribute its services in fifteen-minute increments.

Needless to say, these questions are not exhaustive. However, they may provide a helpful way to begin thinking about the appropriateness of using a particular distributive unit in order to allocate a particular good.

Using Temporal Units to Distribute Intensive Medical Services

When is it appropriate to use increments of time as a distributive unit in the case of intensive medical care? Addressing this question requires us to conjoin two sets of considerations developed in the foregoing pages: We need, in other words, to apply the analysis about the use of time as a direct or indirect method of distribution to our understanding of the specific nature of intensive care, which is the good to be distributed. As noted above, intensive care involves two of the three aspects of the polyvalent good of health care. Because it frequently involves an all-out effort to stabilize a patient after some sort of crisis, intensive care clearly has the purpose of restoring or preserving the health status of a particular individual in the face of a particular illness and injury. At the same time, because many intensive care patients are sharply confronted with the limits of their physical existence and the inevitability of death, the provision of corporal works of mercy is equally involved (or ideally, should be viewed as equally involved) in intensive care medicine. I believe that time is not an appropriate direct distributive method to use for either of these aspects of intensive health care.

With respect to intensive health care understood as having the purpose of restoring an individual's functioning, it is arbitrary to divide and distribute the skill, attention, and resources that are necessary to respond to an immediate medical crisis in units of time. In some persons, the crisis may take longer to resolve than in others. From the perspective of the patients receiving the good, the appropriate description is "they brought both my next door neighbor and me through heart surgery," not "they gave me three days of intensive care, and my neighbor got four days in the unit." By attempting to use time as the direct method of division, we obscure the fact that from a morally salient perspective based on the nature of the good distributed, both neighbors received precisely the same thing: restored physiological functioning and the ability to resume their day-to-day lives.

What about the aspect of intensive health care that is (or should be) understood as an aspect of corporal works of mercy? A key element of this aspect of health care is a resolve not to abandon the vulnerable person for whom one is caring. In this context, telling a person (or her loved ones) that she has a day, or a week, of intensive care is essentially equivalent to giving them an advance announcement of the date on which you will abandon them. (I am assuming here that discontinuing futile intensive care in favor of comfort care is not abandonment; but that discontinuing intensive care that is not futile and that is desired by the patient is experienced by the patient as abandonment.)

In addition, telling patients (or their families) that they have been allocated a certain time span of intensive care may make them focus on the wrong things at the time of illness, thereby interfering with both aspects of the good at stake. So doing may increase their anxiety, impeding their ability to get well and to achieve the first purpose of intensive health care. In addition, by calling to their attention the fact that the bond they have with caregivers is limited by a time span that bears no relationship to their need, they may be unable to receive their health care as a work of mercy. That inability may have serious, nonmedical consequences. As noted above, a primary facet of the third aspect of health care is solidarity, which has an essential communal component. One goal of health care as a corporal work of mercy is to affirm that the individuals receiving such care continue to belong to the human community, because their fragile physical state does not compromise their equal dignity as children of God. Moreover, if those who are seriously ill do not receive the gift of health care as a corporal work of mercy, they may not be enabled to undertake the task of setting in order their relationship with God and with other persons.

For all the reasons set forth above, we may concede that time cannot serve as a *direct* method of distributing intensive health care. Nonetheless, we might ask whether it nonetheless provides the best indirect method of distribution available to us at the current time. From my perspective, this shift in the nature of the argument would count as significant moral progress. Nonetheless, it is also important to keep in mind the risks involved in using time as an indirect method of distribution. Particularly in the current era of managed care, the dangers are great that some persons will mistake the good distributed by proxy for the good that is actually at stake. More specifically, the emphasis on efficiency in the delivery of health care may tempt patients and caregivers alike to think that health care is a good that is appropriately divided into temporal (or for that matter, monetary) increments. If things continue in this way, we will begin thinking that we are really distributing time and money (e.g., hours of professional time and insurance funds), not the complex good of health care. But that is not the case. For example, a person who has received an hour of a lazy, incompetent medical professional's time has received nothing, not a thing of inferior quality.

In a related manner, the danger of mistaking the proxy for the actual good raises the possibility that patients and physicians will be led to fundamental misunderstandings about the nature of the good that structures their relationship. When a patient makes an appointment with a physician, she does not make "a fifteen minute appointment"; she is not seeking "all the diagnosis she can get in fifteen minutes," but a careful and accurate diagnosis of her problem. To the extent that MCOs rigidly press physicians to conform to temporal increments in meeting their appointments without informing patients of this fact, the physician-patient relationship is taking root in misunderstanding, if not outright deceit.

Is there a more morally appropriate direct or indirect method to distribute health care that is also workable from a pragmatic perspective? This, of course, is the crucial question. I suggest that the best direct unit would be treatment for a specified medical problem. Each specific patient should receive what intensive care is necessary for *her* heart problem, not the number of days in the unit that the practice guidelines specify for patients in general. Temporal units (and financial units) such as those found in practice guidelines can be helpful benchmarks. The Medicare program's diagnosis-related groups (DRGs), which specify the number of hospital days normally required for particular medical problems, is also a legitimate approach—provided that enough room is left to accommodate "outliers." However, such benchmarks must retain their status as guidelines, and not assume the status of virtually unbendable rules governing medical decision making. The general media and health care trade publications are replete with stories of MCOs that rely exclusively on their own guidelines to determine the amount and intensity of care they provide for particular illnesses.

REDISTRIBUTION OF INTENSIVE MEDICAL SERVICES

The question of what method and unit of distribution is appropriate to a particular good is closely connected to the question of whether it is ever permissible to redistribute that good after an initial distribution. Any good that is not subject to consumption or destruction over time is subject to redistribution; it can be taken away from its initial recipients and given to others, perhaps using a different principle of distribution or employing a different unit of distribution. By redistributing a good, we maintain that our initial distributions are subject to later evaluation and correction in light of additional information.

General Considerations

As described more fully below, there are morally salient questions that arise with respect to the prospect of redistributing certain goods. However, it can be tempting to try to sidestep the special questions that arise in connection with redistribution of a good by deciding to distribute the good in smaller temporal units. Unfortunately, this does not solve the problem; it simply suppresses it. To see how questions of redistribution are routinely hidden by distributing the good in question in time-based units, consider the contrasting policies employed by two U.S. universities in distributing money to graduate students. When I was applying to graduate school, Yale University awarded entering graduate students five-year fellowships; they provided annual stipends for the length of their graduate studies. The University of Chicago, conversely, awarded fellowships on an annual basis; each year, a student was notified of the amount of her stipend for the coming year. Some students made out better as graduate school progressed, others did not do as well academically or financially. Was the University of Chicago, then, redistributing the good of graduate fellowships on a yearly basis? Was it taking fellowships away from some students in order to award them to others? At first glance, no redistribution questions are involved in the Chicago program at all; it appears only that Chicago was allocating its fellowships in smaller increments than Yale. More specifically, Chicago might have claimed that it had simply chosen to allocate its fellowship monies in units sufficient to subsidize one year of academic study, whereas Yale was making its allocations in larger units covering five years of schooling. In other words, Chicago might claim that redistribution was not an issue because it is not taking a fellowship away from one student and giving it to another, but simply awarding fellowships for shorter periods of time.

How do we determine, then, whether we are facing a situation where we need to deal with the moral implications of redistribution, or simply a situation, by now familiar, where the relevant good is being distributed in units measured by time? The by-now-familiar answer is to look to the nature of the good, and determine whether the unit being distributed will confer anything valuable on the recipient. In this case, the salient good is the opportunity to earn a doctorate in a humanistic discipline at a great university. Assuming that most students are not independently wealthy, and that they will not be able to pay off $100,000 in student loans on the salary of an assistant professor, a year's fellowship should be seen as the functional equivalent of the provision of a year's worth of graduate study itself. As we all know, the completion of one year of a Ph.D. program is good for little more than idle cocktail party conversation at the law firm's holiday party. Consequently, using the unit of time (an academic year) to distribute graduate fellowships makes very little sense. In this case, such use is best seen as a way of masking the redistribution questions that are actually at stake.

Accordingly, when we redescribe the policies of the two schools as redistribution questions, the moral issues at stake are sharply highlighted. At Yale, entering graduate students were awarded five-year fellowships that provided annual stipends for the duration of their graduate programs. Generally speaking, the awards were based on the perceived academic potential of the student. The constraints on redistribution were quite stringent. An entering student who received a fellowship did not need to worry about exhibiting the same degree of competence as she passed through the program as a condition of maintaining her funding. As long as she did not fail the program, the fellowship remained hers.[19] In contrast, at the University of Chicago, the students were reranked each year of the program, and their fellowships were readjusted accordingly. Although there was some presumption in favor of continuing financial support at the level the student received in the prior year, redistribution could and did occur.

As the foregoing example illustrates, there are two ethically salient questions that arise in a situation where redistribution of a good is under consideration. First, what types of events will trigger the possibility of redistributing the good? Second, should there be any preference in favor of the person already in possession? Each of these issues will be considered in turn.

Triggers for a Redistributive Decision

The first question that must be asked is what events will trigger consideration of whether or not to redistribute the good in question. Generally, the question of redistribution arises in two ways. First, we can acquire new information about the good or the person to whom we have distributed the good that was true but unknown at the time of distribution. We may discover, for example, that the patient who was admitted to the ICU does not have adequate health insurance. Second, as time goes on, circumstances can change. Sometimes, the change has to do with the recipient of the good, such as a patient who is not benefiting as much from intensive care as was predicted at the time of admission to the ICU. Sometimes, the change relates to the good itself; for example, reductions in health care expenditures could force downsizing in ICUs. And sometimes, the change involves the appearance of a new potential recipient of the good. What do we do, for example, when a new candidate for intensive care presents herself at the doors of a full ICU?

Circumstances continually change, of course, and new information potentially relevant to the distribution constantly becomes available. How do we deal with this phenomenon? One way is to establish a series of intervals at which the option of redistribution will be considered. For example, depending upon the good, one could review a distribution on a daily, weekly, monthly, or yearly basis. Another way is to identify specific events the knowledge of whose occurrence will trigger the possibility of redistribution. In deciding what will trigger that possibility, we need to pay attention to the value of additional information. It makes no sense to redistribute on the basis of information that is not reliable. Most important, in assessing the value of new information, we need to keep in mind the relationship between the good being distributed and the overarching purpose of the distribution.

For example, Yale holds that it is never appropriate to redistribute a fellowship from one student to another as long as the first student remains a doctoral student in good standing. Chicago holds that it is appropriate to do so after one year of study. Why not after a semester, a month, or the first week of class? Clearly, the first week of graduate school does not tell us much about the student's academic potential. But what does performance during the first year in graduate school tell us? Maybe something about how that student will do in this particular program, but not necessarily very much about her future contributions to academic life as a researcher or teacher. Active membership in the academic community is ultimately the purpose of a doctorate in the humanities, which is the good being distributed. Redistribution of fellowships on an annual basis is not likely to serve this goal.

We also need to consider the effects of redistribution upon the value of the good. What sort of influence will the possibility that redistribution will occur, as well as the timing of that redistribution, have on the ability of the initial recipients to make use of the good? Yale graduate students would argue that they are freer to pursue risky research projects and to work in a collaborate manner with each other, because they do not face the pressure of reearning their fellowships annually. They might further contend that redistribution of fellowships would force them to hide the fact that intellectual growth does not take place in a linear manner that is easily graphed, but by fits and starts. Chicago students might respond that such pressure concentrates their minds, forcing them to prove their mettle. From their perspective, the predictable redistribution of funds means that everything does not ride on the pattern of fits and starts that had demonstrated itself before they applied to graduate school.

Advantage to the Person in Possession

The second basic question that must be asked in face of the possibility of redistribution is what sort of advantage should be given to the person currently in possession of the good? Several issues are salient here. First, there is the matter of whether the person who received the good through the initial distribution has come somehow justifiably to rely on that good. Has she understandably restructured her life plans in a way that depends upon that good, which would be difficult to undo if the good were suddenly removed? Second, there is the question of whether the distributor has behaved in a way that implies a promise to continue furnishing the good. Third, there are issues pertaining to the broader relationship between the distributor and the initial recipient. In the course of the time frame spanning the initial distribution, has a relationship of trust and fidelity developed that would be violated if the good were reallocated? Fourth, there are issues of justice arising from shifting power relationships that need to be taken into account. At the time of the redistribution, is one party markedly more vulnerable and the other considerably more powerful, than was the case at the time of the initial distribution? If this is the case, then there may be an additional reason to limit the possibility of redistribution.

As anyone with some familiarity with legal concepts probably recognizes by now, the questions and categories I have just invoked to guide our thinking on the question of redistribution are drawn largely from the domain of contract law.[20] Legal scholars have commonly distinguished among a range of relationships according to the ability of the parties to redistribute the good that mediates that relationship. At one end of the spectrum, we find contractual relationships. The parties themselves form an agreement that specifies how long, and on what terms, one party is obliged to provide a good or service to the other. You and I may enter into a long-term output contract that requires me to sell you all of the tomatoes I grow for the next twenty years. In effect, entering into a contract to provide a particular good limits one's power of redistribution with respect to that good, according to the terms agreed upon by the parties. The general rule is that absent such a contractual relationship, the goods or services in question are freely redistributable. Absent a legally enforceable agreement, the fact that I sell you my crop of fresh tomatoes today generally does not mean that you have a claim on the tomatoes I harvest next month.

Nonetheless, contract law has developed certain other doctrines that set limits upon the power of one party to redistribute the good in question at the expense of another party, particularly in the context of an ongoing relationship. Some of these doctrines include *promissory estoppel*, which takes into account the reliance that one party has placed on the other's express or implied promise to continue providing the good in question; substantive and procedural unconscionability, which takes into account the fairness of decisions to alter previous patterns of providing a good; and public policy, which considers the social importance of the relationship and the good in question.

At the other end of the spectrum of the possibility of redistribution, we find what have come to be called (in legal parlance) status relationships. Society has decided that some relationships mediate goods that must be preserved from redistribution in virtually all circumstances. In American culture, marriage used to be such a relationship; perhaps the parent-child relationship still is one. In other words, one way of thinking about the goods involved in marriage and parenthood is in terms of the constraints that both institutions place on redistribution. After making an initial choice to marry this particular person, or to bear this particular child, an individual cannot decide five or ten years later to "trade in" her spouse or her child and redistribute her marital or parental affections in an entirely different direction. Marriage and parenthood are (or used to be) known as "status" relationships, rather than contractual relationships, precisely because once distributed, the goods they mediate cannot be taken away and redistributed.

How do we decide where a particular good belongs on the spectrum from liberal redistribution to restricted redistribution? The factors set forth in the context of the graduate fellowship example possess significant explanatory power for settled cases, and provide helpful guidance for situations we have yet to consider. For example, to support the traditional view of marriage as a "status" relationship, one might argue the good of fidelity, a key element of marriage and parenthood, is thoroughly undermined by the creation of an opportunity for redistribution. Furthermore, at the time a redistribution is desired by one party, the other is likely to be far more vulnerable and to have relied to a greater extent on the initial distribution (in marriage, this party is usually the woman).

Application to Intensive Medical Care

How do these general reflections on the factors involved in redistributing a good bear on the specific questions of whether and when redistribution is appropriate with respect to the good of intensive medical care? As a preliminary matter, we should emphasize that the question of the moral permissibility of *redistribution* of intensive care resources is distinct from the issue of what principle of distribution should be applied to determine initial admission to the ICU. One can decide that patients must achieve a certain score on the APACHE III index or other scale in order to receive a bed. In and of itself, however, that decision says nothing about whether redistribution should be permissible, and if so, what the criteria should be.[21] This separate issue should be analyzed in terms of the two general redistribution questions outlined above.

First, what types of events are likely to trigger the possibility of redistribution? In some cases, the answer is absolutely clear, such as when a patient dies or when intensive care is medically futile.[22] But in other cases, we need to formulate an answer to this question. Do redistribution possibilities arise after a set period of time, such as a day or a week, in which we gather and assess a patient's progress? Are they triggered by a particular event intrinsic to the patient's condition, such as when her status takes a sudden, marked turn for the worse? Or are they raised when an event external to a patient's condition occurs, such as the arrival of a new patient who needs the bed?

The second set of questions involves what type of preference the patient already occupying the bed, already in possession of the good, should receive. One could say that, like Yale, a very high score is required to receive the good, and a very bad performance is required to lose it. With this approach, a patient admitted to an ICU bed would be virtually guaranteed to keep it, as long as the care she received was not futile. In effect, she would be protected against the vicissitudes of her performance on the scales of medical progress, and the competition of others who seek the same attention. Or one could adopt Chicago's approach, giving the patient currently in possession of the bed little or no preference at the time of redistribution. A third approach would be to develop a hybrid framework. For example, we could require a certain score on APACHE III or similar index for initial admission to the ICU. Furthermore, if there are two patients presenting for initial admission and only one available bed, we could award the bed to the person with the better score (rather than by lottery). However, once a patient has gained admission to the ICU, she would not be deprived of her bed simply because someone comes along with a better score. To lose her bed, a patient would need to fall below a minimum cutoff score (which might be the same or lower than the cutoff score required for initial admission) and have a score that is substantially lower than a new person presenting for care.

What are the salient factors in formulating answers to the foregoing two redistribution questions? First, we need to assess how knowledge of the possible redistribution will affect the patient's ability to reap the benefits of intensive care. Will redistribution on a rigidly scheduled basis (e.g., daily) impede the ability of patients to benefit medically from intensive care by creating anxiety about whether or not they will pass the next text? Will redistribution on a scheduled basis focus the attention of patients and their families away from other matters that merit their concern (e.g., coming to grips with mortality)? Will the implementation of a schedule of redistribution prevent caregivers from appropriately investing themselves in the welfare of patients currently in their charge?

Second, we also need to consider how the equitable issues fall out in this situation. Does the patient or her surrogate decision maker "rely" on the prospect of continued intensive care in making the decision to submit herself and her family members to the physical and psychological battles associated with such care? What types of promises, express or implied, have the caregivers made to the patient and her family in order to elicit the best response to intensive care? How does the redistributive scheme affect the trust and confidence necessary to establish a successful caregiver-patient relationship? Will the prospect of redistribution erode that trust? Will a patient who has been and wishes to continue receiving intensive care experience involuntary removal as abandonment? Finally, we need to consider all of these questions in light of the change in the relative balance of power between the distributor and the recipient of the good of intensive care. It seems that after a patient has suffered the ordeal involved in intensive care as part of the battle to save her own life, she is far more vulnerable than she was before making the emotional and physical investment in that particular fight. Such a patient is subject to the pressures and disappointments of being forced to relinquish a half-completed project that has already required a substantial degree of her courage and integrity. In developing the answers to these questions of equity, it might be fruitful to place them in a broader context by asking a more holistic question. Where on the spectrum from contractual to status relationships do we believe the bond between the givers and the recipients of medical care should be located?

A responsible exploration of the questions identified in the foregoing paragraphs would need to draw upon empirical data as well as philosophical and theological reflection, and is beyond the scope of this essay. Let me express, however, my own intuition that such an exploration will support the judgment that we should greatly limit opportunities for redistribution in intensive care medicine, other than in cases of medical futility.[23] Put another way, we should be very hesitant before allowing MCOs to institute a series of timed reviews that routinely provide them with opportunities for redistribution, as well as the authorization to deprive patients of intensive care that they are currently receiving, continue to want, and arguably benefits them.

CONCLUSION

This essay has attempted to consider the role played by time in questions of distributive justice. I have argued that the choice of the method and unit of distribution always has an ethical dimension to it. More specifically, I have contended that there are significant reasons to be worried about the use of time as either a direct or an indirect method of distributing the good of intensive medical care; such use can distort our understanding of the nature of this good and warp the relationships among the patients and caregivers that are created around its distribution. Furthermore, I have contended that the moral appropriateness of redistributing a good involves questions distinct from, although superficially similar to, the choice to make the initial distribution of that good in terms of temporal units. I believe that a policy allowing redistribution of intensive medical care is fraught with moral danger, particularly when considered in light of the equitable considerations articulated by contract law to guide the redistribution of goods.

Medical ethicists have long worried about the contours of the fidelity owed by physicians to their patients. In some instances, the virtues embodied in a physician's fidelity to a particular patient are depicted as conflicting with the claims of distributive justice, and in particular with the claims of other patients who might be able to make more cost-effective use of the physician's talents. One way of construing the objective of this paper is as attenuating, if not dissolving, this apparent conflict between fidelity and distributive justice. As this paper has argued, questions of time are central to the problem of distributive justice. We frequently must decide whether a particular good (such as intensive care) can appropriately be divided into temporal units, or whether that good is a suitable candidate for redistribution once a particular number of hours or days have passed. Time is also central to fidelity, which is after all, the virtue that assures the presence of a good throughout the vicissitudes of time and change. From this perspective, it becomes clear that, far from being in competition with distributive justice, fidelity to the nature of the good being distributed and the relationships mediated through that good is at its very core.

NOTES

1. The "we" in this question, of course, is ambiguous. On the one hand, each nation needs to develop general policies that will help constitute the standard of care within its borders. On the other, each health care institution needs to set specific policies that are consistent with its own particular values. For an argument that insufficient attention has been made to the institutional context in which allocation decisions are made, and a call for religious institutions to pay more attention to their own ethos in making them, see the essay in this volume by Khushf.
2. Pope John Paul II held that "Not only must human life not be taken, it must be protected with loving concern" (1995, para. 81). In his essay in this volume, Seifert explores the connection between respect for human dignity and the negative moral absolutes forcefully articulated by the pope (John Paul II 1993, 1995).
3. See David Hollenbach, S.J.: "[Social justice] calls for the creation of those social, economic and political conditions which are necessary to assure that the minimum human needs of all will be met and which will make possible social and political participation for all" (Hollenbach 1979, 152). See the essay in this volume by Honnefelder for a discussion of the right to health care within the context of other human rights, as well as a discussion of what respect for human dignity (the foundation for all rights) requires in the case of patients in a persistent vegetative state.
4. "Basic justice demands the establishment of minimum levels of participation in the life of the human community for all persons" (U.S. Conference of Catholic Bishops 1986, para. 77).
5. Of course, the translation of a moral right to health care into a politically enforceable right in a particular society is a complex process. First, it should be noted that Catholic political theory does not limit the role of government to protecting negative rights; it understands the purpose of the political state as fostering the common good—defined by the Second Vatican Council as "the sum total of social conditions which allow people, either as groups or as individuals, to reach their fulfillment more fully and more easily" (Flannery 1988, *Gaudium et Spes* §26).

    Second, because of the great emphasis placed on participation in community, the principle of subsidiarity directs that issues be dealt with by the smallest and most local social unit capable of handling the problem. Larger social units should step in only if their breadth and strength of influence is necessary in order to secure an aspect of the common good that cannot be secured in another way. Consequently, although it would be ideal if smaller social or political units could ensure persons access to basic health care, Catholic thought imposes no theoretical barrier to the implementation of a national health care policy if smaller and more localized approaches prove ineffective. Third, the nature and scope of the obligation of a particular political regime to provide health care will of course vary, depending upon its resources and the weight of securing other elements of the common good for its citizens.
6. A pressing question that Catholic moralists have only begun to explore is how govern-

ments can rightly raise the funds they need to make goods such as health care widely available. See the essay in this volume by Wildes.

7. Indeed, if the community is not meeting the other basic needs of its population, it has an obligation to do so before subsidizing more advanced levels of health care.

8. The Roman Catholic casuistical tradition has not thus far focused on the question when patients may legitimately be *denied* medical treatment that they would prefer to receive. Instead, its focus has been on a different issue: when patients may legitimately *refuse* medical treatment that they do not wish to receive. In his essay in this volume, Boyle develops the Catholic tradition to shed light on questions of limiting access to medical care. See the essay in this volume by Rössler for a Lutheran perspective on this issue, which is skeptical that the conflicting interests of patients, physicians, and social institutions endemic to distribution problems can ever be resolved in this fallen world.

9. The Medicare program now ensures that no one who needs kidney dialysis will be excluded for financial reasons from obtaining it. It does not afford such blanket access to other types of life-saving treatment. For an argument that society chooses a few discrete cases to affirm symbolically its conviction that human life is priceless, while subjecting the vast majority of measures to preserve life to an economic cost-benefit analysis, see Calabresi and Bobbit (1978).

10. I am pondering the possibility that "to each according to need" may not be the only principle we need in order to distribute health care justly. As discussed below in the text, health care is a polyvalent good. Some aspects of health care (i.e., caring for those who cannot be cured) clearly should be distributed according to need. Other aspects of health care (i.e., measures designed to improve the health of populations) might appropriately be distributed according to the principle "to each according to what will most benefit the whole." Health care designed to cure or ameliorate the health problems of particular individuals may be a more complicated case, requiring a multitiered analysis. We should probably put our money into developing cures for those diseases that most impede the common good, considering both the severity of the disease and the number of people who suffer from it. (From the perspective of the common good, it may be more important to develop a cure for the common cold than for certain lethal, rare, and highly publicized diseases.) After a treatment protocol has been developed, it should be distributed to those who suffer according to the criterion of need.

11. Looking back at the discussions of distributive justice in U.S. medical ethics during the past thirty years, it is understandable that the ethical relevance of the unit of distribution chosen and of the permissibility of redistribution have not received sustained consideration. These discussions have frequently focused on the microallocation question of how we should distribute a limited number of donor organs among the greater number of persons who need transplants. This issue creates a deceptively simple model of the decision-making process. First, in the case of organ distribution, it is easy to sidestep the question of how to *divide up* the thing to be distributed. The answer is so obvious as not to merit explicit discussion. We know that we must distribute the whole organ to one person; we cannot give one third of it Moe, one third to Larry, and one third to Curly. Second, the organ-distribution question also allows us to sidestep redistribution questions. It would be unthinkable to give Moe the heart for a year, then remove it and give it to Larry for the next year, and then remove it a second time and give it to Curly for the third year; the question never explicitly arises.

12. It may be that the specification of the polyvalent good of health care must take into account cultural differences in a way that is beyond the scope of this paper. In his essay in this volume, Heisig reminds us that Catholic moral vision cannot simply accept the in-

evitability of the model of health and well-being on which the most highly developed medical techniques and equipment rest, and then do its best to get a hearing at the highest levels when it comes to the question of how to use the tools. "At some point this will mean shifting the weight of its tradition and its resources toward protecting and encouraging alternative models of the healthy person and the medical vocation" (301). Distinctively Catholic resources have the most to offer with respect to the third aspect of the good of health care, which focuses upon its role as a corporal work of mercy.

13. For an exposition of the virtue of solidarity from the perspective of the Louvain personalist school, see the essay in this volume by Schotsmans.

14. For Christians, the time of illness and the prospect of impending death have a theological meaning, rooted in Christ's own suffering and death. For a theological analysis of the Christian meaning of suffering and its implications for contemporary Western medicine, see the essay in this volume by Hughes. Not surprisingly, the Christian belief that Christ overcame sin and death through his own suffering and dying relativizes the value of earthly life. Compare Hughes's view with the value of human life from a Jewish perspective, as articulated in the essay in this volume by Rie.

15. As Taboada notes in her essay in this volume, a major study (SUPPORT) has demonstrated that far too many Americans die in a way that is deeply inconsistent with the Christian vision of dying well, in part because physicians do not respect their wishes to decline measures such as cardiopulmonary respiration.

16. Other units of distribution are conceivable. For example, sometimes, a lottery can be a *principle* of distribution. At other times, however, dividing a thing into chances at having the whole thing can be a way of coming up with a *unit* of distribution when every other way will destroy the good to be distributed. Examples include the last seat on the plane out of Casablanca, and old movies about which cowboy gets to marry the only girl in town.

17. Sometimes, of course, time and money can both be direct units of distribution. To draw again upon an example noted above, when we distribute a toy among toddlers by giving each one a specified period to play with it, we are using time as a direct unit. When we divide a certain amount of scholarship funds among qualified candidates, we are using money in that way.

18. An example of a good that meets this criterion and therefore is suitable for division in temporal units is property, where the law allows one person to have a life estate in a piece of land, which after her death reverts in fee simple to another person.

19. At the same time, a student who does better than was predicted at the time of her entry to the program generally could not acquire a better fellowship for the remainder of her course of study.

20. For an explanation of these principles, see Farnsworth 1999.

21. The academic institution of tenure is a vivid example of this point.

22. I realize, of course, that the concept of futility is not unproblematic. The Society for Critical Care Medicine's Ethics Committee recommends defining futile treatment narrowly, as a treatment that will not accomplish its attended goal. It cautions against the temptation to use the term "futile" to mask moral and financial judgments about the desirability of treatment (1997, 887–91).

23. The prospect of redistribution in other than cases involving futile care also seems to be problematic from a Jewish perspective. See the essay in this volume by Dagi, in which he contends that the Jewish tradition of medical ethics would endorse the principle that "measures intended to save the life of one individual are not to be compromised in order to rescue another" (230).

BIBLIOGRAPHY

Boyle, J. 1987. The concept of health and the right to health care. In *On Moral Medicine*, edited by Stephen E. Lammers and Allen Verhey. Grand Rapids, Mich.: Eerdmans.

Calabresi, G., and P. Bobbit. 1978. *Tragic Choices.* New York: W. W. Norton.

Farnsworth, E. A. 1999. *Contracts,* 3d ed. New York: Aspen Publishers.

Flannery, A., ed. 1988. *Vatican Council II: The Conciliar and Post Conciliar Documents.* Northport, N.Y.: Costello Publishing Co.

Hollenbach, D. 1979. *Claims in Conflict.* New York: Paulist Press.

John Paul II. 1993. *Veritatis Splendor.* Boston: Pauline Books and Media.

———. 1995. *Evangelium Vitae.* Boston: Pauline Books and Media.

Knaus, W. A., D. Wagner, E. Draper, J. Zimmerman, M. Bergner, P. Bastos, C. Sirio, D. Murphy, T. Lotring, and A. Damiano. 1991. The APACHE III prognostic system: Risk prediction of hospital mortality for critically ill hospitalized adults. *Chest* 100: 1619–35.

Outka, G. 1987. Social justice and equal access to health care. In *On Moral Medicine*, ed. by Stephen E. Lammers and Allen Verhey. Grand Rapids, Mich.: Eerdmans.

Society for Critical Care Medicine Ethics Committee. 1994. Consensus statement on the triage of critically ill patients. *Journal of the American Medical Association* 271 (15): 1200–1203.

———. 1997. Consensus statement of the Society for Critical Care Medicine's Ethics Committee regarding futile and other possibly inadvisable treatments. *Critical Care Medicine* 25: 887–91.

U.S. Conference of Catholic Bishops. 1986. *Economic Justice for All.* Washington, D.C.: U.S. Catholic Conference.

Walzer, M. 1983. *Spheres of Justice.* New York: Basic Books.

Creating Critical Care Resources: Implications for Distributive Justice

Kevin W. Wildes, S.J.

Intensive care medicine is, in many ways, an icon of contemporary Western, scientific medicine. In the last half of the twentieth century, modern medicine was transformed in its self-understanding and public perception. Unlike medicine of the past, contemporary medicine defines itself, and is defined by the curative goal. Western societies have come to expect that medicine will cure diseases and illnesses. And, in both the popular and professional imaginations, medical cures are linked with sophisticated technological interventions. Intensive care medicine embodies both the hope for cure in the face of life-threatening sickness and the use of sophisticated technological intervention to achieve the cure. They are the place of many modern medical miracles.

These expectations, of cure with the aid of medical technology, embodied in the intensive care unit (ICU), carry a dark side, however. When facing death, medicine has no cure to offer. Death is a defeat for medicine in a model of curative medicine. When death looms, the temptation is to bring to bear medical technology, even when cure is impossible or there is no hope of any meaningful recovery. In this way, defeat is put off. But such interventions are costly. They consume resources and other opportunities and can exact a human cost from those patients and families directly involved.

The allocation of resources for intensive care medicine poses an important set of ethical questions. How these questions are answered will have a very direct impact on those who might benefit from such medical interventions. Furthermore, the answers to these questions are important because intensive care medicine can easily consume a great deal of a society's medical resources and has implications for the development and distribution of other goods. Developing ethical policy for allocating these resources is important because it has a very direct impact on the lives of patients and on the practice of health care in general.

One way to approach the question about allocating ICU resources is to consider how to develop criteria that establish limits on what amount of resources can and cannot be distributed to patients. On the local level, the question needs to be asked: How should ICU resources be distributed? One finds this approach embodied in the attempts to develop futility policies. Such policies attempt to articulate principles that govern the use and distribution of our resources.

Another approach is to ask what principles should govern the development of resources for critical care medicine. On the national level, the question needs to be asked: How much of the national resources devoted to health care should be dedicated to ICU medicine? Decisions about developing resources will shape the criteria for the distribution of the resources to patients. If one begins by asking about the development of resources, one situates the question of distributions in a different context. By framing the question in this way, the Roman Catholic tradition on social justice becomes a rich source for reflection. Yet social justice is a line of thought that is often overlooked or confused with distributive justice. However, rather than address the questions of distribution, the category of social justice asks questions about how a society, and the distribution of goods, ought to be organized.

In addressing issues of allocation, one element that must be taken into consideration is who, or what organization, has authority over the resources that are to be distributed. There are at least three levels of organization that are important for this approach to allocation. In some way, each level gives different criteria and guidance on limiting resources that might be useful to thinking about intensive care medicine. One level is the personal level. How much of my own resources ought I use for intensive care? This level has been richly addressed in the church's traditional distinction of ordinary and extraordinary means. This tradition, however, will be of limited use in shaping social policy. I have argued elsewhere that the distinction is a personal one and that it is patient centered (Wildes 1996, 1998; Meilaender 1997). The distinction is helpful in addressing the question of allocation insofar as it reminds us that any treatment, ordinary or extraordinary, must offer some "hope of health." However, beyond this necessary condition, determining if a treatment is ordinary (morally required) or not turns on a weighing of the benefits and burdens of the treatment that must be done by a patient or his surrogates. This distinction is not, I would argue, a place to find guidance on the issue of allocating intensive care resources within Catholic thought.

A second level of organization is that of institutions such as hospitals and health care systems. At this level, decisions about how to allocate resources will turn on at least two key elements. One key will be the social and political context of an institution. The other will be the mission and identity of an institution or organization. How an institution understands itself, and its mission, will shape the way it uses its resources. An institution dedicated to the care of the poor, for example, may decide to use none of its resources for intensive care medicine (Wildes 1997).

A third level of organization for the question of resources is that of public policy for civil society and the decisions made by civil society in developing resources for intensive care medicine. This level is the focus of this essay. In this area, the church's social teaching and its assumptions will give some general guidance about the development and distribution of intensive care resources. This essay argues that, although the tradition gives some general guidance, it will not give much specific guidance regarding the allocation of such resources. Indeed, the tradition will leave open the question of whether or not a society should even develop such resources. This essay argues that the social teachings give great flexibility to a society and how it might develop and deploy its health care resources. (In point of fact, one could well argue within the Roman Catholic tradition that a society ought not invest in critical care resources while there are populations of human beings who do not have access to basic medical resources.) This essay examines Catholic thought and how it might guide a society's decisions to put resources into health care in general and intensive care in particular. The essay argues that Roman Catholic reflections on taxation, the common good, and social justice give guidance to a society in developing and allocating goods in health care.

This essay argues that the moral justifications for the development of such resources in some way directs how they are distributed. The essay examines the moral justification for the development of public resources for health care and what guidelines for distribution might be gleaned from the development of resources. What gives societies and governments the moral justification to impose taxes? What are the proper ends of taxation? Is health care such an end? What guidance, if any, do the theological arguments about taxation and health care give to arguments about the distribution of resources? One could argue that we need to ask what is an appropriate use of a society's resources and what is an appropriate use of individual and personal resources. What guidance can the Roman Catholic tradition give to those thinking about these questions?

THE DEVELOPMENT OF PUBLIC GOODS AND THE JUSTIFICATION OF TAXES

It is important to remember that Roman Catholic thought has long recognized a distinction between the state and civil society. Civil society logically precedes the state, and the state is to serve the needs of civil society. For this essay, because we are concerned with developing policy for allocating critical care resources, I am assuming that a crucial element in the development of health care resources will be the efforts of the government working on behalf of civil society.[1] Such theological reflections on taxation can be helpful in focusing questions about the appropriateness of developing critical care resources. These reflections give guidance about why taxes can be levied and the limits to taxation. In Catholic thought, the redistribution of wealth through taxation depends upon an appeal to basic human goods and needs that is embedded in the discussion of the common good. Second, a justification of taxation makes certain assumptions about the nature and function of the state. Third, it embodies some understanding of justice. Taxation can take place in different forms. It can be by direct taxation but it can also take place by indirect public investment such as tax exemption for nonprofit entities.

Basic Human Needs

Roman Catholic moral thought has argued consistently, although in different moral languages, for the dignity of the human person. The anthropological assumptions of Roman Catholic moral theology and social teaching are central for understanding the argument supporting the development of health care resources. Health care is viewed as one of the basic human needs or goods that are required for men and women to live with human dignity.

Roman Catholic thought has worked out of a philosophical anthropology, which has supported, in turn, different ethical methodologies. The tradition assumes that there is a basic human nature that can be known by reason. Furthermore, there are obligations, on the part of society, to respect the basic human nature. Catholicism supports at least two complementary forms of discourse in ethics. Traditionally set in the language of natural law, Catholic views of human nature, though articulated in diverse ways, lead to both negative proscriptions and positive duties for human behavior. There is a positive duty to preserve one's health, for example. Natural law does not exhaust, nor is it the only language used to frame discussions of basic human nature found in the Roman Catholic tradition. The tradition has also deployed the language of virtue to articulate a vision of what are the basic parameters of human flourishing and acting. The virtue of charity supports the obligation to see that the basic needs of others are met. The social justice tradition attempts to move the discussion in a somewhat different direction insofar as it asks about the basic conditions that are necessary for human flourishing and society's responsibilities to men and women in realizing these basic conditions. Social justice builds on the natural law tradition in that it develops the assumptions about the need for basic human goods. This development in the tradition has found expression in the language of human rights.

The social justice tradition in Catholic thought assumes that there are basic human needs and these needs create moral obligations on the part of society toward members of the society. It must be noted that this language of "needs" is open to many different interpretations. One must make certain assumptions about what it is to be human in order to identify those needs that are *basic*. Within the tradition itself there are different accounts of natural basic needs of men and women (e.g., Grisez 1974; John Paul II 1995; Ashley and O'Rourke 1997).

Saint Thomas Aquinas gives a simple classification of these basic human needs (1951; *ST* I-II, q. 94, a. 2). There is the need to preserve life. There is the need to procreate. There is the need to know truth. Finally, there is a need to live in society. It should be noted that this list represents a mixture of needs for the human race as a species and as individuals. In the modern papal encyclicals and episcopal statements on social issues, there has been a further development of the category of basic human goods. In recent years, the Roman Catholic tradition has been quite at home with a tie between human rights, as expressed in the United Nations general declaration (1940) and concerns expressed in the language of basic human needs/goods. One could argue that the language of human rights is based on a set of assumptions about basic human needs (Ashley and O'Rourke 1997, 114).

The anthropology used in Roman Catholic thought supports the idea that we can discover the basic, essential nature of what it is to be human. As such, we can identify basic human needs. In light of these assumptions, the virtue of charity helps to articulate an obligation of society to meet the basic needs of the members of a society. Within this tradition, there is the view that governments should act when the actions of individuals are not sufficient to meet the basic needs of all men and women.

The Common Good

The notion of the common good in Catholic thought is rooted in the ancient world. Most notably, it is found in the work of Aristotle and Cicero, who argued that for the polis to flourish there needs to be more than minimal cooperation. Indeed, Cicero spoke of the *res publica* as a partnership for the common good. In Catholic thought, Augustine and Aquinas take the notion and expand on it. They give the notion of common good a theocentric interpretation. The commandment to love one's neighbor is a commitment to the common good that goes beyond any particular polis.

Within the social justice tradition, there is an ongoing assumption about the common good, and the appeal to the common good has played an essential role in thinking through the obligations of civil society in meeting the basic needs of men and women (Quinn 2000). The idea of the common good balances the insights of modern liberal thought and communitarianism. It supports the liberal view of individual freedom. However, it situates that freedom within the context of a community. The notion of common good requires the community to meet the basic needs of the individual in order to assure the exercise of liberty. David Hollenbach has argued that contemporary talk of the common good, in the Catholic tradition, has taken place within the language of human rights (Hollenbach 1989).

In recent official writings, one finds two interpretations of the common good at work. The first, clearly stated in *Gaudium et Spes* (Abbot 1966b), is that human beings were created by God for the formation of social unity (#32). They were not created to live in isolation. The common good is a social reality in which all persons should participate. There is a theme of the participation of all in the benefits of the common good. The common good is the set of conditions that facilitate social living, by which persons are enabled to more fully and readily achieve their perfection (*Mater et Magister* #65 [John XXIII 1995a] and *Gaudium et Spes* #26 [Abbot 1966b]). In more recent writings, the language of human rights has been used to define participation in the common good. In *Pacem in Terris,* John XXIII (1995b) clearly sees medical care as part of the common good. He writes: "Beginning our discussion of the rights of man, we see that even man has a right to life, to bodily integrity, and to the means which are suitable for the proper development of life; these are primarily food, clothing, shelter, rest, medical care, and finally the necessary social services" (#11). John Paul II reaffirms the vision of John XXIII in *Pacem in Terris* when he speaks about the right of working people to health care which is cheap (#19). He then goes on to tie medical care within the context of labor. In 1981, the U.S. Catholic Conference (1981) called health care "a basic right which flows from the sanctity of human life" (#2).

The Goods of Creation

The link between basic human goods and civil society's obligation to meet these needs is further supported by a theology of creation that shapes the tradition's views about private property. The tradition makes an assumption about the commonality of the creation that is central to its reflections on topics such as basic human needs and private property. Since the nineteenth century, the Catholic tradition has supported a notion of private property but always understood private property within limits and never as an absolute. In *Rerum Novarum*, Leo XIII (1995) wrote: "For every man has by nature the right to possess property as his own. This is one of the chief points of distinction between man and the animal creation. For the brute has no power of self-direction. . . . It is the mind, or the reason, which is the chief thing in us who are humans . . . it is this which makes a human being human and distinguishes him essentially and completely from the brute" (#5). Citing Thomas Aquinas, Leo holds that private property is not only lawful but necessary (1995, #20; Aquinas 1951, *ST* II II, q. 66, a. 2). Nonetheless, the right to private property is not an absolute right. It is limited by the needs of others. A society is required to see that others have access to the basic human goods and the right to private property can be limited by this more basic right. Again, the starting point is the dignity of the human person and what is needed for a minimally decent human life. It is the obligation of society to ensure that all humans have the minimum necessities required for human existence.

One should be careful not to assume that because there is a commitment to basic human needs and goods, that a society must have a large governmental structure. Indeed, the tradition is flexible. It repeatedly speaks of the need to consider the context of time and circumstances. The principle of subsidiarity, emphasizing the importance of local action and the obligation of general structures to assist the local structures, implies that the first responsibility in meeting human needs is with the free and competent individual, then with the local group. Other, more complex levels of community and society must contribute when local levels cannot assume its duties or refuse to do so.

The picture that emerges in the Roman Catholic tradition is that there are certain needs that are basic to all human beings and there are obligations to see that these needs are met. In *Dignitatis Humanae* (Abbot 1966a), the Second Vatican Council wrote: "The common welfare of society consists in the entirety of those conditions of social life under which men enjoy the possibility of achieving their own perfection in a certain fullness of measure and also with some relative ease" (#6). Many such needs can be met at levels of the family or voluntary association. However, such groups may not be able to meet these needs and require assistance of others or society as a whole. Governmental structures grow out of these natural associations and respond to the need to meet basic human needs.

The Nature of the State

A central assumption in Roman Catholic thought is that the state, though it may take different forms, is "natural." The state is not established simply because of humanity's fallen nature. Instead, the state, as part of the social, associational life of human beings, is part of the natural order of creation. The end and purpose of the state is to promote the welfare of its citizens. Thomas Aquinas writes that "Laws are said to be just, from the end, when, to wit, they are ordained to the common good—and from their author, that is to say, when the law that is made does not exceed the power of the lawgiver—and from their form, when, to wit, burdens are laid on the subjects, according to an equality of proportion and with a view to the common good" (1951, *STI*, q. 96, a. 4). Elsewhere, Thomas speaks of the "community of the state" (*STI*, q. 96, a. 1). The purpose of the social order is not order for its own sake but for those who are ordered. "The state exists and functions for the sake of human beings. It attains this end primarily by safeguarding those interests that are *common* to all persons under its jurisdiction" (Ryan and Boland 1950, 127).

The Roman Catholic position on the state can be described as a "middle of the road" position between collectivism and individualism. Individualism, on many accounts, does not give enough importance to the social nature of human beings. At the same time, collectivism does not pay sufficient attention to the individual. Nor does it take into account the different groups that exist in society. Charles Curran has written that "human society is unique because it is a whole made of by other wholes" (Curran 1987, 99). Within this tradition, there are important natural associations and communities like the family and voluntary communities. These natural associations form boundaries for the authority of the state and, as we shall see below, direct certain positive duties of the state.

The measure of state functions, therefore, is to be found in the necessities of the human and the inability of the individual or the family to provide these necessities. Anything, therefore, which is necessary, whether for the individual or for society at large, and which the individual or the family is not in a position to supply, may legitimately be regarded as included in the end of the state. This is again an appeal to the principle of subsidiarity.

In this view, the state is justified to act on behalf of the *common good*. In so doing, it safeguards those interests that are common to all the persons in its domain. It is the pursuit of the common good that justifies the need for taxation to pay for necessary expenditures (Curran 1987). It is this line of argument that supplies the *just cause* for the taxation. That is, a tax needs to be for the common good and not the private good of the ruler or some segment of a society or private interest. Insofar as possible, taxes ought not to be on necessities but in support of necessities. Furthermore, the beneficiaries of tax should bear the burden proportionately.

Taxation: What Type of Justice?

Within the tradition, there has been an ongoing argument about the type of justice that underlies the practice of taxation. There has been a transition in the ethical framework used for understanding taxes. A long-standing view on taxes has been that taxes do not oblige in conscience, but merely by coercive power. So tax laws are merely penal laws and tax evasion was not a sin that demanded restitution. One of the earliest proponents of this view was Blessed Angelus of Clavisio (1411–95),[2] who treated tax laws as penal laws. This position is one that was widely held through the nineteenth century. E. Genicot (1856–1900), for example, argued that while there was an obligation to support the state, most tax laws were purely penal. He argued that this position was the opinion of the tradition, that many taxes are probably unjust and that for a tax to be morally obligatory it must clearly support the common good (Genicot 1927, vol. 2).

At the same time, there was another line of thought that understood taxes as imposing a moral obligation in conscience. Saint Antonius (1389–1449) held the view that if a tax law is just then it is binding in conscience in virtue of commutative justice (Antonius 1581–82, II). This view was expanded and supported by moralists such as Louis Molina (1536–1600) and Francisco Suarez (ca. 1486–1546). In his lengthy analysis of taxes, Antonius writes: "tax laws are not *per se* penal laws . . . nor are they made purely penal by the fact that they have a penalty attached to them . . ." (1581–82, V, c. 8, no. 3). He argues that the matter of such laws are matters of commutative justice. A tax is the just stipend to be given to the ruler. Saint Alphonsus Liguori (1696–1787) takes a similar position: "Just as the King is bound to work for the good of the people by administering justice and performing other duties, so, on the other hand, are the people bound from justice and the natural law to pay taxes for the maintenance of the prince" (Liguori 1905, III, 616).

Gradually, one finds a shift in the tradition to a more positive view of taxation and moral obligation. This shift comes, in part, to the need to have the state involved in areas like health care and education, which have grown more and more complex. For those who take the position that taxes are morally obligatory, there are different views as to what forms the basis for such obligations. One argument appeals to commutative justice as the basis of taxation. Taxation is part of the relationship between the individual and the ruler (society). This view of taxation argues that evasion of taxes was binding in conscience and involved theft and restoration. They argue that there is a just stipend to be given to rulers, so that they may carry out their offices (rulers as ministers of God).

The transformation of the state in the modern age seems to move the argument about taxes in another direction. It moves away from the basis in commutative justice (as a contract between subject and ruler) to legal justice. For example, H. Noldin (1838–1922) argues that tax laws should be judged by the same norm as other laws: legal justice. This is not a surprising shift as the model of the state moves away from the prince and what is owed to a person in virtue of the office to a more complex, bureaucratic structure. A. Tanquerey (d. 1932) argued that, because people are born to live in society, they have an obligation to supply whatever is necessary to preserve the good order of society. Because the state is involved in mutual obligations to work for the common good, tax laws, like other laws, oblige in legal justice (Noldin 1939).

The understanding of taxes was transformed further in the twentieth-century discussion of social justice. The term, used by Pius XI (1995) in *Quadragesimo Anno* has more to do with social organization (the common good is effected through social organization). The term "social justice," used by Pius XI, is never clearly defined. It is used to emphasize government and citizen responsibility to build a social order that sustains the common good. The common good "embraces the sum total of those conditions of social living whereby men are enabled to achieve their own integral perfection more fully and more easily" (John XXIII 1995a, #58). In Pius XI's writings, the notion of social justice is considered in relation to the aspects of the common good of the whole social order. The term is primarily applied to the socioeconomic order. Distributive justice in concerned with the role of the state in distributing social goods, whereas social justice is concerned with the social organization and participation in the social and economic orders.

Summary

The concept of basic human needs is tied to an assumption about a basic human nature. Health is understood to be one of the basic human needs. Within the context of Roman Catholic thought, human beings are naturally part of civil society. It would be inconceivable to think of men and women apart from society. This assumption shapes the view that society has certain obligations to all of its members, especially with regard to obtaining the basic human needs. Furthermore, men and women commonly share the gift of a common creation. Although there is an important role for private property, it is not an absolute. Rather, private property is limited by the mutual use of a common, created world and by the needs of others. Civil society's obligations to see that the basic needs of all members are met imposes a limit on private property. There is also an assumption, within the tradition, that these obligations are best met at a local level and that government is best used, morally, when it assists local communities in meeting basic needs. On this account, the tax policy of the state is to guide the creation and distribution of the basic goods needed by all men and women. The proper moral end of taxation by the state is to assist in the common good. Taxation cannot be confiscatory, because there is a right to private property, and it is in the common interest that there is fair economic distribution and productivity. If one assumes that the goal of society is to support human flourishing (dignity) by supporting the common good as the condition for realizing that dignity, then we can begin to develop a number of questions about the development and use of health care resources.

COMMON GOOD, TAXATION, AND HEALTH CARE

To this point, the essay has been exploring the broad outlines of basic human goods, the common good, and society's obligation to provide basic goods to men and women. Now, in light of this exploration, we want to see what light, if any, these reflections can shed on the questions associated with using resources for critical care medicine. What direction are we given by the tradition in terms of the development of health care resources and their distribution? One limit in resources for critical care medicine is the limit that comes with taxation in general. That is, societies are admonished by the Roman Catholic tradition not to make tax burdens oppressive or confiscatory.

There are two lines of argument at work in the tradition that can be helpful to questions about developing resources for health care and critical care medicine. First, there is one argument that is tied to basic human needs and goods and the purpose of society. The purpose of the state is to promote the welfare of its citizens, and the bases of that welfare are basic human necessities. In light of these assumptions, one can argue that health care is a basic necessity for human existence and, as such, falls under the promotion of the common good. This line of argument gives a direction (goal) but not a means. That is to say, the tradition speaks of the importance of health care (not exclusively medicine) and the importance of some kind of social security as men and women face sickness.

One could easily imagine that a society could decide to promote health by providing better water, sanitation, and police protection, while limiting investment in expensive medical care. Health care is part of the common good. It is limited by the basic finitude of creation, the need to provide other basic goods (education, family, food, shelter), and the right to private property. These competing needs create limits for a society's investment in health care. The Catholic tradition is similar to the Jewish view that saving lives must be balanced against other values and goods. In the Roman tradition, it is a balancing of basic goods. The social obligation is to provide basic goods. This obligation to provide basic goods gives a first limit to taxation and resources. That is, a society is concerned to provide, as best it can, all of the basic resources (food, education, health care, shelter).

The tradition has always allowed for flexibility in culture, place, and time in meeting basic needs. A society is not obliged to do what cannot be done. It would not be surprising to find differences between states and the care of health; nor should it be surprising to find variation and change in the history of a state and society. The tradition leaves open a variety of ways to interpret how health care should be provided. Health care need not be equated exclusively with medical care. One could imagine easily that the provision of basic health care might involve improvement in education, roads, housing, food (i.e., other basic human needs). One might well imagine a model of health care that focused principally on public health (sanitation, inoculation, drugs, food, etc.) and that asked what will best serve the health of the whole. Indeed, one might think of a society that devoted none of its common resources to critical care medicine.

However, if a society decides to tax for medical care and invest common tax resources in its medical infrastructure, then one could easily see the importance of the second argument from social justice. The category of social justice examines the structure and organization of society. If a society is organized in such a way that it invests social resources in health care (e.g., medical education and research), then all its members ought to have some access to health care.

Roman Catholic social thought gives some further guidance as to how we might examine justice and social organization in relation to health care. One of the first principles that is important is the principle of subsidiarity. This principle supports the importance of *local* action in addressing social issues. The duty of higher, central state authorities is to help when the local level is unable to meet basic needs. Help need not be understood strictly in terms of taxation. It can be understood in terms of coordination of efforts (e.g., clean water, inoculations).

In summary, basic human dignity is at the heart of the Roman Catholic moral tradition and social teaching. The common good is the set of necessary conditions for the realization of this dignity. Health care can be understood as an element of the common good. The resources that are devoted to health care are limited by the realization of other basic needs and the access of all men and women to those basic goods. One could well imagine, within these parameters, a society in which there is no public investment in the development of intensive care resources. In such a society, the personal use of one's resources to pursue the goods of critical care medicine would be addressed by the ordinary-extraordinary means distinction.

CONCLUSION

In the Roman Catholic tradition, one can argue that health care is a basic human good. Insofar as it is possible, a society has an obligation to meet the health care needs of its members. Furthermore, insofar as a society invests in health care, then social justice requires some access for all its members. The tradition recognizes that there are differences between societies and their ability to support health care. It also recognizes that there are differences within a society. Hence, the importance of the principle of subsidiarity. On a macroeconomic level, there are limits to the resources a society should develop for health care. Those limits come from the need to ensure other basic human goods (e.g, housing, food, education) and the need to ensure private property and, with it, individual freedom. A balance must be struck between taxation that is oppressive and providing others with basic human goods. Also, it should be noted, in light of other basic human goods, that medical care is not the only way to deliver health care. It is, perhaps, not even the best way to deliver health care.

In terms of resources, society's first obligation is to provide basic human needs in some way. The amount of public resources dedicated to health care at the macro level will depend on meeting the other basic needs and a society's resources. Furthermore, in distributing health care resources in a society, one need not assume that critical care medicine ought to be a part of the basic care available to all. To the extent that resources are available for critical care medicine, the tradition of ordinary-extraordinary means will be helpful in guiding individual choices in this area (see the essay by Boyle in this volume).

It is clear that ICUs save lives (see the essay by Rie in this volume). But the Roman Catholic tradition has long made a distinction between our absolute duties (e.g., not intentionally taking innocent human life) and imperfect duties (e.g., the preservation of human life). In thinking about how a society might develop and allocate resources, we engage in a threefold balancing act. First, in general policy questions of taxation, there needs to be a balance between the individual's rights to property and social needs. Taxation policy ought not stifle the freedom and creativity of individuals. Second, society must balance the goods of medicine and health care against other basic human needs, such as housing, food, and education. Third, there needs to be a balancing within those resources allocated to medicine. Critical care resources must be balanced against such areas as primary health care.

NOTES

1. Contemporary Catholic writings would cast the net even further and argue that the question of allocating resources for basic human needs is a global question and not a national one.
2. He was one of the most popular pre-Reformation theologians. His work appeared in 1476 and had gone through thirty-one editions by 1520. His book was one of the first burned by Luther.

BIBLIOGRAPHY

Abbot, W., ed. 1966a. *Dignitatis Humanae.* In *The Documents of Vatican II.* New York: Guild Press.

———. 1966b. *Gaudium et Spes.* In *The Documents of Vatican II.* New York: The Guild Press.

Aquinas, T. 1951. *Summa Theologiae.* Matriti: La Editorial Catolica.

Antonius. 1581–82. *Summae Sacrae Theologiae: Iuris Pontficii et Caesarei* (4 volumes). Venetiis: Apud Iuntas.

Ashley, B., and K. O'Rourke. 1997. *Health Care Ethics,* 4th ed. Washington, D.C.: Georgetown University Press.

Cronin, M. 1917. *The Science of Ethics,* New York: Benzinger Brothers.

Curran, C. 1987. *Toward an American Catholic Moral Theology.* Notre Dame, Ind.: University of Notre Dame Press.

Genicot, E.-S. 1927. *Institutiones Theologiae Moralis.* Brussels: Albert Dewitt.

Grisez, G. 1974. *Beyond the New Morality: The Responsibilities of Freedom.* Notre Dame, Ind.: University of Notre Dame Press.

Hollenbach, D. 1989. The common good revisited. *Theological Studies* 70.

John XXIII, Pope. 1995a. *Mater et Magister: Christianity and Social Progress.* In *Catholic Social Thought: The Documentary Heritage,* ed. by David O'Brien and Thomas Shannon. New York: Orbis.

———. 1995b. *Pacem in Terris.* In *Catholic Social Thought: The Documentary Heritage,* ed. by David O'Brien and Thomas Shannon. New York: Orbis.

John Paul II, Pope. 1995. *Laborem Exercens: On Human Work.* In *Catholic Social Thought: The Documentary Heritage*, ed. by David O'Brien and Thomas Shannon. New York: Orbis.

Leo XIII, Pope. 1995. *Rerum Novarum: The Condition of Labor.* In *Catholic Social Thought: The Documentary Heritage*, ed. by David O'Brien and Thomas Shannon, New York: Orbis.

Liguori, A. 1905. *Theologiae Moralis.* Rome.

Meilaender, G. 1997. Ordinary-extraordinary treatments: When does quality of life count? *Theological Studies* 58: 527–30.

Noldin, H. 1939. *Summa Theologiae Moralis.* Insbruck: Schmitt.

Pius XI, Pope. 1995. *Quadragesimo Anno: After Forty Years.* In *Catholic Social Thought: The Documentary Heritage*, ed. by D. O'Brien and T. Shannon. New York: Orbis.

Quinn, K. 2000. Viewing health care as a common good: Looking beyond political liberalism. *University of Southern California Law Review* 73 (2): 277–375.

Ryan, J., and Boland, F. 1950. *Catholic Principles of Politics.* New York: Macmillan.

Ryan, J. 1950. *Catholic Principles of Politics.* New York: Macmillan.

Tanquerey, A. 1937. *Synopsis Theologiae Moralis et Pastoralis,* 10th ed. Toraci: Desclee et Soc.

U.S. Catholic Conference. 1981. *Pastoral Letter on Health and Health Care.* Washington, D.C.: U.S. Catholic Conference.

Wildes, K. Wm. 1996. Ordinary-extraordinary means and the quality of life. *Theological Studies* 57: 500–512.

———. 1997. Institutional identity, integrity, and conscience. *Kennedy Institute of Ethics Journal* 7: 413–19.

———. 1998. Quaestio disputata: When does quality of life count? *Theological Studies* 59: 505–08.

PART VI

From a Different Point of View: Jewish, Orthodox, and Protestant Perspectives

Allocation of Scarce Medical Resources to Critical Care: A Perspective from the Jewish Canonical Tradition

Teodoro Forcht Dagi

This essay explores the Jewish perspective on limiting access to scarce medical resources. In general, the Jewish canonical tradition is not sympathetic to the idea that medical care be restricted intentionally, if the result of such restriction is to shorten the life of a
patient. It views life as sacrosanct and regards the preservation of human life as a central and
incontrovertible obligation incumbent upon all members of the Jewish faith. This obligation is accompanied by rewards for those who respond to it punctiliously and sanctions for
those who do not.

Four abiding principles govern the behavior of caregivers and patients:

1. Any intervention possessed of a reasonable likelihood of prolonging life must
   be implemented.
2. Interventions to prolong and preserve must be effective, or at least not harmful.
3. There is no requirement to implement futile therapy.
4. Quality-of-life issues do not play a prima facie role in the decision process.[1]

These four principles, which emanate from a strict interpretation of the canonical tradition
in Jewish law, embody the most traditional views of the faith. They would be acknowledged
as dispositive by Orthodox Jewish scholars. Adherents of the other branches of Judaism—
Conservative, Reform, and Reconstructionist—might take issue with the fourth principle,
but probably not with the first three.

The canonical tradition relies upon biblical sources, upon Talmudic texts dating
from the second to the sixth centuries C.E., upon commentaries and codifications of Jewish
law that were compiled in medieval times, upon rabbinical *responsa* dating from Talmudic
times to the present, and upon other, more interpretive writings. The canonical tradition is

fundamentally scholastic: Later ideas must be reconciled to earlier authority, and the writings closest in time to the canonical Talmudic texts are ranked more authoritative.

The structure of Jewish law is based on rules called *mitzvoth*, religious obligations, and *responsa*, which constitute the equivalent of common law in the Anglo-American tradition. What is relatively absent is the equivalent of legal policy. Binding legal opinion is triggered on a case-by-case basis, a response directed at the petitioner for the purpose of clarifying points of law applicable to a problem and defining the governing rules and obligations. The responsa are directed at actionable questions rather than broad policies.

This does not mean that general principles may not be inferred—or perhaps, more correctly, induced from the particular cases in the responsa literature. In the traditional Jewish legal system, these principles have no intrinsic legal authority, though they may well carry a contextual authority.[2] In the nontraditional view of Jewish law, these inferred principles carry significant weight.

There are three major American Jewish movements at the present time: Orthodox, Conservative, and Reform. They are differentiated by the extent to which they believe the practice of Jewish ritual and the application of Jewish law should follow canonical Jewish texts. They also differ in the extent to which they teach the traditional rabbinical model of textual interpretation and deem themselves bound to it; the manner in which they follow the teachings of certain sentinel legal, theological, and philosophical authorities; the degree to which they are influenced by individual conscience; and the ways in which they are responsive to external political, social, and philosophical influences.

THE HISTORICAL CONTEXT

The split between the Orthodox and the Reform movements began in early-nineteenth-century Germany and was exported to, or spread to, much of Western Europe, the British Commonwealth, and the Americas. The Conservative movement is a twentieth-century, quintessentially American religious phenomenon, whose adherents are centered primarily in North America.

Religious Authority in Jewish History

Those less familiar with Jewish practice are often perplexed by the diversity of opinion within the religion, and equally puzzled by the seeming lack of a central religious authority. The reasons for decentralized authority may be found in the history of Judaism after the destruction of the Second Temple in Jerusalem and the fall of the Second Jewish Commonwealth around 70–72 C.E. From the earliest Talmudic times, there existed an established legal system that included courts, attorneys, judges, and rules of evidence, rules for sentencing, and rules for settling jurisdictional disputes.[3] Like canon law in the Catholic and Muslim traditions, Jewish, or Talmudic, law did not distinguish clearly between civil, criminal, and religious matters. The law dealt with all three.

The Beth Din

Central to the system was the Jewish court, or Beth Din. The Av Beth Din (*Av* meaning father, whence the cognate *abbot*) was a rabbi who had achieved the status of *dayyan* or judge, and who was recognized as a Talmudic authority in both the legal and the spiritual sense.[4] Overseeing the entire legal system was the Great Sanhedrin, a body that possessed unique authority to legislate and change existing laws, and dismiss or modify the effect of precedent.[5]

With the exception of the Great Sanhedrin, Jewish communities replicated most elements of the Jewish legal system throughout the diaspora after the end of the Second Commonwealth. In the Roman Empire, particularly after Constantine, Jewish courts acted as courts of arbitration, and decisions could be referred to the Roman judiciary for enforcement.[6] In Babylonia, between the first and eleventh centuries, the Jewish community flourished, and the exilarch was granted considerable autonomy and even ruling lieutenancy by the king.[7] As a result, Jewish law was exercised in the Jewish community, and a body of Jewish legal commentary and Jewish legal precedent evolved.[8]

Prior to Constantine's Edict of Toleration (313 C.E.), the Jews in the empire were fairly protected. This status diminished significantly as restrictions against the Jews were incorporated into various legal codes including the Code of Theodosius and the Code of Justinian. The Germanic juridical system, superimposed on the western part of the Empire after the fall of Rome, allowed Jews to continue an independent legal tradition. In his Breviary, Alaric modified the anti-Jewish statutes imposed by earlier codes. In Visigoth Spain, Jews were less free, and in Byzantium, forced conversion of the Jews was decreed by Heraclius, and the practice of the religion was outlawed in 629 C.E.

In the wake of Islamic conquests, Jews and Christians in Mohammedan lands were compelled to convert. Ironically, the Islamic onslaught diverted attention from the Jews in Byzantium and left them free to worship. Islamic rulers also came to tolerate nonbelievers in their midst.

Both Christian and Muslim rulers eventually allowed Jews a lowly but stable status as a subject nation with many legal encumbrances and disabilities. Curiously, the institution of the exilarchate was tolerated, and the Babylonian Talmudic academies flourished. Despite intermittent periods of intense persecution, Jews migrated from the Near East to regions under Islamic rule in Spain and North Africa, where Jewish scholarship was permitted and Jewish communal life was encouraged.

The Talmud as Canon

The Talmud was, by this time, widely disseminated and studied as a canonical text. As a systematic legal document, however, its organization left much to be desired. Many matters were addressed in more than one place. No index existed to guide the scholar through the various discussions. As a result, the Talmud could only be studied and used for reference once it had already been mastered in its entirety by the scholar.[9] The Talmudic heuristic, furthermore, could only be learned by long apprenticeship.

Codifications of Jewish Law

During the eleventh and twelfth centuries, Jewish scholars began codifying Talmudic law.[10] The codifications became, ipso facto, interpretations because they required the authors to decide which legal precedents and rabbinical rulings would be deemed authoritative. The three most important codes were the *Sefer Halachot*[11] of Isaac ben Jacob, also known as the Rif (1013–1103; born in Algeria and lived in Morocco and Spain); the *Mishneh Torah*[12] of Moshe ben Maimon, also known as Maimonedes (1135–1204; born in Cordoba, Spain, and lived in Morocco and Egypt); and the *Arba'ah Turim*[13] of Rabbi Jacob ben Asher, also known as the Tur (1280–1340; lived in Toledo, though of German origin).[14] Even these works did not altogether satisfy. They remained terse and indicial, rather than expository or explanatory, and presupposed a high degree of legal and textual competence.[15]

In 1522, Joseph Karo (1488–1575, also spelled Caro), a refugee from the Spanish Inquisition in Toledo, who settled with his family in Turkey and later moved to Safed, in Palestine, undertook a thirty-year project: a total review of *Halachah* (practical Jewish law), including both its origins in the Talmud and conflicting interpretations. This work, the *Beth Joseph,*[16] was designed to be comprehensive. Karo based his work on the *Turim,* and provided both an encyclopedic bibliography and a set of normative Halachic prescriptions. A later, simplified version, the *Shulchan Aruch,*[17] omitted the analysis and simply advanced a code of Jewish law and the norms of religious practice. It was intended as a vade mecum and was meant to be memorized by students.

Another scholar, Moshe ben Israel Iserles, known as the Rema (ca. 1525–72; born in Poland), also sought to comment on the *Turim.* A jurist and rabbinic commentator in Cracow, he had been criticized, in his youth, for issuing opinions based directly on the Talmud and its classical exegesists, who were primarily of Sephardic (Spanish and North African) origin, without reference to contemporary scholars of the Ashkenazi (German, Polish, and Eastern European) tradition. After the publication of the *Shulchan Aruch,* the Rema devoted himself to a gloss on this book. This work, called the *Mappah,*[18] was meant to match Karo in its scholarship, to summarize the voluminous material in the *Shulchan Aruch,* to represent the Ashkenazi custom and precedent, to emphasize in practical terms more recent decisions and local custom, and to respond to Isereles' earlier critics by referring to and citing the Ashkenazi authorities of the time. Together, the *Shulchan Aruch* and the *Mappah* constitute one of the very few central and authoritative reference texts in Jewish law.

One of the most enduring themes in the rabbinic literature is the tension between codification and simplification on the one hand, and interpretation and analysis on the other. This tension, notes Twersky, is "catalytic." "No sooner," he writes, "is the need for codification met than a wave of noncodificatory work rises. A code could provoke guidance and certitude for a while but not finality" (1979 [1967], 361).

The dialectic of Talmudic scholarship in the Talmudic academies in the patriarchate and the exilarchate was communal, transtemporal, and transgeographic. The dialectic among the codifiers was solitary and scholastic. Over time, a third legal tradition known as the responsa literature developed among the Jews.[19] The responsa literature represents the body of written rabbinic responses to personal lay and rabbinic queries in search of definitive Halachic answers to issues that could not be answered easily by local authorities. The responsa literature normally addresses individual questioners, not with general rules or principles, and is directed to the petitioner rather than to any broader audience.[20] Freehoff links the term to the practice in Roman history in which a specialized group of experts in Roman Law and tradition, referred to a *iuris consulti* or *iuris prudentes,* were authorized to issue responses called *responsa prudentium* carrying imperial authority. These responsa were recorded, and, by the time the process fell into disuse at the end of the third century, they had achieved significant legal authority (Schreiber 1979, 366). The existence of responsa prior to 200 C.E. is documented in the Talmud, but correspondence flourished more actively after the prohibition on reducing the Oral Law to writing was overcome. Few examples remain. The authorities in Babylon, known as the *gaonim* (Eminences), clarified questions emanating in many far-flung communities where knowledge of Jewish law was quite sparse. The responses were preserved not by the gaonim themselves, but by the recipients of the decisions, for whom they served as texts for study as well as practical guidelines. Responsa were terse and undecorated. The earliest responsa literature was composed primarily in Arabic. Later responsa were composed in Hebrew.

The nature of the literature changed around the twelfth century with the responsa of Jacob ben Meir Tam, also known as Rabbenu Tam (1100–71; born in France), the greatest Talmudic scholar of his time and an accomplished poet; and of Solomon ben Abraham Adret, also known as the Rashba (ca. 1235–1310; born in Barcelona), an equally eminent jurist and author of novellae. Writing in pure Hebrew or mixed Aramaic-Hebrew, Rabbenu Tam and the Rashba both composed lengthy and erudite responsa, which they themselves preserved and published. This evolution also reflected the increasing erudition of the petitioners, for whom the Talmudic texts and earlier commentaries were no longer arcane.

In each century, several major centers of Jewish learning emerged. During the late Middle Ages and Renaissance, Ashkenazi responsists worked primarily in the Rhineland, Germany, and France, and later Austria. Important responsa emanated from Italy as well.[21] After the destruction of Jewish communal life in Portugal and Spain during the Inquisition, scholars of Sephardic origin migrated to the Levant. The North African school was the first to consolidate after the expulsion of the Jews in 1492, but within a century its influence was eclipsed by scholars in Turkey, Salonika, Constantinople, and Cairo.

The Ashkenazi community also migrated. Through the works of Isserles and others of his generation, Poland assumed preeminence. By the late seventeenth century, the center of scholarship shifted back to Germany and Bohemia, and then grew to embrace the Low Countries. It then moved to the Austro-Hungarian Empire during the nineteenth century, and then to Russia and Lithuania.

Innumerable responsa have been composed during the past millennium. But when one looks at the authorship of these responsa, only some 75 to 100 individuals met the bar of true authority. The contemporary evolution of Jewish legal scholarship continues to find its voice primarily in the responsa literature.

The Emergence of Liberalism

The liberal tradition is very influential in North America and arguably has the highest number of followers. In this essay, the doctrines of the liberal tradition will not be analyzed. A brief note about its origins will help explain its differences from traditional orthodoxy and why I have elected not to comment on its teachings in this context.

Little is known of movements to reform or liberalize Judaism prior to the eighteenth century. What is now known as the Liberal or Reform movement (sometimes also called Progressive Judaism)[22] can be traced to Germany at the turn of the nineteenth century. Some link the movement to the work of Moses Mendelssohn (1729–86), a rabbi in Berlin who was also a philosopher of the German Aufklärung, and became a friend of G. E. Lessing. Mendelssohn translated the Pentateuch into German written in Hebrew characters and compiled a modern commentary that was strongly contested by traditional rabbis. In his *Biur*,[23] Mendelssohn emphasized the aesthetic aspects of Judaism as well as its canonical and religious aspects.

The first true reforms centered on the liturgy. In 1819, a group of laypeople in Hamburg adapted a prayer book to conform more to the style of the Lutheran Church. In the United States, the synagogue in Charleston, South Carolina, introduced an organ into the service at about the same time, thereby earning the distinction of becoming the first Reform congregation in North America.

During the next twenty years, a number of rabbis became leaders in the movement, which increasingly presented doctrinal and ideological challenges to the traditional Orthodox rabbinate. In particular, the Reform movement attacked the liturgy, which was deemed "irrelevant" and "archaic"; raised objections to the use of the organ during the service;[24] opposed the strictness of religious observance required by the Orthodox; and objected to the continuation of practices considered "obsolete" or "unnecessary," such as the observance of Jewish dietary laws and certain theological doctrines.

The Reform movement took early root in the United States. Rabbi Stephen Isaac Meyer Wise (1819–1900) emigrated to the United States from Bohemia in 1846 and introduced mixed pews, choral singing, and confirmation ceremonies. In 1856, he published *Minhag America*, a modification of the liturgy for American Reform congregations. And in 1875, he became the president of the Reform Hebrew Union College in Cincinnati. He later helped found the Union of American Hebrew Congregations and the Central Conference of American Rabbis, which became the voice of the U.S. progressive movement.

Reform doctrine was compiled in the Pittsburgh Platform of 1885 and the Columbus Platform of 1937. Among other changes, the Pittsburgh Platform abolished the dietary laws, Jewish dress codes, and the idea of priestly purity. The platform also denied the idea of bodily resurrection, though it affirmed the idea of the immortality of the soul.

The Conservative Movement

The Reform movement was fundamentally German, and consequently Western European, in origin and outlook. It found fertile ground in the German Jewish population that constituted the majority of the Jewish immigrants to the United States in the mid-nineteenth century. By the 1880s, however, a different group of Jews—different religiously and culturally—began immigrating to the United States. These Jews were Yiddish-speaking Eastern Europeans, more parochial in outlook and more isolated from Western European thought. To the rabbis trained in Eastern Europe, even to those with modern views, the changes advocated by the Reform movement in the Pittsburgh Platform were exceedingly radical. These rabbis almost universally had been trained in traditional rabbinical academies. In reaction to the Reform movement, and in an attempt to achieve an acceptable middle ground, there emerged a Conservative movement that was tolerant of some change in the liturgy and in practice, but much closer to traditional Judaism in its exegetical tradition and identity. The Jewish Theological Seminary was founded in 1887 and became the intellectual home of the Conservative movement. In 1913, the United Synagogue of America was established as the central agency of the Conservative movement, and in 1924, the Rabbinical Assembly of America was constituted as its central rabbinical organization. The Conservative movement satisfied a very particular American need. Although there are congregations outside of North America, it remains a preeminently American institution, and its heuristics reflect its particularly North American concerns.

Post-Holocaust Jewish Scholarship

In the wake of the Holocaust, Jewish scholarship in Europe was thrown into disarray. A number of important Talmudic academies had been established in the United States and in England during the late nineteenth and early twentieth centuries. These now attracted surviving European scholars. Within two decades, their students went on to found new Jewish institutions of higher learning across North America. Other scholars migrated directly to the newly founded state of Israel. By the end of the twentieth century, two epicenters of Jewish scholarship could be identified: North America and Israel.

The second half of the twentieth century also saw the emergence of an identifiable Conservative and Reform scholarly tradition. Most scholars are identified as such. Conservative and Reform scholarship was published in both the academic and lay press somewhat earlier than similar work from Orthodox academic circles.

THE CURRENT SITUATION

The central claim of Orthodoxy is adherence to the traditional, scholastic, rabbinical model of canonical and textual exegesis, and an accurate understanding and representation of the outcome of this heuristic. Religious practice based on this model is considered orthopraxis. The reverse, however, does not necessarily apply: Orthopraxy alone does not entail adherence to the canonical tradition from an exegetical or philosophical perspective. Some orthopractic Jews profess non-Orthodox, even secular, exegetical traditions but choose to practice according to Orthodox teachings.

As noted above, the Orthodox impute incontrovertible authority to certain canonical Jewish texts and sources. Conservative and Reform congregations dispute this claim. Adherents of the Conservative and Reform movements feel less reluctance to seek inspiration in extracanonical material, including secular writings or material from other philosophical traditions. Because the Orthodox scholar would be reluctant to grant such material legal authority in the sense of having standing as, or contributing to, the formulation of legal precedent, the Conservative and Reform responsa are not deemed dispositive in the traditional sense.

A notable example is the role played by individual conscience in the three major branches of Judaism. The Orthodox bestow qualified weight but not unqualified moral authority upon individual conscience. The Conservative, in general, are not unsympathetic to the idea that individual conscience may assume a highly influential role. They, however, differ as to the extent of authority conscience ought to assume. The Reform movement holds that tradition, as well as teachings of traditional authority, are open to review and reinterpretation in the light of individual conscience.

The leaders of the Conservative and Reform movements have sought equal standing in courts of Jewish law unsuccessfully for years. As a result, in some locations, parallel courts have been established. The Orthodox rabbinate disputes the legal authority of these courts. The Orthodox rabbinate technically has legal standing in the Conservative and Reform movements, but not vice versa.[25]

Outside North America, orthopraxy prevails, irrespective of the extent to which individual Jews practice their religion or consider themselves affiliated.[26] The Orthodox canonical tradition holds sway in civil matters such as marriage, divorce, and conversion, and the vast majority of rabbis are trained in the Orthodox tradition.

In none of its forms does Judaism lay claim to a monolithic tradition. A robust and nuanced exegetical tradition leads to a range of approaches to, and a range of opinions regarding, many difficult matters. The responsa tradition is inherently individualist and casuist. Nevertheless, and notwithstanding the absence of a monolithic tradition, traditional Judaism holds little tolerance for relativism. What may appear to be relativism proves to be, in almost all instances, an indication of tolerable differences of opinion,[27] of unresolved difference of interpretation, or of imperfect or naive attempts to reconcile expressions of conscience or external philosophical influences with the traditional Jewish canonical tradition.

At the end of the day, the three major movements share a fundamental exegetical tradition and set of received and revered canonical texts. The divisive issues center upon the extent to which the traditional exegetical methods and the traditional exegetical conclusions are theologically and morally compelling, and historically and legally dispositive.[28]

DEFINING "TRADITIONAL JEWISH LAW"

For purposes of this essay, "traditional Jewish law" is defined as the body of law, exegesis, precedent, and interpretation that would meet the standards for evidence and precedent required by an Orthodox Beth Din, or court of Jewish law. I also focus on the traditional interpretations of the value of human life as expressed in this tradition. Jews who profess more liberal philosophies may consider these interpretations to be overly narrow. They may be parochial, but they are not narrow if what one seeks to understand is the traditional Jewish view.

The debate between the traditional and the more liberal schools of Jewish thought turns on the influence of post-Enlightenment, Western political and social philosophy. Traditional Judaism is positivist, and positivist Judaism is wary of this influence. Liberal Judaism embraces it, incorporating themes, icons, and philosophies that will be quite familiar to the Western intellectual, though problematic to the strict traditionalist.

In the wake of the Enlightenment, liberal Jewish thought shifted the emphasis of the religion from personal obligations to personal rights. Traditional Judaism defined virtue in terms of fulfillment of sacred and inseparable religious and moral obligations. More liberal, humanist visions of Judaism changed this focus from the sacred to the virtuous; from the fulfillment of Divine obligations entailing *pari passu,* commitment to the welfare of one's fellow humans, to the idea that virtue, and perhaps even worship, might be defined in humanist, even anthropocentric terms; and that this vision of virtue might concentrate chiefly on concerns about the welfare of society and the protection of human rights. In an effort to represent the traditional voice of Jewish philosophy, this essay dwells on the canonical, rather than the humanist, movements in Jewish thought.

PRICE ELASTICITY AND THE DEMAND FOR HUMAN LIFE

The global demand for health care services always exceeds supply, so that supply becomes, by definition, a scarce resource. How should such resources be allocated? The disciplines of medical ethics, religious ethics, public policy, and law have struggled to formulate a cogent answer. The debate can take place at many levels, ranging from the allocation of money for biomedical research to the training of health care personnel, from the provision of universal insurance to the imposition of price controls, and from centrally planned public policy to free market decisions. It is a daunting task.

Rationing

Sometimes, an attempt is made to simplify the issues by framing them in methodological terms: How should one ration health care? This question is in itself problematic. It assumes that rationing—the grant of limited or gated access to goods and services in accordance with certain rules or formulae—is the answer.[29] On what basis, if any, may rationing be advocated, and what reach may the rationing process be allowed?[30] If one does not allow rationing, access may be determined by chance events. If one does allow rationing, the rules under which access is permitted are subject to ethical scrutiny. But the debate over whether to allow rationing or not must be resolved prior to addressing the methodological issues of how to establish rules and how to impose them.

Although not all issues of scarce-resource allocation can be reduced to a debate about the monetary value of human life, many can. With respect to those that do, the issues may be framed as an exercise in conjoint analysis. What is to be preferred: (1) that person A[31] be treated, or survive, in the knowledge that another (or another population) goes untreated when there is an opportunity to substitute one for the other or affect the allocation of care, or (2) that another path of action[32] be *actively* pursued,[33] assuming that economic resources alone serve as the limiting factor.[34] This is the question on which Jewish law has focused with particular clarity.

The Value of Human Life

Traditional Jewish law stipulates that the value of human life cannot be measured and that the demand for human life should be inelastic.[35] It views human life as an objective good; one requiring no external defense or justification, and one completely independent of an individual's personal estimate of the value of his or her own life.[36] Human life is not to be disparaged for any reason.

The obligation to preserve human life derives its importance from two sources: a vision of the intrinsic value of human life and a perception of the value of the obligation to save human life. The fulfillment of this obligation is so highly valued that it is said "if any man saves alive a single soul Scripture imputes it to him as if he saved alive a whole world" (*Sanhedrin* iv, 5, see also Jakobovits 1959, 45 ff.; Bleich 1979, 1–44). The force of this obligation is also reflected in a parallel duty to undertake substantial economic sacrifice to discharge it. And yet, the objective value of human life in Jewish law explains this obligation only in part. The obligation stands independently, as a positivist legal principle.[37]

The Obligation to Rescue Human Life

Because the worth of a single life has been equated metaphorically with the life of an entire world, no lesser effort may be exerted on behalf of a single life than on behalf of a community (*Sanhedrin*, iv, 5). This legal finding excludes a utilitarian, greater-good-argument justification that pits the benefit of the collective against the benefit of the individual.[38] *Pari passu*, the obligation to preserve human life stands supreme above virtually all other obligations.[39] The exchange of scarce resources for the preservation of human life is considered a rational, as well as an obligatory, trade. This line of reasoning confounds attempts to justify the rationing of life-saving interventions on economic grounds: As a general proposition, Jewish law prohibits using economic cost as a reason not to fulfill an obligation.[40] To the extent that one might seek a corresponding, deontological moral imperative, such an imperative would be derived from the legal statute.

The scope of the obligation is not limited to medical intervention. *All* life-saving interventions should be provided to all threatened individuals, irrespective of the society or community to which they belong, and medical methods of preserving or saving human life merit no inherent moral preference over other methods of preserving or saving human life. For this reason, they deserve no preferential economic treatment; but neither may they be dismissed.

LIMITS TO THE OBLIGATION

The emphasis on the obligation to rescue human life notwithstanding, some limits to the allocation of resources to this purpose seem to be permitted under very restricted circumstances. Four considerations are salient:

1. the immediacy and specificity of the threat to life;
2. the existence of a plausible remedy;
3. priority, in very specific situations; and
4. other special circumstances.

The Immediacy and Specificity of the Threat to Life

The more immediate the threat, the more compelling the obligation to meet it, and the stronger the obligation to expend resources to meet the threat. When danger is relatively remote, the pressure to respond is far less evident. The legal metaphor that is used is the metaphor of Sabbath violation. Public and purposeful violation of the Sabbath is a capital offense according to biblical law. Sabbath observance becomes a bar according to which the seriousness of a situation, and its potential to threaten life and limb, are measured. One would violate or suspend observance of the Sabbath to respond to immediate life- or limb-threatening danger, or a cogent suspicion that such danger might arise. One would not suspend observance of the Sabbath for a more remote threat, such as an environmental hazard, if the threat could be contained until the end of the Sabbath without violating it. Even so, one would seek the least degree of Sabbath violation consistent with meeting the threat (Jakobovits 1959, 45–53, 67–68, 77–81). At the same time, in order to trigger suspension of the Sabbath, it is necessary that a specific threat to a specific victim be identified. The Sabbath may *not* be violated to contend with a vague or an unidentifiable threat, or a threat whose target cannot be specified or delineated precisely. From these rules, the circumstances that limit the obligation to rescue may be inferred (Jakobovits 1959, 68–71).

The Plausibility of the Remedy

The obligation to intervene depends on the existence of a plausible remedy. And conversely, futility, defined as the condition of having no effective remedy, modifies the obligation to intervene. Even futility, however, does not entirely vacate the obligation. There remains a residual mandate to prolong life, even in the event that no definitive cure or effective remedy is believed to exist.[41]

How concrete must the possibility of a remedy become before it triggers the obligation to intervene? The framework favored in Jewish law prefers to put the question the other way around: To what extent must the possibility of a remedy (not a cure, but a remedy) be attenuated before the obligation weakens? Jewish law does not consider quality of life or length of life to be important modifying issues in considering this question. Permission to retreat from the obligation is based on the certainty, not on the likelihood or even the overwhelming likelihood, that any known remedy will be ineffectual. In case of doubt, the requirement to intervene stands unqualified.

There is one important exception. Jewish law recognizes a category called *goses*, loosely translatable as moribund. The *goses* will be dead in three days. The obligation to intervene is lightened if someone can be certified to be *goses*. This is, however, only a theoretical construct. This diagnosis can be framed with certainty only after the fact. Because any intervention that abridges even these three days is considered to be murder, neither the codes nor the responsa literature seriously contemplate exploiting this legal concept for purposes of diminishing the force of the obligation. More recently, it has been suggested that patients satisfying brain-based criteria for death may qualify as *goses* almost in an "*ex conditio*" or inherent fashion (Jakobovits 1959, 121; Bleich 1979, notes 118 and 120). The concept is applied in the following way. If during the management of a patient dependent upon life support it is necessary to disconnect the life-support system for routine care—for example, to provide pulmonary toilet for an intubated, ventilator-dependent (and brain-dead) patient—there is, arguably, no obligation to reconnect the life-support device. This approach is applicable only to patients with whole brain death, who are then deemed not dead, exactly, but *goses*; because of the criteria for that diagnosis and the proven irreversibility of the process, the obligation to intervene, therefore, is thought to disappear.[42]

Priority

By a doctrine of priority, I refer to a doctrine of relative social worth. The basis for allocating scarce resources according to a doctrine of priority in Jewish law is derived from a Talmudic discussion about the obligation to ransom captives. The ransom of captives is considered a very powerful prima facie legal obligation. The issue on which the Talmud dwells is in what order captives are to be freed:

> If a man and his father and his teacher were in captivity, he takes precedence [in procuring his ransom] over his teacher, and the latter takes precedence over his father, while his mother takes precedence over all of them [because her dignity is at stake]. A scholar takes precedence over a king of Israel, for if a scholar dies, there is none to replace him, while if a king of Israel dies, all Israel are eligible for kingship. A king takes precedence over a high priest. . . . a high priest takes precedence over a prophet. . . . (*Horayot* iii, 7)

The passage describes a very particular situation: the treatment of individuals, all of whom are threatened identically and simultaneously, but who can be rescued only seriatim. It is an extreme situation so framed in order to explore the issues.

Despite the plain meaning of this passage, this source is not interpreted to suggest a doctrine of priority, even for the teacher, the scholar, or the very pious. Although Jewish tradition recognizes an areteic quality known as *tzedek*, or righteousness, attained through humility, scholarship, piety, charity, and good works, the tradition teaches that the life of every individual is equally worthy. While the *tzadik* is recognized as deserving special deference, every individual is understood to possess an equal measure of divinity. Indeed, every individual may lay equal claim to life and is entitled to an equal part of the communal resources available to sustain life (Rosner 1979, 346–52). Although the *tzadik* may have attained a high level of righteousness, *every* Jew is exhorted to pursue righteousness. The *tzadik* is recognized for having succeeded.

That the *tzadik* deserves reverence and admiration is not at issue. The questions center on issues of privilege and the doctrine of priority: Does (or should) the *tzadik* have greater claim on communal resources than others do or others should?[43] Is the *tzadik* to be rewarded on earth on in heaven? Does the quality of righteousness inherently justify a greater share of communal resources?[44] Although Jewish tradition accords tremendous respect to the *tzadik*, opinions regarding the doctrine of priority, even if based upon this exalted state, differ widely.

One fundamental Talmudic tenet holds, for example, that one life may not be sacrificed for another.[45] If as a result of a man saving himself, his teacher, his father, or his mother were to perish, that tenet would have been violated, albeit perhaps indirectly, and certainly unintentionally. Perhaps in consequence, but also for other exegetical reasons, this passage is generally not construed literally. It seems more plausible to interpret the discussion first as a reference to the obligation to save one's self; and second, as a reference to the respect due a great scholar. It is far less plausible to derive a doctrine of priority from this passage. At best, this doctrine is accorded only a grudging tolerance in Jewish law.

Futility

Futility refers to the inability to change the natural history of an illness or an injury. A treatment is deemed to be futile when it has no bearing on the patient. *Ceteris paribus,* futility suspends the obligation to intervene. It may be necessary to *prove*, however, that no treatment is effective. In the event a *treatment* proves ineffective, there is no obligation to continue or repeat the treatment. In the event no treatment is effective, the patient is deemed incurable. The diagnosis of incurability requires a logical transition from the observation that no treatment has been effective to the prediction that no treatment shall be effective. That transition captures the essence of futility. The "potential for cure" is what actually matters. A patient "with potential for cure takes precedence in the allocation of scarce resources over a patient whose illness would at best be only controlled" (Rosner 1979, 349). The diagnosis of futility is rarely invoked.

Debates on futility in Jewish law have not risen to the level of detail encountered in the world of twentieth-century bioethics, perhaps because the tradition requires that the diagnosis be rendered on an individual basis, and decisions about futility to be made on a case-by-case basis. The public policy dimensions are not really emphasized. As a result, legal precedent, of which there is not a huge repertoire, prevails when public policy issues are encountered.

Medical and Nonmedical Models of Rescue

The fact that no special importance is accorded to the saving of a life threatened by disease or injury (medical rescue) as opposed to the saving of a life endangered by other hazards should not be interpreted to mean that medical rescue is accorded no special value. On the contrary, there does exists a special obligation to treat illness and relieve suffering. The treatment of the sick receives specific mention as a compelling example of virtuous behavior. Nevertheless, the satisfaction of this obligation holds no priority over other forms of rescue. It is the rescue of human life from threat that matters, rather than the means through which this is accomplished, or the nature of the threat.

Summary: The Issues from the Judaic Perspective

The issues that matter most from the Judaic perspective are reflected in four questions:

1. Can the victim or potential victim be specified? A victim is deemed to be specific when he or she can be named and immediately located. A victim must be specifiable in order to assert a claim upon resources.
2. How many souls are at immediate risk? The greater the number of *identifiable* souls at *immediate* risk, the more stringent the requirement to see to their rescue and allocate resources to that task.[46]
3. Is the remedy proven, or only theoretical or supposed? The more concrete and proven the remedy, the more powerful the imperative to intervene by utilizing it.
4. Is the threat concrete? Can it be articulated, described, and measured, or is it only theoretical and immeasurable? The more concrete the threat, the more material it is deemed to be and the more compelling the imperative to intervene.

The Jewish tradition regards the obligation to rescue human life as inelastic, especially with respect to cost. This obligation embodies two distinct and important values. The first is the value of the obligation itself. Satisfaction of the obligation bestows merit on those who satisfy it. The second reflects the constant and inelastic value of human life in Jewish law, which stands independent of the persona that is saved.

Thus, even though one might gain great personal merit from saving the life of a righteous individual or a saint, neither the strength nor the value of the obligation to save a life, nor the merit accorded the satisfaction of the obligation, can be enhanced or depreciated by the philosophical, religious, moral, or physical qualities of the life that is rescued. Equal merit is accorded the rescue of a saint and the rescue of a sinner. Even in the event that one could conclude that the value of a particular human life were worth less than the value of another (an extraordinarily debatable premise in Jewish law), the strength of the obligation would not be diminished.[47]

ALLOCATION DECISIONS IN THE INTENSIVE CARE UNIT

The principles that govern the allocation of resources in the intensive care unit (ICU) do not vary from the principles that govern the obligation to rescue in other contexts. Whatever means may be required to save lives should be provided. Economic constraints are given very short shrift, particularly a priori. There are compelling obligations to rescue; obligations to conserve resources are less compelling. When there is competition among means, resources, or funds, Jewish law directs that the means most likely to succeed be selected, without concern for cost. Saving one life is good. Saving many lives is better still. Nevertheless, keeping in mind the overarching framework of the obligations and constraints of Jewish law,[48] the obligation to rescue is unique and specific to each life, rather than to a population or a group. One may not lessen the chances that one soul will survive in order to rescue others.[49] Souls are not fungible. What counts as important in Western philosophical traditions does not always carry the same weight in the Judaic tradition. The Judaic tradition, for example, is not Cartesian in its view of life.

In Jewish philosophy, there is no requirement that one think, or be fully capable of acts of mind, to be alive or meaningfully to live. The value of life may be derived from (or simply expressed in terms of) benefits to others, even in terms of allowing others to fulfill their obligations, rather than to the individual whose life is at stake. Thus, the idea of a life not worth living is simply alien to the Jewish tradition. For this reason, decisions about resource allocation based upon quality-of-life considerations are extremely difficult to defend.

Life is considered worth living always and categorically for two reasons: because life ought to be theologically and philosophically significant to the individual, and because life *is* theologically and philosophically valuable to the community. No category of life is deemed to be irrelevant or insignificant, if for no other reason than that continued existence ipso facto satisfies a legal and theological obligation. Cognitive activity is not deemed a requirement for valued life, because the world of the mind is perceived to be only one dimension of human activity. Human beings can influence the world in ways other than thought. The ability to inspire or cause fulfillment of *mitzvoth* (theological and legal obligations) by others suffices to justify existence. My obligation to preserve the life of another is not linked to the value of that life to the individual concerned nor to its value to society. The value of a given life may be framed in terms of its provision to others of an opportunity to meet higher religious obligations. These obligations arise from a direct and personal connection to the Divine, and can be satisfied, at least in part, through obedience to revealed commandments.

The obligation to rescue is special. It emphasizes the relationship between two individuals (the soul rescuing, and the soul rescued) in terms of the benefit to an entire world. It assures the rescuer of a reward in the next world as well as this world. And it emphasizes the obligation to attempt the rescue rather than to succeed.

In general, it is taught that God values the attempt to meet the Divine obligations imposed upon them by Divine decree. The effort alone has value and may induce God to intercede and assure the success of the attempt independent of its "natural" likelihood of success. Prayer for divine intercession represents a dimension through which humans can affect the fate of their world. The work of trying to fulfill an obligation translates into a "prayer in action." Insofar as it relates to the rescue of human life, the attempt is conceived as an invocation of God's merciful and healing nature. It is seen as capable of inducing recovery through Divine intercession. Hence the importance of trying and the *lack* of emphasis on the dimensions of futility. Futility is acknowledged to be a condition of human existence, but certainly not of the Divine.

The more mystical side of the tradition motivates adherence to Divinely imposed obligations, to obedience to the Divine, through ideas of *imitatio dei* (hence the metaphor between the creation of humans and the rescue of an entire world), and of "*ichud,*" or metaphorical union with God through prayer and good works. Humans are elevated more closely to the Divine through obedience. Each attempt to serve God and fulfill the commandments results in the addition of "sparks of holiness" that improve the world and bring it closer to the Divinely inspired and Divinely decreed ideal. Each act of fulfillment is taken to represent an act of holiness, of Divine provenance. Each is also perceived as an objective good.

FINDING LIMITS

With this background, is it possible to define the limits to an obligation to rescue? Two ideas begin to help answer this question. The first is the idea of competition for resources. *A priori*, on a public policy basis, it is reasonable to derive from the concepts of rescue an obligation to pursue the most pressing needs and the most efficient use of resources. This means only that a decision among several options may be decided on this basis, *ceteris paribus*. It does not mean that the care given to a specific, named individual with specific needs growing out of a specific threat at a specific moment in time may be compromised because of a theory of greater or community need.

The second idea that helps begin to answer this question is the idea of futility. Because futility, defined in the economic sense as "ineffectual" or "irrelevant as to outcome" does not coincide with or track the concept of futility in the Jewish theological sense, it is difficult to extrapolate from one use to the other. Proof that an intervention does not change the outcome (effect a rescue) eliminates the obligation to attempt that particular intervention, but not others. Proof that *no* intervention will change the outcome still does not eliminate the obligation to maintain life or pray for rescue. It does eliminate the obligation to attempt any particular technological intervention. On a case-by-case basis, certainly, the obligation to institute new interventions may be limited.

To emphasize this point once again: The limitation is based on the ineffectiveness of the interventions at hand relative to the individual at risk from the problem at hand. It is not based on abstract public issues when the problem at hand relates to a specific individual. To put it differently, there is no good global precedent or authority in Jewish law through which to reconcile the problem of a preexisting public policy intended to allocate resources rationally and equitably confronting a situation in which life-threatening needs of an individual might realistically be met at the expense of a more remote public policy goal. Where the needs of a community are specific and as immediate as the needs of an individual, and when the issue becomes one of numbers on one side or another of the equation, community needs do override private needs.

Neither of these ideas should be understood to suggest that the obligation to attempt to preserve or rescue life, either on an individual or a community basis, is suspended by the failure of existing technologies or interventions.

When faced with allocation decisions, the Jewish tradition directs that the decision be made along the following axes:[50]

1. immediate and measurable, rather than theoretical, threats to life;
2. identifiable endangered individuals;
3. specific remedies with predictable effects;
4. maximum number of souls rescued; but
5. measures intended to save the life of one individual are not to be compromised in order to rescue another or others.

For these reasons, the problem of the allocation of scarce resources in the ICU cannot be addressed on a pure policy level in Jewish law, For the resolution of specific crises on a case-by-case basis, qualified rabbinical expertise is sought.

CONCLUSION

The Jewish tradition frames allocation decisions of this sort in terms of strong obligations to save, or attempt to save, human lives. The obligation devolves both on individuals and communities. Although overarching public policy concerns do play a role in allocation decisions, their role is limited to situations in which the immediacy of an identifiable threat can be compared with respect to the numbers of identifiable individuals who are likely to be rescued, and the likelihood of rescue given the means at hand. The tradition is indifferent as to what types of interventions are used, and whether they are particularly "medical" or not.

This framework results in the following conclusions.

1. The obligation to care for an individual patient in the ICU is not strongly affected by overarching public policy concerns.
2. The obligation to admit a patient who is unlikely to recover is less than the obligation to admit a patient much more likely to recover, presuming that both are identified at the same time, they compete for the same bed, and all other factors are equal.
3. Projects may certainly compete for resources on the basis of merit and need. The decision matrix includes five elements: the immediacy and level of need,

the number and identifiability of those affected, and the likelihood of success given the best available data.

4. Acute needs may override public policy decisions, which, in any event, are not capable of overriding obligations incumbent upon individuals faced with a life-threatening situation.

There is another dimension to this discussion that has not been pursued here. This has to do with the relationship of small moral communities to larger ones. Like the Amish, Muslim minorities, or specific Christian and Jewish sects, to what extent should the exacting needs of particular moral communities compel the planning of the community at large? This topic—cooperation and competition for moral suasion among amicable, but not entirely compatible, groups—requires further exploration. From the strictly Jewish perspective, the obligation to fulfill Divine commands is independent of the behavior or subsidy of the community at large.

The unstinting obligation to rescue human life is based less on rational analysis than on Jewish legal exegesis and what may be most correctly termed mystical ideas about the fulfillment of Divine purpose. The rational for enacting limits a priori is weak. The rational for modifying not the obligation, but its application on a case-by-case basis, has been described. After the fact, there is, perhaps, more tolerance for a wider range of decisions than *a priori.*

NOTES

1. For example, the Talmud dictates that an individual trapped under a fallen wall must be rescued even if his ultimate survival will be prolonged only by seconds. *Yoma,* 85a. In a responsum cited by J. David Bleich, Rabbi I. Y. Unterman, former chief rabbi of Israel, ruled that "medical risks are warranted 'when there is a hope of a cure . . . even if in most cases [the procedure] has not been successful and will shorten life'" (Bleich 1979, 28–33, especially n. 105).

2. It would be the authority of the scholar citing the principles, as well as their context, that conveys the authority of the citation rather than the principle or the citation itself.

3. See, in general, Baron (1957, vols. III–VIII). For a detailed exposition of methodology in and the history of Jewish law, see Elon (1975, 1–149).

4. There are, traditionally, four levels of rabbinical ordination. The lowest is akin to a certification of competence in teaching, granted upon graduation by a number of Jewish seminaries, none of which considers itself Orthodox. The next, which is the most common Orthodox ordination and earned by examination, certifies the holder competent to decide on potentially difficult matters of Jewish ritual (e.g., the preparation of kosher food) and on matters of Jewish law not requiring a court. The third level is the level of *dayyan* or judge, earned by exceedingly few rabbis, which permits them to participate in or to preside over a Beth Din, or Jewish court. The fourth level would permit the holder to participate fully in a Sanhedrin, were it in existence today. This level of certification has not been given in any traditional sense at any time during the past 1,000 years.

   Under the Roman Emperor Hadrian (ca. 150 C.E.), Jewish courts were entirely abolished and ordination proscribed. Both the ordainer and the ordinand were subject to execution. Nevertheless, about a century later, Origenes, in his *Epistula ad Africanum,* section 14, refers to a Jewish court in Palestine hearing and sentencing capital offences:

"trials are conducted according to the Torah in private, and some are condemned to death, but not, however, completely in public, but yet not without the knowledge of Caesar" (cited in Schreiber 1979, 229 and n. 7).

5. See, e.g., Schreiber (1979, 226–49).

6. Schreiber (1979, 248). A similar system prevails today in, e.g., New York state, where Jewish courts ruling on civil matters are treated as courts of arbitration whose jurisdiction is agreed to by all parties to a dispute.

7. A majority of world Jewry resided in Parthian and Persian Babylonia and became the most influential influence on the development of Jewish law. The community actually predated the end of the Second Commonwealth by 500 years, when King Yehoyachim of Judah was exiled to Babylon. After the second century C.E., the most famous Talmudic academies grew in Babylon, and gave rise to a compilation of Aramaic glosses on the Mishnah (the Oral Law and commentary on the Bible reduced to writing by Judah HaNasi, Judah the patriarch, ca. 200 C.E., in response to Roman persecution and a prohibition on Jewish legal study and rabbinic ordination) and on Jewish Canon Law. This gloss became known as the Gemarah. The Mishnah and the Gemarah together were called the Talmud.

   A parallel Talmud evolved under the authority of the patriarch (*Nasi*) in Jerusalem. The original term for this position was "ethnarch"; it was first conferred upon John Hyrcanus by Julius Cæser in 47 B.C.E. Later, the Latin "patriarch" was preferred, and the rule of the Nasi referred to as the patriarchate. In 140 C.E., Emperor Antoninus Pius appointed Shimon ben Gamliel as the first ethnarch following the fall of the Second Commonwealth, and bestowed upon him great power as the representative of the Jewish community to the Roman government, and the leader of the Jewish community in both civil and religious matters. He headed the Academy and was given the right to appoint or depose judges and other officers. Jews throughout the empire were assessed a tariff of one-half shekel yearly to support the Nasi. It was the Nasi Judah, around 200 C.E., who overcame the prohibition against reducing the Oral Law to writing and compiled the Mishnah. In 212 C.E., Emperor Caracalla conferred Roman citizenship on all freemen in the Empire, including Jews, through the *Consitutio Antoniniana*. The position of Nasi was abolished by Rome in 429 C.E. as an anti-Jewish act. The funds collected for support of the ethnarch were converted by the emperor to his own use. The community in Palestine was eclipsed in most respects, from that point onward, by the Babylonian community.

   The Babylonian Talmud is considered more authoritative than the Jerusalem Talmud, though both are studied and cited in precedent. There has been a resurgence of academic interest, recently, in reevaluating the actual import of the Jerusalem Talmud, which may have been greater than traditionally believed. For references to the prohibition against reducing the Oral Law to writing see, principally, *Gittin* 60b, *Temurah* 14b, and *Eruvin* 21b; Azulai (1783), *inyan* (*in res*) 49; and Elijah of Vilna: notes to the *Shulchan Arukh*, *inyan* 49. See also, more generally, Baron (1942).

8. See Schreiber (1979, 183–225). The community in Babylon declined when the Caliphate, begun by Omar around 630 C.E., disintegrated into rival hegemonies in Baghdad, Cordoba, and Cairo at the end of the twelfth century, after which the Mongols invaded and, in 1258, conquered Babylonia. See Schreiber (1979, 283–91) and Baron (1957, vol. 1, 216 ff.), for more detailed treatment of the history that follows. This discussion closely follows their analysis.

9. See Feigenbaum (1988, 3–8); also see Schreiber (1979, 191–205).

10. Jewish law recognized 613 biblical commandments: 365 prohibitions and 248 positive

precepts. These commandments were perceived as overly cryptic to constitute a basis for practical law. They were, however, directly addressed in various forms in the Talmud. The codes were intended to distill the Talmudic discussion into a set of operative principles governing all aspects of Jewish legal concern and religious life, and transforming concepts into normative rules.

11. Literally, *Book of Laws.*
12. Literally, *Teachings of the Torah.*
13. Literally, *The Four Rows*: an allusion to the *ephod* or breastplate worn by the high priest in the Temple, whose twelve stones, each representing one of the twelve tribes of Israel and arranged in three columns and four rows, were deemed to manifest oracular powers. They were also called simply *Turim*, or rows. Rabbinical authors were often known by the title of their most significant work; hence, Jacob ben Asher is also called the *Ba'al HaTurim*, the "master of the rows," or simply the *Tur*, "the row."
14. The works differed in several important respects. For example, the *Mishneh Torah* made no effort to differentiate between laws that were primarily of theoretical interest, such as the laws regulating sacrifices in the Temple in Jerusalem, and laws of practical and current interest. The *Arba'ah Turim*, in contrast, addressed practical and concrete matters. Both works strove to create new classifications of *Halachah*. Maimonedes worked by topic and concept, and intended his work to be used for education. The Tur was guided by practicality. Both works, however, offer no lack of extra-Halachic comments, *obiter dicta*, ideological advice, and philosophical ideas.
15. This section is adapted from Twersky (1979 [1967], 357–66).
16. Literally, *The House of Joseph.*
17. Literally, *The Set Table.*
18. Literally, *The Table Cloth.*
19. See, e.g., Freehoff (1955).
20. Jakobovits (1959, xxxvi).
21. Notably Joseph Colon, 1320–1480.
22. "Liberal" is used in the British Commonwealth; "Reform" is used in the German tradition, most prominently represented in North America. They are not entirely the same, religiously, politically, or philosophically, for reasons beyond the purview of this discussion, but they stem from the same roots, address the same issues, and share a number of similarities. The term "Progressive Judaism" is also used to denote the same movement.
23. Literally, "explanation."
24. Instrumental music had been part of the liturgy at the time of the Temple in Jerusalem but was banned in commemoration of its destruction starting in the first century C.E. The Reform movement argued that the prohibition was obsolete, and that the Jewish liturgy ought to be beautiful and inspiring in the same ways the Christian liturgy could be. It emphasized the use of the organ in the service. The use of the organ and the translation of the liturgy from Hebrew into the national language became icons of Reform Judaism.
25. Admission to the rabbinate is akin to admission to the bar: The academic degree in law does not necessarily admit one to practice in any given jurisdiction. Traditional Jewish sources establish specific criteria for admission to the rabbinate, which the Conservative, Reform, and Reconstructionist movements do not necessarily deem dispositive. The Orthodox require a rabbi to achieve at least the second level of ordination (*vide* note 4, *supra*). The Conservative, Reform, and Reconstructionist movements hold that graduation from a seminary acceptable to their movement—and generally resulting in certification at the first level of ordination—suffices.

The relationship of authority and ideology is complex. A set of responsa, or answers to questions regarding permissible or advisable behavior in Jewish law—intended to be legally binding but promulgated by an Orthodox rabbi—would not necessarily be considered binding by a Conservative or Reform rabbi. Conversely, a traditionally ordained Orthodox rabbinical court would not deem a Conservative or Reform decision to have prima facie legal relevance.

For example, in matters of divorce, these issues take on critical importance, because adultery is considered an extremely serious offence, and the children of an adulterous relationship are considered irremediably illegitimate. To an Orthodox court, a divorce granted through the Reform rabbinate has no validity; as a result, a woman so divorced cannot remarry without appropriate legal remedies.

26. There is a growing Conservative tradition in South America, however, and a strong Liberal tradition in the British Commonwealth.

27. For example, based in casuistry, or conditioned upon specific interpretations of concepts, words, or idioms that might be taken to be indistinguishable except for revealed knowledge or received wisdom.

28. There are, nevertheless, certain beliefs that might be deemed heretical. Such aspersions have almost never been invoked. Thus, the Orthodox might judge the radically secular Jew to be mistaken or untutored, but under no imaginable circumstance heretical.

29. There are two aspects that make up rationing: limitations on access beyond limitations such as scarcity or price created by market conditions, and the establishment of rules for gaining access. In the event resources are scarce, the limitation on access becomes a means to assure directed distribution of goods and services and, as a separate matter, a means to control price. The idea of rationing in pursuit of fairness is well known. In the absence of free access, limited resources may go to the highest bidder, or to those who exercise other forms of economic power. That outcome may or may not be consistent with a particular vision of justness, fairness, or incentive. Rationing may also be used as an incentive (e.g., access to computer games in a boarding school granted as a function of good grades).

30. For example, does the rationing decision allow for a top-down debate on budgetary allocation? Should agricultural subsidies eclipse hospital subsidies in priority? Is there a limit to acceptable profits within the health care services industry? Should budgetary surpluses be earmarked for medical research rather than education? What is the role of government, or other central-planning authorities, in making allocation decisions?

31. This could as well be stated in terms of "group A" (a few people) or "population A" (many people) or AIDS victims, or newborn infants, or wounded soldiers on the battlefield (a few or many).

32. A decision or other mental act is included.

33. Actively pursued, as opposed to simply wishing that alternatives existed or suggesting that, had one the opportunity, one would have chosen differently. Thus, a decision *not* to ration or to direct the allocation of health care resources actively would count as an active choice.

34. The more global question of how to develop a long-range public policy approach when economic resources are not the limiting factor in any immediate sense, but priorities need to be established and budgetary policy implemented, is beyond the scope of this discussion.

35. The concept of price elasticity relates demand to price. In a fully elastic system, demand ranges from 0 to infinite, depending on price. In an inelastic system, demand is not influenced by price at all.

There is no attempt in Jewish law to engage in descriptive ethics. What matters is not whether the value of human life is or is not elastic in practice, but whether it ought to be. Jewish law concludes that it had ought to be, irrespective of what society at large might do.

36. The status of autonomy as moral imperative, in contrast, is decidedly inferior.

37. Positivist in the sense of its validity not being subject to external scrutiny or validation.

38. The suggestion that "good" means the greatest good for the greatest number is not accepted in Jewish law.

39. One might debate whether to say "*pari passu,*" "in consequence," or both. There is no doubt about the priority of this obligation or its categorical nature. Nonetheless, for two reasons, I hesitate to say "in consequence." The first reason is that there exists an important principle in Jewish law that admonishes against attempting to delineate justifications for obligations, at least in any simplistic way. The second is subtler. It is not altogether clear that obligation to save human life arises as a consequence of the value of human. There are instances in Jewish law in which the logic is precisely the opposite: The value of the good pursued is defined in terms of the power of the obligation.

40. *Ethics of the Fathers,* II: 1.

41. The obligation to save a life suspends the obligation to observe the Sabbath, an obligation that, when publicly transgressed, carries the death penalty. By what instrument the life is threatened, or by what means the rescue is effected, has no bearing on the matter. The fact that a physician is permitted to transgress the Sabbath day in order to save the life does not distinguish him or her. Anyone is permitted to do so.

42. Jewish law recognizes brain-based criteria for death only with certain stipulations (Rosner 1979, 241–51).

43. Legends regarding the behavior of such individuals during the Holocaust and during other catastrophic periods in Jewish history abound. The legends emphasize that the *tzadik* in his humility and humanity refused special treatment and shared the fate of the common man. Nevertheless, the *tzadik* has always been accorded deference, reverence, and privilege. See, e.g., Helmreich (1982); see also Birnbaum (1993, 29–46).

44. Although this discussion focuses on the *tzadik*, it could as well focus on any other quality or status that might rewarded by social privilege.

45. "The blood of one is no redder than another's. . . ." *Pesachim,* 25 b.

46. The idiom, "to see to their rescue" is intentionally ambiguous. It is intended to describe two broad, separate, but, in the Jewish tradition, overlapping obligations: the obligation to *personally* rescue a victim at risk and the obligation to participate in communally, or even to facilitate a rescue impersonally. The first is a *personal* obligation. The second is a specific embodiment of the separate obligation to tithe to communal charity. *Communities* then have a separate obligation to "see to the rescue" of individuals and charitable donations are appropriately used for this purpose. One implication of this tradition is that a community may, conceivably, exhaust its resources and thereby have reached the limits of its obligation to underwrite the rescue of a group or an individual, but the *personal* obligation incumbent upon members of the community may not have been satisfied. The reverse may also hold true. Conceivably, an individual may be impoverished and therefore have satisfied the *personal* obligation, but the community, out of its (still ample) coffers may have a separate and as yet unsatisfied obligation to aid the victim.

47. The strength of the obligation does not depend on the merits of those endangered.

48. It is important, however, to distinguish between the utilitarian view that defines good in terms of some vision of the greatest good for the greatest number, and the traditionally deontological Jewish view, which is based in obligation. The Jewish tradition is sensitive

to the need to assess the outcome of the satisfaction of an obligation: If the rescue of one life is good, the rescue of many lives is better. But Jewish law sees the good defined in the satisfaction of the obligation rather than just in the number of lives that have been saved. It is based in process as well as in outcomes.

49. Another theme in Jewish law teaches that one may not sacrifice one life for another under ordinary circumstances, and certainly not because of economic considerations. One may not remove what has been committed to one individual in order to meet the needs of another *even when the other may appear more likely to survive.* The examples of military heroism or self-sacrifice in battle are exceptional. See, e.g., *Sanhedrin* iv, 5; Maimonedes, *Hilchot Yidoei HaTorah,* 5: 5; Rosner (1979, 47–50).

50. These rules are extrapolated from the rules that govern when Sabbath observance may be suspended in order to save lives.

BIBLIOGRAPHY

Azulai, H. Y. D. 1783. *Responsa Birkei Yosef.* Livorno.

Baron, Salo Wittmayer. 1942. *The Jewish Community.* Philadelphia: Jewish Publication Society.

———. 1957. *A Social and Religious History of the Jews,* 2d ed. New York: Columbia University Press.

Bleich, J. David. 1979. The obligation to heal in the Judaic tradition: A comparative analysis. In *Jewish Bioethics,* ed. by Fred Rosner and J. David Bleich. New York: Sanhedrin Press.

Birnbaum, Meyer (with Yonason Rosenblum). 1993. *Lieutenant Birnbaum.* Brooklyn: Mesorah Publications.

Elon, Menachem. 1975. *The Principles of Jewish Law.* Jerusalem: Keter Publishing.

Feigenbaum, Yitzchalk. 1988. *Understanding the Talmud. A Systematic Guide to Talmudic Structure and Methodology.* New York: Philipp Feldheim.

Freehoff, Solomon. 1955. *The Responsa Literature.* Philadelphia: Jewish Publication Society.

Helmreich, William B. 1982. *The World of the Yeshiva.* New York: Free Press.

Jakobovits, Immanuel. 1959. *Jewish Medical Ethics.* New York: Bloch Publishing Company.

Plato. 1992. *The Republic,* trans. by A. D. Lindsey. New York: Alfred A. Knopf.

Rosner, Fred. 1979. The physician and the patient in Jewish law. In *Jewish Bioethics,* ed. by Fred Rosner and J. David Bleich. New York: Sanhedrin Press.

Rosner, Fred, and J. David Bleich. 1979. *Jewish Bioethics.* New York: Sanhedrin Press.

Schreiber, Aaron. 1979. *Jewish Law and Decision Making.* Philadelphia: Temple University Press.

Twersky, Isadore. 1979 [1967]. *The Shulhan Aruk: Enduring Code of Jewish Law.* Reprinted in Aaron Schreiber, *Jewish Law and Decision Making.* Philadelphia: Temple University Press.

The Current Medical Crises of Resources: Some Orthodox Christian Reflections

Very Reverend Edward Hughes

The moral issues raised in considering limiting access to medical treatment due to limited resources are of pressing interest in industrial countries today. It has been, in the United States at least, also an issue of some political importance. How our cultures and countries deal with these issues will reflect how we feel about life and its meaning, as well as death and its meaning.

In a discussion of the Roman Catholic perspective on limiting access to medical care, it might be asked what an Orthodox Christian might contribute. Pope John Paul II's apostolic letter of May 2, 1995, *Orientale Lumen*, speaks directly to such a question. To begin with, he says,

> Since, in fact, we believe that the venerable and ancient tradition of the Eastern Churches is an integral part of the heritage of Christ's Church, the first need for Catholics is to be familiar with that tradition, so as to be nourished by it. . . . Our Eastern Catholic brothers and sisters are very conscious of being the living bearers of this tradition, together with our Orthodox brothers and sisters. The members of the Catholic Church of the Latin tradition must also be fully acquainted with this treasure. (§1)

> I listen to the churches of the East, which I know are living interpreters of the treasure of the tradition they preserve. . . . It is earnestly recommended that Catholics avail themselves more often of the spiritual riches of the Eastern Fathers which lift up the whole man to the contemplation of the divine mysteries. (§5)

The Pope of Rome is aware that in the study of revealed truth East and West have used different methods and approaches in understanding and confessing divine things. This is quite important in a discussion such as ours. Because the Orthodox tend to use different approaches and methodology, very often Western philosophers have difficulty in appreciating their point of view. It may appear unintelligible because it is not couched in the familiar cat-

237

egories of Western philosophical discussion. As the Patriarch of Constantinople, Bartholomew, pointed out in his address at Georgetown University on October 21, 1997:

> The Orthodox Christian does not live in a place of theoretical and conceptual conversations, but rather in a place of an essential and empirical lifestyle and reality as confirmed by Grace in the heart. This grace cannot be put in doubt either by logic or science or other type of argument. . . . Holy Tradition for the Orthodox Christian is not just some collection of teachings, texts outside the Holy Scriptures and based on their oral tradition within the Church. It is this, but not only this. First and foremost, it is a living and essential imparting of life and grace, namely, it is an essential and tangible reality, propagated from generation to generation within the Orthodox Church. This transmittal of the faith, like the circulation of the sap of life from the tree to the branch, from the body to the member, from the Church to the believer, presumes that one is grafted to the fruitful olive tree, the embodiment in the body.
>
> Membership in the Church is not an act of cataloging a person as a member of a group but it is the true rebirth of this person in a new world, the world of grace. From that moment forward, he or she is nourished and grows a new body which is of different substance than the body of the flesh, and is joined with the body of Christ through baptism.
>
> The relevant baptismal hymn, "Whoever is baptised in Christ, has been clothed in Christ" is not simply symbolism or a poetic allegory. It is a real fact that brings change in the substance of the human being.
>
> Those baptised as infants, whose Orthodox parents grafted them into the body of the Church, are unable to express in words the change that took place in them, but they feel it. However, those present at the moment of baptism who have purity of heart see the grace that surrounds them. Those baptised at a more mature age and with depth of faith are able to describe the liberating feeling of renouncing the devil and joining Christ.
>
> This ontological view of the life in Christ entails a substantial element of the experience of the Eastern Orthodox Church. The glow of its light illumines all facets of our ecclesiastical and personal life in the Church and disposes of the need for foolish inquiries. (Bartholomew, Patriarch of Constantinople 1997)

This point of view, which seems so distant from traditional Western academics, is the view of the ancient church fathers and doctors that Roman Catholics and Orthodox have in common. It is the view from the time of the Holy Apostles through the undivided church, the age of the great councils in which the definitions of our faith were formulated and our liturgical traditions took form. One might term it, in Western categories, the ascetical/mystical tradition; in the West, perhaps, one among others, in the East, perhaps, the only tradition. Because the ideas involved are not commonly taken for granted in the religious and ethical discussions of today, it is absolutely necessary to present a significant amount of material toward understanding these ideas in order to see how widespread and deep these ideas are within the tradition. As is customary, I will present excerpts from texts taken from the liturgical books, the great church fathers, as well as some contemporary theologians and historians.

I will be speaking from within the ancient common Tradition, not as an outside observer of the Roman Catholic tradition, but, rather, as a participant in a common stream flowing from our jointly venerated font of faith. The unavoidable differences in our current doctrinal positions will necessarily appear only when trying to explain particular facets of the tradition, as the differences regarding original sin, or the connection between Baptism, Christ's Resurrection, and our own immortality. I will not be trying to present an "Orthodox point of view" to be observed next to a "Roman Catholic perspective." I am seeking to point out sources of understanding and of action found within our common heritage, and calling for their restoration as the basis of moral action.

Moreover, I will regard such questions from a pastoral point of view. For more than twenty years, I have been involved in pastoral, hospital, and institutional ministry in the church. I have worked in mental homes, terminal care centers, hospices, small local hospitals, and large teaching institutions. I have tried, as much as possible, to be present with the families, or occasionally without them, when my spiritual children have "given up their spirits." I have prayed with them and for them as they have passed away in hallways, emergency rooms, wards, private rooms, intensive care units (ICUs), and their own homes. My understanding of the tradition of the church with regard to end-of-life issues is based on the teachings of the fathers and of the tradition, as well as my own personal clinical and pastoral experience.

In this volume, Dr. Rössler and I together focus more on the "victims" personally rather than the institutional and political mechanisms of allocation issues. Not all of us are in positions of institutional responsibility or political influence such that we can affect these situations. We must deal with those who are within the system, on the bottom, as it were. We identify with those who are suffering at this very moment, not with the reasons for their suffering (although some of that must be dealt with). Professor Kaveny, Reverend Professor Wildes, and Professor Honnefelder are more poised to handle such issues. Professor Rie is perhaps most effective in challenging the status quo. We, for ourselves, must be resigned to the system as it is developing. Although I do have strong views on how things should or could be, this is not the thrust of my essay. For my part, my attitude is formed from my beliefs, which I perceive coming from the authentic tradition of the church: Death no longer exists, suffering is not worth considering, or perhaps is a desirable good to be used for the good of others, and God Himself will not allow any of us to be taken from this life before we are ready. With these in hand, I can perhaps be of some help to those who are closing their lives in ICUs and to their families standing prayerfully around them.

We have been given, as a point of departure for this discussion, an essay by H. T. Engelhardt, Jr., in which he introduces some ideas on the topic at hand. He presents a moral position that Plato advanced in his *Republic*, in which he makes observations on Herodicus. Plato writes:

> For all well governed peoples there is a work assigned to each man in the city which he must perform, and no one has leisure to be sick and doctor himself all his days. . . . Will you not establish by law in your city such an art of medicine . . . [which] will care for the bodies and souls of such of your citizens as are truly well-

born. But those that are not, such as are defective in body, they will suffer to die, and those who are evil-natured and incurable in soul they will themselves put to death. This certainly, he said, has been shown to be the best thing for the sufferers themselves and for the state. (409 c–d)

I do not think it a coincidence that Plato's observations on Herodicus touch upon our contemporary concerns. He writes as a pagan, with a pagan's interest in this present physical life. He very clearly sees the value of life tied to productivity and service to society. These are essentially the same values in evidence in much present-day discussion of euthanasia. It would seem shocking and distasteful to state with Plato, who says of Asclepius, that "If a man was incapable of living in the established round and order of life, he did not think it worthwhile to treat him, since such a fellow is of no use either to himself or to the state" (407e). Yet "quality-of-life" discussions often are based upon these same presuppositions and values. Popular folk definitions of "suffering" lately all seem to assume that inability physically to enjoy normal activities constitutes "suffering." As Plato says: "A life of preoccupation with illness and neglect of the work that lies before him is not worth living" (406d). Such an attitude, focused entirely upon the external aspects of this physical existence, if allowed to grow and spread, would allow individuals the freedom to end such useless and intolerable lives at any point that it appeared that they could not tolerate contemplating such a future. It would also give moral authority to cultural institutions and governments to encourage individuals to end such lives, to help them to do so by providing means and support, and even to intervene and end such lives by external fiat without the will or consent of the unfortunate victim who would at least then be "freed from all his troubles" (406e).

It seems that this is precisely the materialistic modern attitude against which the church must speak. We are not created merely to "live in the established round and order of life." We, as Christians, believe in a personal and loving God, Who created humans to share the whole of creation in relationship with Him, Who created all just expressly for that purpose. It is the relationship with the Creator that makes us truly human, and which gives life meaning. To try to judge a person's life in the light of his "functioning" in the physical world without reference to relationships with other people and with his Creator is totally materialistic and, as such, truly inadequate to evaluate what is essentially a spiritual reality. It is the great tragedy of our age that materialism has become the predominant philosophy throughout the world, depriving both life and death of any real meaning.

Traditional Christianity, concerned primarily with man's relationship with God and tied directly to that with other persons, must necessarily value life and individual lives differently. Each life is an opportunity for some individual to enter into relationship with God, Who reveals Himself to that living soul in a variety of ways in order to initiate and enlarge a personal relationship. It also represents an opportunity for other individuals to enter into relationship with that individual both as a response to their relationship with God and in order to enlarge and deepen that relationship. For God has revealed that there is a link between our relationship with Him and our relationship with each other, as He clearly defines in the Gospel according to Saint Matthew: "Verily I say unto you, Inasmuch as ye have done it unto one of the least of these my brethren, ye have done it unto me" (Matthew 25:40). And, as Saint John writes in his first letter: "If a man say, I love God, and hateth his brother, he is a liar: for he that loveth not his brother whom he hath seen, how can he love

God whom he hath not seen? And this commandment have we from him, That he who loveth God love his brother also" (1 John 4:20–21).

As all humans share the same nature, we can be said to be consubstantial with each other, each of us being created in the image and likeness of God. We are all united in one humanity in the same way that the Holy Trinity is united in His Godhead, all three Persons sharing the same nature. Since Christ has become incarnate, He has become consubstantial with us, sharing completely our human nature, taking on the image and likeness of the created. In the Liturgy, when we cense each of the people present, we are censing and paying honor to the presence of God in each of them, exactly as when we cense a relic, the Gospel, or an icon. When we kiss the hand of a bishop or a priest, we are paying honor to Christ, whose icon and objective presence they are. So it is with our service to each other. As we help, support, console, and comfort one another, we are giving service and honor to Christ, Whose image we are, as He Himself taught. The incident in the life of Saint Martin of Tours is characteristic. After he divided his cloak with the freezing beggar, Christ appeared to him and said to His Angels: "Martin is only a catechumen, and see, he clothes Me in his garment!" The same thing occurs many times in the history of the saints.

As we love, care for, forgive, support, and encourage each other, we draw ever closer to God, Who loves us, cares for us, forgives us, supports us. and encourages us both directly and through the ministrations of others. In this light, a life lived in isolation, especially in self-centeredness or in materialism, is a tragic loss to all of humanity; whereas a life lived in love and care for others, in a close relationship with God, is a life fulfilled—indeed, a real life.

It is important that such a life of love and caring for others must be for the sake of love of God, or it fails still to have real meaning. If our love and service do not have God as their ultimate focus, then however beautiful they may seem, they cannot transcend this physical world. In this case, the life itself was meaningful only in relationship to this temporal world. Only in God can we transcend the boundaries of temporality and join with Him in eternity. Indeed, Traditional Christianity holds that a loving and caring person is not even limited by death from continuing to practice love and care for others.

FOR THE CHRISTIAN, THERE IS NO DEATH

The mystery of Christ's death and Resurrection allows individuals to continue to show care and love to others without hindrance beyond the falling asleep of the physical body. The liturgical hymns sung on the feasts of the saints make this clear:

> The God-given grace of thy miracles, O martyr Theodore, thou dost grant to all who turn to thee in faith. We therefore praise thee saying: Thou dost deliver prisoners and heal the sick; thou givest riches to the poor and guardest those who sail the seas. Thou restrainest slaves from useless flight, and showest robbers what their punishment will be; thou teachest soldiers to abstain from plunder. In thy loving compassion thou dost grant the prayers of children, and thou art the fervent protector of all who keep thy holy memory. With them we also sing the praises of thy martyrdom, O saint of God: pray to Christ that He may show us His great mercy.
>
> O martyr Theodore, thou art a matchless gift from God; for after thy death as during thy lifetime, thou dost grant the petitions of those who turn to thee. Thus

once it happened that the son of a poor widow was carried off by soldiers of another faith; and she came weeping to thy shrine. Mounted upon a white horse, in loving compassion thou hast defended her child with thine invisible protection. And, now as then, never dost thou cease from working wonders: pray to Christ our God, for the salvation of our souls. (Vespers; Friday of the first week of Lent; Mary and Ware 1977, 274)

Who will not marvel, who will not render Glory, who will not hymn with faith the miracles of the wise and all-glorious unmercenaries? For even after their holy repose, they richly impart healings with all who have recourse to them with faith, and their precious and holy relics pour forth the grace of healings. . . . (Menaion, month of July, 1st day, Saints Cosmas and Damian, Matins; Lambertsen 1991, 5)

Even after thy repose hast thou been shown to be an intercessor for suffering and sorrowful men. For thus the people beheld thee issuing forth from thy tomb and praying in the midst of the church with angels. O truly most glorious wonder! O joy and confirmation of the faithful! (Menaion, month of October, 28th day, Saint Job of Pochaev, Matins canon ode 5; Lambertsen 1991, 7)

Saint Augustine, on preaching about the multitudes of miracles worked by Saint Stephen's relics, said "Though dead, he raises the dead to life, because in reality he is not dead" (Guéranger 1983, vol. XIII, 250). Here is precisely stated the point which is clear in the liturgical hymns. Saint Stephen, the martyrs, and actually all those fallen asleep in Christ, though no longer having the use of their bodies, in reality are not dead.

When Saint Seraphim of Sarov was nearing his death in 1833, he gathered his spiritual children to say good-bye to them. He said: "When I am no longer with you, come to my grave often, and bring me all your sorrows and sufferings. Talk to me as though I were still living, for I shall always be with you" (Zander 1968, 45). He was not teaching anything new or surprising, rather, he was speaking from the accepted Tradition. Perhaps in the West, this was not as common, but it exists nonetheless. According to Peter-Thomas Rohrbach, O.C.D., in his book, *The Search for Saint Thérèse*, Saint Thérèse of Lisieux, beginning in July of 1897, two or three months before she gave up her spirit,

became suddenly convinced that a world wide mission was soon to begin for her after she died. "I feel my mission is about to begin, my mission of making souls love God as I love Him, my mission of teaching my little way to souls. If my desires are fulfilled, I shall spend my heaven upon earth until the end of the world. Yes, I shall spend my heaven in doing good upon the earth." As the weeks and months passed, her statements became more firm, more absolute. "I know the whole world will love me." "I will send down a shower of roses." "Will you look down?" she was asked. "No, I will come down. . . . I will begin my mission. I will come down to aid missionaries and to obtain the baptism of pagan children before they die." Pauline told her they would put a palm branch in her hand after her death. "Yes," Thérèse said, "but I will have to let it slip from my hands because I will use them to shower graces." (Rohrbach 1961, 190–91)

What she said caused some problems for her canonization in the Roman Church because it sounded presumptuous. Yet, in the light of the full tradition, Saint Thérèse is not outside normal Christian expectation. Indeed, in the Christian East, it has always been the custom to encourage orphans to pray to their deceased parents for guidance and protection.

This continued fellowship of love in Christ is, in fact, central to the revelation of the meaning of life and death. If the death of the physical and material body does not hinder the practice of what might be called "practical Christianity," the practice of charity, then materialism is manifestly empty, and real meaning lies in the Christian way.

All of this is, according to the traditional teaching of the church, the result of Christ's Resurrection. The destruction, the annihilation of death which was accomplished through Christ's Resurrection, has set the human race free, not just from the fear of death, but from death itself. This profoundly alters the ways in which we view life, sickness, and the final falling asleep of the body. If this life is a complete and finite reality that ends at death, whether it is followed by some kind of afterlife or not, this only slightly alters the fact that this experience irrevocably ends. If, however, death does not exist, if we leave our bodies only temporarily, and if we remain vitally connected with our loved ones and indeed the whole Christian community through the Resurrection of Christ, then the focus of life must be on those things that are eternal, but the experience of those things now "in this life" continues uninterrupted into "the next life." For, in fact, they are the same life, life in Christ, which—because of His Resurrection—is endless.

Some discussion here is necessary on Christ's destruction of death and the meaning of Christian Baptism. The Orthodox Church sings throughout the forty days of Pascha: "Christ is risen from the dead, trampling down death by death, and upon those in the tombs bestowing Life!" By "trampling down death by death" the church means the destruction and abolition of death itself through Christ's life-giving death. Father Alexander Schmemann (1921–83), the late dean of Saint Vladimir's Seminary and a world-renowned theologian, wrote of Christ's death:

> "Death reigned from Adam to Moses" (Romans 5: 14), the entire universe has become a cosmic cemetary, was condemned to destruction and despair. And this is why death is "the last enemy," (1 Corinthinas 15:20) and its destruction constitutes the ultimate goal of the Incarnation. This encounter with death is the "hour" of Christ of which He said that "For this hour have I come" (John 12:27). (1982, 6)
>
> Now this hour has come and the Son of God enters into Death. The Fathers usually describe this moment as a duel between Christ and Death, Christ and Satan. For this death was to be either the last triumph of Satan, or his decisive defeat. (1982, 6–7)
>
> It was essential that death be not only destroyed by God, but overcome and trampled down in human nature itself, by man and through man. "For since by man came death, by man came also the resurrection of the dead" (1 Corinthians 15:21). (1982, 8)
>
> Such is the meaning of Christ's descent into Hades, of His death becoming His victory. And the light of this victory now illumines our vigil before the Grave [of Christ on Pascha eve]. (1982, 9)

O Life, how canst Thou die?
How canst Thou dwell in a tomb?
Yet by death Thou hast destroyed the reign of death, and raised all the dead from
hell (Lamentations of Holy Saturday Matins, stasis 1:2). (1982, 9)

In a tomb they laid Thee,
O Christ the Life.
By Thy death Thou hast cast down the might of death and become the font of life
for all the world (Lamentation of Holy Saturday Matins, stasis 1:7). (1982, 9)

This joyful song is captured well by the Paschal homily of Saint John Chrysostom, which is
read on Pascha night:

> Let no one fear death for our Saviour's death hath set us free! He that was taken by
> Death has annihilated it! He descended into Hades and took Hades captive! He em-
> bittered Hades when it tasted His Flesh! Anticipating this, the Prophet Isaiah ex-
> claimed, "Hades was embittered when it encountered Thee in the lower regions."
> Hades was embittered for it was abolished! Hades was embittered for it was
> mocked! Hades was embittered for it was purged! Hades was embittered for it was
> despoiled! Hades was embittered for it was bound in chains! Hades took a body and
> met God face to face! Hades took Earth and encountered Heaven! Hades took what
> it saw, but crumbled before what it had not seen! O Death where is thy sting? O
> Hades, where is thy victory? Christ is Risen, and you are overthrown! Christ is
> Risen, and the demons are fallen! Christ is Risen, and the Angels rejoice! Christ is
> Risen and life reigns! Christ is Risen, and not one dead remains in the tombs! For
> Christ being raised from the dead has become the first-fruits of them that slept! To
> Him be glory and dominion unto ages of ages! Amen.

This is also expressed in the hymnology of the West, most powerfully in the antiphon *O
magnum pietatis opus,* "O mighty work of mercy! Death then died, when life died upon the
Tree" (*Breviarium Monasticum* 1930, 608).

It is through baptism that the Christian participates in this victory of Christ. The
Catechism of the Catholic Church states, "According to the Apostle Paul, the believer enters
through Baptism into communion with Christ's death, is buried with him and rises with
him."

> Do you not know that all of us who have been baptized into Christ Jesus were bap-
> tized into his death? We were buried therefore with him by baptism into death, so
> that as Christ was raised from the dead by the glory of the Father, we too might
> walk in newness of life (Rom. 6:3–4 cf. Col. 2:12). (1994, 315, para. 1227)

Saint Cyril of Jerusalem, (ca. 315–86), declared a doctor of the church by Pope Leo XIII in
1882, writes in more detail:

> After these things, ye were led to the holy pool of Divine Baptism, as Christ was car-
> ried from the Cross to the Sepulchre which is before our eyes. And each of you was

asked, whether he believed in the name of the Father, and of the Son, and of the Holy Ghost, and ye made that saving confession, and descended three times into the water, and ascended again; here also covertly pointing by a figure at the three-days burial of Christ. For as the Saviour passed three days and three nights in the heart of the earth, so you also in your first ascent out of the water, represented the first day of Christ in the earth, and by your descent, the night; for as he who is in the night sees no more, but he who is in the day, remains in the light, so in descending, ye saw nothing as in the night, but in ascending again, ye were as in the day. And at the self-same moment, ye died and were born; and that Water of salvation was at once your grave and your mother. And what Solomon spoke of others will suit you also; for he said, There is a time to bear and a time to die (Eccl. 3:2); but to you, on the contrary, the time to die is also the time to be born; and one and the same season brings about both of these, and your birth went hand in hand with your death. . . . Let no one then suppose that Baptism is merely the grace of remission of sins, or further, that of adoption; as John's baptism bestowed only the remission of sins. Nay we know full well, that as it purges our sins, and conveys to us the gift of the Holy Ghost, so also it is the counterpart of Christ's sufferings. (1977, 60–61)

As recently as the 1860s, Dom Prosper Guéranger wrote in his *Liturgical Year*:

Thrice then, has the catechumen entirely disappeared under the water: it has closed over and shrouded him. We have the explanation of this given us by the great apostle: the water of Baptism is the tomb, in which we are buried together with Christ; and, together with Him we rise again to life: the death we had suffered, was the death of sin; the life we are henceforth to live, is the life of grace. Thus is the mystery of Jesus' Resurrection repeated, with all its fullness, in them that are baptized. (1983, vol. VI, 617–18)

Even though we see this truth affirmed in the church from the beginning, and reaffirmed by the Roman *Catechism* so recently, still it is not widely understood. As Schmemann wrote, there is an

inability of modern post-patristic theology to explain the relationship between Baptism and the Death and Resurrection of Christ, a relationship clearly affirmed by both liturgy and Tradition. Not only do they affirm it, but they make this relationship the very content and meaning of the sacrament. We are baptized "in the likeness of the Death and Resurrection of Christ . . . that being buried, after the pattern of Christ's death, in baptism, we may, in the like manner, be partakers of His resurrection" (Rom 6:5). Hence the emphasis, in the liturgical tradition, on the organic connection between Baptism and Pascha; hence the paschal character of Baptism and the baptismal content of Pascha in the early Church.

This clear affirmation did not remain central, however, when theology began to be understood and developed as a rational explanation and interpretation of the Christian faith. One continued to pay lip service to the baptismal "symbolism" of death and resurrection but the real meaning of the sacrament shifted elsewhere. In virtually every manual of our "systematic" theology the two essential references in explaining Baptism are original sin and grace. Baptism, we are told, removes from man and liberates him from the original sin, and it also bestows upon him the grace necessary for his Christian life. As all other sacraments, Baptism is defined as a "means of grace," as a "visible sign of an invisible grace." It is absolutely essential, to be sure, for our salvation; but in these definitions and explanations, it is no longer presented as being truly—in essence and not only in external symbolism—death and resurrection.

Baptism being performed "in the likeness" and "after the pattern" of death and resurrection therefore is death and resurrection. And the early Church, before she explains—if she explains them at all—the "why," the "what," and the "how," of this baptismal death and resurrection, simply knew that to follow Christ one must, at first, die and rise again with Him and in Him; that Christian life truly begins with an event in which, as in all genuine events, the very distinction between "form" and "essence" is but an irrelevant abstraction. . . . Baptism is what it represents because what it represents—death and resurrection—is true. (Schmemann 1974, 54–55)

At least part, if not the root cause, of this problem is a simple problem of translation. Father John Meyendorff writes in *Byzantine Theology*:

The scriptural text which played a decisive role in the polemics between Augustine and the Pelagians is found in Romans 5:12, where Paul, speaking of Adam, writes: "As sin came into the world through one man, and through sin, death, so death spread to all men because all men have sinned [*eph ho pantes hemarton*]." In this passage there is a major issue of translation. The last four Greek words were translated in Latin as *in quo omnes peccaverunt* (in whom [i.e., in Adam] all men have sinned"), and this translation was used in the West to justify the doctrine of guilt inherited from Adam and spread to his descendants. But such a meaning cannot be drawn from the original Greek—the text read, of course, by the Byzantines. The form *eph ho*—a contraction of *epi* with the relative pronoun *ho*—can be translated as "because," a meaning accepted by most modern scholars of all confessional backgrounds. Such a translation renders Paul's thought to mean that death, which was the "wages of sin" (Rm 6:23) for Adam, is also the punishment applied to those who, like him, sin. It presupposes a cosmic significance of the sin of Adam, but does not say that his descendants are "guilty" as he was, unless they also sin as he sinned. (1983, 144)

A number of Byzantine authors, including Photius, understood the *eph ho* to mean "because" and saw nothing in the Pauline text beyond a moral similarity between Adam and other sinners, death being the normal retribution for sin. But there is also the consensus of the majority of Eastern Fathers, who interpret Romans 5:12 in close connection with 1 Corinthians 15:22—between Adam and his descendants there is a solidarity in death just as there is a solidarity in life between the risen Lord and the baptized.

This interpretation comes, obviously, from the literal, grammatical meaning of Romans 5:12. *Eph ho*, if it means "because," is a neuter pronoun; but it can also be masculine, referring to the immediately preceding substantive *thanatos* ("death"). The sentence then may have a meaning which seems improbable to a reader trained in Augustine, but which is indeed the meaning which most Greek Fathers accepted: "As sin came into the world through one man and death through sin, so death spread to all men; and because of death, all men have sinned. . . ."

Mortality, or "corruption," or simply death (understood in a personalized sense), has indeed been viewed, since Christian antiquity, as a cosmic disease which holds humanity under its sway, both spiritually and physically, and is controlled by the one who is "the murderer from the beginning" (Jn 8:44). It is this death which makes sin inevitable, and in this sense "corrupts" nature. (1983, 146)

Father John then goes on to show Cyril of Alexandria, Theodoret of Cyrrhus, and Theodore of Mopsuestia in agreement and representative of Eastern thought on this matter.

There is indeed a consensus in Greek patristic and Byzantine traditions in identifying the inheritance of the Fall as an inheritance essentially of mortality rather than of sinfulness, sinfulness being merely a consequence of mortality. The idea appears in Saint John Chrysostom, who specifically denies the imputation of sin to the descendants of Adam, as well as in the eleventh-century commentator Theophylact of Ohrida and in later Byzantine authors, particularly Gregory Palamas. Maximus the Confessor, when he speaks of the consequences of the sin of Adam, identifies them mainly with the mind's submission to the flesh and finds in sexual procreation the most obvious expression of human acquiescence in animal instincts; but as we have seen, sin remains, for Maximus, a personal act, and inherited guilt is impossible. For him, as for the others, "the wrong choice made by Adam brought in passion, corruption, and mortality," but not inherited guilt:

> In this perspective, death and mortality are viewed, not so much as retribution for sin (although they are also a just retribution for personal sins), as means through which the fundamentally unjust "tyranny" of the devil is exercised over mankind after Adam's sin. From this, baptism is a liberation, because it gives access to the new immortal life brought into the world by Christ's Resurrection. The Resurrection delivers men from the fear of death, and, therefore, also from the necessity of struggling for existence. (Maximus the Confessor 1984, Quaest. Ad. Thal., 90: 408BC)

This is the central point on which traditional spirituality, morality, and ethics turn. Some have questioned why it is necessary to explain original sin in a discussion such as this, but this point is the crucial center of everything, most especially of medical and end-of-life ethics.

This means that all aspects of everyday life are transfigured by the experience of the Resurrection. How we live and relate to others is determined by the fact that we are living in the Resurrection now, living the life in Christ which will endure eternally. All of our choices, conversations, and activities have eternal ramifications. Those choices and actions that are consistent with life in Christ contribute to our eternal well-being. They constitute, to use the scriptural phrase, our "treasure in heaven," which will always be there for us. Choices and actions that are at variance with life in Christ detract from that well-being, and could actually contribute to everlasting discomfort.

PAIN AND DEBILITATION ARE POSITIVE GOODS TO BE DESIRED AND ENJOYED AS A MEANS OF COMMUNION WITH CHRIST

This, however, is only one direction to take in regard to this topic. The other important consideration is the Christian attitude toward bearing sickness and preparing to lay down the body in an act of trust in God.

> O Mighty Prince Who wast born of a Virgin:
> In the depths of passionlessness,
> I beseech Thee to drown the tripartite soul;
> That to Thee as with Tympani
> In the mortality of the body,
> I may sing a victory song. (Paraklitiki 1984, 191; my translation)

This ancient hymn speaks very eloquently to the Orthodox Christian attitude toward the mortality of the body. It is often stated that the Orthodox Church has preserved itself throughout the centuries through the Liturgy. In fact, the Liturgy has been an important locus for the expression and explanation of the Faith in general, along with specifics on dogmatics and the spiritual life. As part of the Tradition, the liturgical texts hold a place alongside the canonical Holy Scriptures, the ecumenical councils, and the writings of the great church fathers. They are not simply pious devotional pieces, but are a full and rich expression of the content of the Faith.

Of course, it is understood that the entirety of the Tradition is a single whole. Each element of the Tradition is a different expression of the same content. Icons, poetry, sermons, canon law, and Holy Scripture each and all express the fullness of the same faith and Way.

That having been said, this hymn which is of apparent antiquity, being certainly earlier than the seventh century, and probably later than the third century, speaks pointedly to the problem at hand.

The "mortality of the body" is precisely the problem of sickness and death, the special provenance of the health care industry. The phrase, in fact, is probably a quote from the physician Galen, who uses these exact words several times in his works—which probably predate this hymn. The mortality of the body: sickness, increasing weakness, and eventual death all can be an ultimate terror, or perhaps something else. In light of the Christian tradition, the mortality of the body holds terror only for those whose lives were lived outside of Christ, or in rejection of Him and His Way. For the faithful believer, the mortality of the body leads only to a temporary separation of soul and body, in the loving care of God, and not a separation from Him or from the Christian community. This hymn writer would have us celebrate this gift in the sickness and dying itself. The hymn writer says that we are to create a victory song out of our mortality. The writer uses an ancient allusion to pre-Christian worship in the mention of tympani. Ancient sources attest to the use of tympani in the rites of worship of Cybele and Bacchus; in the case of Bacchus, probably associated with his festal processions, which were common and popular throughout the Greek world. Perhaps this is exactly the image that the writer has in mind: a festal procession, a victory procession in honor of Christ, Who Himself is victor over death. (In Orthodoxy, the phrase IC XC NIKA, which is stamped even on the bread to be consecrated at the liturgy, always means Jesus Christ conquers or is victorious over death.) The idea of the process of mortality as a festal, victory procession is one of powerful beauty. In recent lectures, Matushka Juliana Schmemann has referred to the death of the well-known theologian, Father Alexander Schmemann, as "the feast of my husband's passing." She speaks about it as an event of profound spiritual beauty. This is, in fact, the tradition of the church. Each Christian must prepare himself in such a way as to be able to make of his own mortality a festal, victory procession in praise and honor of Christ.

It is through the body that we ourselves benefit from our love and care of others. Each moment given us is precious as an opportunity to advance in virtue and in relationship with God. The body itself is a gift from God for our use in His service. Nevertheless, there is a tradition of those who bore lengthy sicknesses with patience, being examples for others, and even turning their sicknesses into a means of ministry.

Saint Poemen, the much-ailing of the Kievan Caves Monastery in Russia, was remarkable for his patience in bearing sickness. He had been sickly since childhood, and in his enforced quiet, he began to desire the monastic life. Finally, he was taken to the Kievan Caves for healing and was left there, where he remained until his death. He lay sick for twenty years, working wonders and miracles until the time of his death. His sickness was horrible to see, including open sores and a foul smell that made it difficult for the other monks to care for him. As a result, he often was without care for days at a time. He was always patient and kind and never blamed the others for their lack of care and compassion. He was healed and rose from his bed only the day he died, as had been foretold to him by angels. He has continued actively to work miracles and is popular among the Kievan saints for his wonders.

A Bishop Steven wrote down his experience once in a communist labor camp in the 1930s. He was facing a fifteen-year extension of his sentence and was advised to pray to Matrona, a holy woman living hundreds of miles away at the time. He did, and found himself released shortly. He journeyed to meet this woman, and found her tiny and deformed, without arms or legs, and blind. She was kept in a box on a table in a room. She knew him and called him by name at his approach even though they had never met. He found that she had been abandoned in a church while still a baby, and that the Christian congregation had cared for her there, in the church, until she was older. She foretold the future, worked miracles by her prayers, and guided pious people in their lives. She died in a communist prison soon after this meeting.

In 1993, a Mother Macrina reposed in Russia. She had been paralyzed since childhood, and was twisted into an uncomfortable position, from which she could not even sit up. She became a great wonderworker and spiritual guide from her sickbed, healing many people who asked for her prayers. She eventually died from abuse at the hands of her caretakers.

These are only three examples of this type of holiness; many others can be found in both traditions, such as Saint Theresa of the Child Jesus in France, who died at the age of twenty-four from tuberculosis, and Saint Jean Vianney, who suffered considerable pain and physical debilitation for years, but in fact continually increased his labors until his death. These remarkable Christians are filled with peace and confidence in God, which makes their sufferings not only bearable, but precious to them.

Two very recent Greek elders, who have only reposed in this decade, Fathers Paisios and Porphyrios, are also important in this regard. These remarkable fathers are renowned as wonder-workers and healers in Greece and on Mount Athos. Father Paisios reposed in 1994 at the age of 70. He suffered from cancer of the bowel, which had metastasized to the lungs and liver. His pain was extreme, as were his weakness and fatigue due to loss of blood. When pressed to receive treatment for his disease, he said: "My health's condition is a great benefit to my spiritual life and I do not really wish to alter it. . . . At least, let me suffer from cancer as a consolation to people in distress. Now, thank God, everything is just fine. . . . I had asked God to make me suffer from cancer" (Christodoulos 1998, 19). Father Porphyrios reposed in 1991 at the age of 85. He had been chaplain at the Polyclinic in Athens for many years. At one time speaking to his friend Dr. George Papazahos, an assistant professor of cardiology at the University of Athens, he said:

> I have cancer in the pituitary gland . . . you should know that when I was a monk, maybe 16 years old, on Mt. Athos, I felt so elated especially after receiving Holy Communion . . . that I cried out: "Glory to you, Lord . . . What do I do for you? What pain do I suffer for you? Lord send me a cancer!" But now He sent me the cancer. Do you understand what a good turn it is? Even though it is late, I will suffer together with Him a little. (Ioannidis 1997, 266–67)

Dr. Papazahos wrote: "It is the first time in my medical career that I had heard such an expression, 'Thank God, I've got cancer!'" (Ioannidis 1997, 266–67).

A priest once visited Father Paisios and told him that he had been suffering from terrible headaches for many years. On being healed before a miraculous image of the Virgin, he had come to share his joy with Father Paisios. Father replied to him: "I cannot understand your way of thinking. You just asked the Virgin Mary to 'relieve' you of the only 'bank book' you had, where you could constantly make spiritual deposits, and you are happy about it" (Christodoulos 1998, 113)!

Obviously this is a special calling and gift from God, and not the case for everyone. However, every Christian should strive to attain to at least some measure of such peace and confidence. As many pious writers have explained, we have much time in our lives to prepare ourselves for our final act of faith. Most of us squander that time and reach our end quite unprepared. But it does not need to be so. We need to be reminded by our spiritual guides to work at being prepared spiritually for that day, which will surely come to all of us. As Saint John Chrysostom wrote:

> What then? Are we to give thanks for everything that befalls us? Yes; be it even disease, be it even penury. For if a certain wise man gave this advice in the Old Testament, and said, "Whatsoever is brought upon thee take cheerfully, and be patient when thou art changed to a low estate" (Eccles. 2:4); much more ought this to be the case in the New. . . . But if thou give thanks when thou art in comfort and in affluence, in success and in prosperity, there is nothing great, nothing wonderful in that. What is required is, for a man to give thanks when he is in afflictions, in anguish, in discouragements. Utter no word in preference to this, "Lord, I thank thee." And why do I speak of the afflictions of this world? It is our duty to give God

thanks, even for hell itself, for the torments and punishments of the next world. . . . Let us therefore give thanks not only for blessings which we see, but also for those which we see not, and for those which we receive against our will. (Homilies on Ephesians, Homily XIX, Eph 5:21; Schaff 1976, 137)

Even more, the church has always held the possibility of making spiritual use of our sufferings. Pious nuns in parochial schools all over the world used to remind their young students to never miss an opportunity to "offer up" their sufferings on behalf of others. In the present time, we have lost some sense of that. It goes all the way back to the age of the great martyrs, who prayed for others and healed the sick at the very time of their own sufferings and torments. Father Paisios in Greece said: "God is deeply moved when someone, who has cancer or some other serious problem, does not complain about it, but instead prays for his fellow men" (Christodoulos 1998, 19). Anyone familiar with the hagiography of the Roman Church is aware of the many saints who transcended their own personal suffering in order to intercede for others. Nearly twenty years ago, just after he was elected, Metropolitan Theodosius of the Orthodox Church in America wrote: "The elderly especially, with the shut-ins and the infirm, are urged to a special ministry of prayer" (1980, 4). For those who are personally prepared and at peace, they can and need to move on to this step and begin praying for others and for the community.

The Christian support community must be aware of this ideal and sensitive to the individual's progress toward it. Times of sickness, especially serious sickness, must be times of reflection focused on the ultimate course of life. Neither lightheartedness nor frantic, desperate denial is appropriate to the Christian life, and neither tends toward the necessary goal. Here the support of the Christian community, especially the clergy, is critical for those who are spiritually aware and well prepared. They can say with Saint Paul:

> Christ shall be magnified in my body whether it be by life or by death. For to me to live is Christ, and to die is gain. But if I live in the flesh, this is the fruit of my labour: yet what I shall choose I would not. For I am in a strait betwixt two, having a desire to depart, and to be with Christ; which is far better: Nevertheless to abide in the flesh is more needful for you. And having this confidence, I know that I shall abide and continue with you all for your furtherance and joy of faith. (Philippians 1:20–25)

I knew two sisters, both in their eighties at the time. One had lead a "tragic" life. In midlife, she had found her daughter murdered with an axe in the family store. After this trauma, she lost the ability to speak. Later, Parkinson's disease took away almost all her movement. This woman lay for more than twenty years mute, paralyzed, and confined to bed, only able to move her face. Nevertheless, visiting her was a joy. He family had made her the center of their family life. Grandchildren brought their friends to sit and chat, watch television, or play games around their grandmother's bed. She took a lively interest in life and was joyful, peaceful, and deeply devout. She looked forward to visits from the clergy, to prayers, to blessings, and to the Sacraments. In spite of her bodily limitations, she was filled with joy and was a joy to those around her. In contrast, her sister had lived a normal, happy life up to old age. Her husband had been a successful businessman; her children were healthy, happy, and well married; and her grandchildren were a source of comfort and pride. Yet when she began to show symptoms of Parkinson's disease, the whole family went into mourning. Shades were drawn, people spoke in strange subdued murmurs, and everything was overcast and darkened with gloom. The poor woman was sick for perhaps eight years, and was able to walk with help and get around for most of that time, yet she and all around her were quite overcome with her suffering. What made the difference? Clearly, the older sister had suffered so much more, but she and her family had surely overcome these sufferings. "Suffering" is a matter of attitude more than anything else, an outlook, perhaps a philosophy of life.

This is not to say that we may not seek, expect, or pray for healing. Obviously, God has given us the means and opportunities for healing. Neither may we seek to hasten our departure from the body either by our own actions or negligence. Certainly, the church does pray for the advent of physical death if someone is suffering terribly at the end:

> O Lord our God, Who in thine ineffable wisdom hast created man, fashioning him out of the dust, and adorning him with comeliness and goodness, as an honorable and heavenly acquisition, to the exaltation and magnificence of thy glory and kingdom, that thou mightest bring him into this image and likeness; but forasmuch as he sinned against the command of thy statute, having accepted the image but preserved it not, and because, also, evil shall not be eternal: Thou hast ordained remission unto the same, through thy love toward mankind; and that this destructible bond, which as the God of our fathers thou hadst sanctified by thy divine will, should be dissolved, and that his body should be dissolved from the elements of which it was fashioned, but that his soul should be translated to that place where it shall take up its abode until the final Resurrection. Therefore we pray unto thee, the Father Who is from everlasting, and immortal, and unto thine Only-begotten Son, and unto thine all-holy Spirit, that thou wilt deliver N. from the body unto repose, entreating, also, forgiveness of thine ineffable goodness if he in any wise, whether of knowledge or in ignorance, hath offended thy goodness, or is under the ban of a priest, or hath embittered his parents, or hath broken a vow, or hath fallen into devilish imaginations and shameful sorceries, through the malice of the crafty demon: Yea, O Master, Lord our God, hearken unto me a sinner and thine unworthy servant in this hour, and deliver thy servant, N., from this intolerable sickness which holdeth him in bitter impotency, and give him rest where the souls of the righteous dwell. For thou art the repose of our souls and of our bodies, and unto thee do we ascribe glory, to the Father, and to the Son, and to the Holy Spirit, now, and ever, and unto ages of ages. Amen. (Office at the parting of the soul from the body; Hapgood 1965, 366)

For those who are unprepared, either for sickness or to leave their bodies, their anxiety can only be eased by entering into a focused relationship with the Living God. If they have regrets, they need to find forgiveness and peace and so begin, however late, to make their victory song and their festive procession.

PRACTICAL AND PASTORAL RESPONSES BY THE CHRISTIAN COMMUNITY

This is a situation in which we may foresee using every resource of medical technology to extend physical life a bit longer if possible. For those who are just making a beginning as they are "at the end," a little more time may be crucial. An increase or extension of physical suffering and pain may be a fair trade-off in light of coming to terms with one's self and ultimate reality. The support of family and the Christian community in such a case would be of inestimable value to the individual concerned.

The sad case is that, under pressure from the secular world, most individuals do not prepare themselves in the way they live their lives for their eventual eternity. Too many distractions and cares keep them from focusing on this important consideration. Only as they lie critically ill do they turn their thoughts toward their approaching end. Nursing homes and hospitals become the first places where many people find the time, the quiet, and the inclination to contemplate their preparedness for the most demanding and important time of their lives. Even then, they must cope with televisions, radios, newspapers, and well-meaning visitors who encourage them to persist in materialistic denial. ICUs become blessed retreats and safe havens away from these distractions. Often there are no televisions or radios and visitation is strictly limited. Even the medical paraphernalia tend to scare away many worldly minded visitors. Although certainly not the ideal (which would to be surrounded by a caring, spiritual Christian support group in prayer and perhaps hymnody), at least being free from anti-Christian worldly distractions is a considerable blessing. It needs to be stated here that some people do not realize that a patient who is unresponsive, and seemingly unconscious, may be still quite spiritually active. Spiritual activity does not depend in any way on mental consciousness; it is accomplished by another faculty entirely. In a spiritual person, the mind, when conscious, can apprehend and be aware of his own spiritual activity; such activity, however, does not originate or take place in the mind, but rather in the "heart." This is such a vast and difficult topic, that—even though incredibly important—it cannot be taken up at this time. For those interested, I would recommend Bishop Hireotheos Vlachos' books on Orthodox spirituality. But I must state quite emphatically that spiritual life can and does persist even when the mind is not at work.

To properly make use of medical interventions in a Christian manner, one probably needs to be aware of what being a Christian is all about and to accept that as one's own way of life. Perhaps evangelization is a necessary precondition to move away from an essentially pagan worldview and the crises that grow naturally from that, to a Christian view and the peace and acceptance that grow naturally from that. The focus of our discussions is supposed to be specifically on the allocation of health care resources in intensive care situations. This is a point at which many themes in the Tradition converge. In many instances, intensive care involves "end-of-life" decisions, and such decisions necessarily require the convergence of all of the Christian tradition, because that is the moment for which we have been living, the culmination and climax of our Christian lives, the ultimate "act of faith." It involves both the Christian attitude toward the suffering of others, sacrificial and complete sympathy and care, as well as the Christian attitude toward bearing one's own suffering, which is undemanding and self-denying, rooted in a radical belief in Christ's Resurrection and destruction of death.

Informed and motivated by these principles, traditional Christians would make distinct health care choices. In general, a Christian focus to life must be on the welfare and well-being of those around us, not on our individual selves. Talk about "rights" and "entitlements" has little meaning when all is a gift from God as He sees fit to bestow. We see only opportunities to love and serve for Christ's sake. Those who are ill or suffering need to be cared for by the community of believers. This is not and cannot be about allocation of public funds and resources. We, as the Christian community, need to care for the needy, the sick, and the suffering because it draws us closer to Christ and fulfills us as His disciples. The "public" or the civil government cannot so benefit, because, in the pluralistic, secular modern world, the State is not Christian, and, therefore, has no conception of specifically Christian virtue or benefit from acts of Christian kindness. However that may have been possible or beneficial in the age of "Christian princes," it is manifestly not the case now. Although the needy and sick may benefit materially from the expenditure of public resources, such benefit is without Christ, and so is merely material and temporal. Having no eternal and spiritual dimension, it cannot fulfill either the giver or the recipient. The Christian community, from the absolute beginning, has provided care for the needy, sick, and suffering. Indeed, it has always been the identifying feature of Christians, that they care for each other and others as well. Father Stanley Harakas, in his *Health and Medicine in the Eastern Orthodox Tradition*, says:

> In the early church caring for the sick and suffering, regardless of their religious beliefs, nationality, and race soon became a hallmark of the Christian life. Dionysius, the bishop of Alexandria, provides a moving example in his description of the Christian response to a great pestilence that fell upon that city about the year 203:
>
> The most of our brethren were unsparing in their exceeding love and brotherly kindness. They held fast to each other and visited the sick fearlessly, and ministered to them continually, serving them in Christ. And they died with them most joyfully, taking the affliction of others, and drawing the sickness from their neighbors to themselves and willingly receiving their pains. And many who cared for the sick gave strength to others [and] died themselves having transferred to themselves their death. . . . Truly the best of our brethren departed from life in this manner, including some presbyters and deacons and those of the people who had the highest reputation; so that this form of death, through the great piety and strong faith it exhibited, seemed to lack nothing of martyrdom . . . But with the heathen everything was quite otherwise. They deserted those who began to be sick, and fled from their dearest friends. And they cast them out into the streets when they were half dead, and left the dead like refuse. . . . (Harakas 1990, 63)

This, in fact, has been cited as a decisive factor in the growth and spread of Christianity. Rodney Stark in his book, *The Rise of Christianity: A Sociologist Considers History* (1996), reminds us of Tertullian's quote of a pagan who said "See with what love these Christians love each other." He also shows how Emperor Julian the Apostate fumed and raged at the pagan priests because they could not compete nor could they get their people to compete with Christians in charity and good works. It also is the first thing that anti-Christian governments have proscribed. Charity by the Christian community has been outlawed by governments, which can see how powerful a witness this is to the faith of the community.

The collection and distribution of specifically Christian resources for the care of the sick and suffering must be organized on both local and higher levels. At one time in the history of the church, this was a very large undertaking, handled by the most trusted staff. It was almost the rule in Rome that the Bishop of Rome be succeeded by his archdeacon, who, because he handled the care of the widows, needy, and sick, was well known to be committed, trustworthy, and competent, having detailed knowledge of every aspect of the church's operations.

Father Stanley Harakas shows from his research and that of Timothy Miller, who published *The Birth of the Hospital in the Byzantine Empire*, that hospitals as we know them as places where the sick are provided with "beds, meals, and constant nursing care . . . while they undergo medical therapy at the hands of professional physicians" (Miller 1985, 4), are a Byzantine invention dating from the fourth century. He says:

> These places of healing were originally expressions of Christian philanthropy for the poor and for strangers (hence their original name *xenones,* meaning "places for strangers"). It was for the medical care of the sick in these institutions that the church of the Eastern Roman Empire (that is, Byzantium) engaged private physicians, organized them, financed them, and thus gave birth to the hospital in history.
>
> Thus, the Byzantine xenones represent not only the first public institutions to offer medical care to the sick, but also the mainstream of hospital development through the Middle Ages, from which both the Latin West and the Moslem East adopted their facilities for the ill. To trace the birth and development of centers for the sick in the Byzantine Empire is thus to write the first chapter in the history of the Hospital itself.
>
> It is critical to note that it was the church in the East that established the xenones and the hospitals, or nosokomeia (literally, "places for the care of the sick"). The church governed the hospitals, financed them, and provided their staffing. It did this as an expression of its Christian calling to "love humanity" and as an embodiment of its calling to become God-like; God was above all *philanthropos,* "One who loves humanity." Thus, after mentioning the "significant roles" of the Cappadocians and Chrysostom in the early years of Christian hospitals, Miller expresses in general terms the intimate relation between the Orthodox Church and the development of the hospital.
>
> As the orthodox church came to exalt the medical profession as the epitome of philanthropia, it in turn felt obliged to make this philanthropia available to all—especially the poor—by sponsoring hospitals. Since most Greek church leaders continued to esteem medicine as one of the best expressions of Christian love until the final days of the East Roman Empire, so too they did not falter in supporting nosokomeia. As late as the 1440s the monastery of John Prodromos in Petra still maintained a public hospital. (Miller 1985, 4)

As this quotation indicates, hospitals in Byzantium were frequently part of monastic establishments. The founding charters of many monasteries included provisions and rules of governance for these hospitals for the general public (which were in addition to the infirmaries devoted to the exclusive treatment of the monks). One of the most famous was the hospital in the twelfth-century Pantokrator Monastery whose charter (typikon) shows a highly professional organization, with administration in the hands of the monastics, the medical care and surgery handled by carefully graded staffs of physicians, and ranks of supportive staff drawn from the monastics. The hospital had specialized clinics and the necessary physical facilities to fulfill its task. (Harakas 1990, 74–75)

Father Harakas also shows that the Islamic Ottoman Empire's destruction of the Byzantine State seriously limited the ability of the Orthodox to continue this tradition of free hospital care for all. Presently, however, the church has allowed the public sector to usurp this role in many modern societies. This is tragic, because the church, in losing its important activity, has also lost much of its voice in society. When she provides the major humanitarian assistance, the church can also set the agenda for moral and humanitarian discussion. Although the church stands empty handed, she also has only empty words to say about anything of importance.

Christian hospitals and hospices need really to be free of any financial restraints; financial realignments must be made to shift funds here rather than to other places of less importance to the core of the church's being. Christians need to be more generous in their giving to such causes within the church. Philanthropists, of which there are many these days, need to direct their funds to such projects that bear the life and presence of Christ. And the vanishing resource, the dedicated, trained, and idealistic monastics, need to be reenlisted to service in the church. In the Acts of the Apostles, we read that the deacons were elected to serve the poor and the widows of the communities. The communities of widows and virgins arose to continue this good work. Until the present age, the church has not wanted for committed monastics to carry on the ministry of love within the community. It must be seen that the social trends that have been allowed to infiltrate the church have not had a positive effect on her life. Monastics once were the normal teachers at Catholic schools and formed almost the entire staff at Catholic hospitals. Obviously, this is no longer the case. Entire orders of nuns have disappeared from Catholic life. The reasons for this are probably quite complex and difficult to trace, making the reversal of the trend very difficult to imagine, let alone implement. Yet this must be done. At the present time, with Orthodox monasticism undergoing something of an increase worldwide, Orthodox theologians frequently speak of monasticism as a sign of the health of the church herself. This may be very true, for healthy monasticism speaks to the vitality of the faith of the community, which can inspire young people to make a life of asceticism and self-denial as a witness to Christ's victory. But this monasticism must also reflect the fullness of the life and faith of the church. Even as the early church saw practical care of those around and even outside of her as an absolutely necessary expression of her being, so must present-day monasticism perform these same services, which express the church's love for humankind, and which monastics once performed with great piety and enthusiasm. It is no good to say that the church and her monastics once did great deeds for the poor and sick, and presently provide nothing. This would be the same as saying that the church once used to believe in the Virgin Birth, the divinity of Christ, and His bodily Resurrection, but presently does not. As we believe, so must we act. The community needs to fight back with vigor and reclaim the hearts, minds, and hands of these armies of holy men and women who can give of themselves for the life of the church. The Christian community, and especially the huge Catholic community, should certainly be able to provide itself with more than enough hospitals, hospices, and the people to staff them from the vast resources that it has on hand.

The Orthodox parish of Saints Peter and Paul in Ben-Lomond, California, forms a very close community. As a matter of course, they help care for the sick and the elderly of each others' families. This provides levels of care far greater and more effective than at most nursing homes. The parish of Saint Michael in Beaumont, Texas, used to have the custom of sitting with the sick of the parish in hospitals and nursing homes. They provided such care as dressing, washing, and feeding, as well as basic company and fellowship. This was not seen as a hardship on anyone, but provided enormous relief for the families as well as comfort for the patients.

In the modern, secular scenario, we have the critical care patient (or his family) demanding heroic, inappropriate medical interventions to extend his life by hours, days, or weeks pitted against a health care industry intent on containing costs and allocating resources to get the greatest return, measured in quality and length of survival. The patient's "rights" are in direct conflict with the "greater good" of the entire community whose resources are being used. In the Traditional Christian pattern, we have the community poised to use every means to alleviate suffering and attain healing with absolutely no limits whatsoever. What? No limits? How can this be? The secular, the worldly mind cannot understand that in such affairs of the Kingdom of God, we are not bound by economic constraints. God Himself always provides the means to accomplish His will. The Eastern as well as the Western traditions are full of stories of saints who spent freely, beyond rational behavior, trusting in God to provide resources. Saint Laurence Justinian, first Patriarch of Venice, even took on debts in order to help the poor. When he was asked on whose help he relied for payment, he answered: "On my Lord's help, and he can easily pay for me" (Guéranger 1983, 142). Saint Jean Vianney did the same with his orphans and their care, and was never left in need by God. Indeed, he was mocked and abused for being impractical and endangering their welfare, but he persevered in faith, and God rewarded him. For those who are believers, this is nothing much; for those who do not believe, nothing can be said to convince them. Only experience can teach such faith. Also, in the traditional Christian pattern, the patient (and his family) is undemanding, being at peace with God and with himself, quietly and joyfully awaiting God's pleasure for him. See how the dilemmas disappear. The community has placed every resource at the patient's disposal, but he is demanding none of it, patiently experiencing the joys of communion with Christ. If there is any conflict whatsoever, it would be that the patient would rather be left alone to be with God and finally to go to God; whereas the community would be anxious to comfort, to heal, to help so much, finally becoming a nuisance to the patient, until sensitivity would force them to back away.

Practically and pastorally, the critical care scenario is really rather rare. Critical care of the type described in our discussions is extremely expensive. The very idea of a one-to-one (or even one-to-two or -three) nurse-patient ratio during three shifts per day is costly. Also include the fact that these nurses must be specially trained and therefore command higher salaries, and the costs do indeed skyrocket. But it is equally rare. Only huge teaching hospitals can afford such critical care nurses. Most communities do not have such hospitals, these being largely confined to the great urban centers. In community hospitals, whether private or public, ICUs are staffed with fewer nurses, who have received less training than that described in our discussions. Also, with the rise of health maintenance organizations, patients no longer have free access to any hospital they might choose. They can only receive care at hospitals that are in their program. Any deviation, such as because of travel emergencies, is subject to approval by company representatives. The result is that such expensive care is absolutely not available to the general population.

The Christian response to this circumstance is twofold. The Christian community can and indeed must operate hospitals at its own expense that provide, at nominal cost or less, the absolute best, top-of-the-line care that is technologically possible to everyone who comes, whether from within or outside the community of faith. To even consider anything less is to betray our very being as Christians.

Conversely, if it is not currently available, and it is not, we do the best that we can. Not only is proper Christian health care not available, but most important, Christians are not properly trained, educated, and prepared for their physical end. To make proper use of medical interventions in a Christian manner, one probably needs to be aware of what being a Christian is all about and to accept that as one's own way of life. Perhaps evangelization is a necessary precondition to move away from an essentially pagan worldview and the crises that grow naturally from it.

Our entire Christian education program needs to focus sharply on the radical nature of Christian life and its meaning. Preaching and teaching from every source need to inform and challenge Christians on these ultimate concerns. Much has been written about the Western culture of denial of death, ignoring it and disguising it so that people do not have to come to terms with it. This, again, is a pagan approach. Saint Paul wrote to the Thessalonians: "I would not have you to be ignorant concerning them which are asleep, that ye sorrow not, even as others which have no hope" (1 Thess. 4:13). The Christian faith provides clear answers and alternatives to the fear and avoidance of death. In Christ, we have absolute freedom from death and all its terrors. If Christians are ignorant of this, then their ignorance must be remedied.

Pastoral care in hospitals and hospices certainly can be greatly improved along these lines. Hospital pastoral care tends to be perfunctory and full of the emptiness of the secular world. Every fashion of popular psychology and self-help is propagated and used rather than the Traditional teachings and prayers of the church.

Those in hospitals and hospices are at an important time in their lives, perhaps the most important. The care, expense, and time we spend on helping adolescents cope with making life decisions we consider well spent, and perhaps insufficient. Christians should see that just as much care, expense, and time need to be spent on those making end-of-life transitional decisions. People in these institutions should see pastoral ministers as much as they see their physicians and nurses. Christian institutions such as hospitals and hospices need to see that pastoral, spiritual care is equal to physical, medical care. Manifestly, at that point, the things of the flesh are passing away, and much more emphasis needs to be placed on the things of the spirit.

Indeed, this is the time to be aggressive in this field. This is precisely the moment to be seized! No more are these people distracted by the cares of this world, making money, establishing businesses, caring for homes and families, and concerned with the physical future. Rather, they have the leisure, even if the time be short, to concentrate on their spiritual health and well-being. They should not be deprived because the focus and concentration of the medical care industry is tragically elsewhere. We ponder who benefits the most from the use of life-extending therapies. We begrudge people an extra hour or day or week in an ICU because, ultimately, they are going to die. Well, ultimately everyone is going to die, at least physically. We need to see why they want this extra time in their bodies. Will they use the time to grow and mature spiritually? Will they use it to prepare themselves with faith to place themselves in the hands of God? Give it to them! Will they spend it merely writhing in pain and crying out in fear against death? Give it to them as well, but spend that time trying to teach and comfort them, praying with them and for them, to help them make the transition in faith. Do they not need it, being already prepared and at peace and in lively expectation of God's mercies? Then do not force it on them. Allow them to press on toward the next step in their continuing life in Christ with eagerness, rather than seeking to keep them in the body beyond their time. The deciding factor is not their Acute Physiology and Chronic Health Evaluation III scores, nor the projected "futility" in keeping them alive, but how prepared they are for their physical end from a Christian spiritual point of view.

It happened recently that I was called upon to be present at the bedside of a dying Roman Catholic. He was eighty years old, had suffered an enormous heart attack, had been without heart function for more than five minutes, and had suffered significant organ and brain damage. It was clear that he was going to die, but by accident he had been put on a ventilator and was receiving high doses of dopamine and lidocaine intravenously. The doctors informed the family that even though he would never come out of this state, nevertheless, the combination of drugs and ventilation would keep him alive for some days. They suggested that after twenty-four hours they would begin, with the family's assent, to withdraw the drugs, and perhaps after that, the ventilator; specifically to hasten the man's death, which, they said, was inevitable. The family had not wanted this medical support in the first place, and they understood and accepted the impossibility of the patient's improvement, but they did not want to initiate the withdrawal of life support. I thought it best to put the problem to the patient himself, since leaving the body is normally an active, not a passive act. Even though he was deemed to be unconscious, I explained to him that he probably did not want to place this burden on his wife and children, and that because he had already received the last rites of the Roman Catholic Church, and was assured of the prayers of his family as well as the community, he could, and ought, to release his body as soon as possible. Surrounded by his loving family praying for him, he "gave up his spirit" perfectly peacefully without having any of his life support decreased. He did it because he was convinced that it was the right and most expedient thing for him to do. He spared his family an agonizing decision, and perhaps years of doubt and regret.

The moment of the end of life can be a time of great personal choice and under personal control. It need not be a time of helplessness or empty waiting. When one is ready, one can die, regardless of the amount of medical intervention. I have seen many cases of this, as have most doctors. There exists the accepted notion that people will die if they lose "the will to live." This is a very negative way of stating it. In fact, people can die whenever they are truly ready. In her essay in this volume, Dr. Taboada refers to this circumstance, that dying as an *acta humanus* is very important to our discussions. Perhaps she had something else in mind, but I take her to mean the patient's conscious and willful participation in his own death.

This can sometimes be truly remarkable. I was with one woman when her doctor informed her that tests showed a malignancy in her lung. As he went on to explain his program for treatment, she turned to me and began to make her funeral arrangements, completely disregarding the doctor as well as my protests. She passed away two days later while her family and I held her hands and her doctor looked on helplessly. (This is not for rhetorical effect; her doctor was actually quite distressed.) I have seen quite a few like her since then. Another woman had a serious stroke and was immediately hooked up to all manner of life support. She showed absolutely no brain activity. Her family gathered one at a time at her bedside in the ICU. After her last brother arrived and spoke with her, she died, life support notwithstanding. I received a call one afternoon from a woman in the hospital saying that she was going to die, would I please come over. I arrived to find her sitting up in bed speaking with her husband, who had just come in as well. She asked me if I was ready. She and her husband spoke for the next hour or so about all kinds of things. Several of her children joined us as time passed. Finally, she said that she was tired and would go to sleep. Shortly, a nurse came in and took her blood pressure. Upon hearing that the diastolic number had dropped to thirty, I suggested to the family that we say a prayer. As I finished the prayers for the departure of the soul some fifteen minutes later, she quietly breathed her last. None of her family had been aware of her phone call to me, why I was there, or that she was dying. They were quite surprised and upset, but she had controlled the entire afternoon as she herself had wished.

We need to shift the focus from being concerned about who gets the best medical care to meeting the needs of every Christian for the best spiritual care. Spiritually mature Christians will not present many intensive care dilemmas. There will not be such competition for extreme intensive care resources, because those seeking them will do so only in cases of real need. If ICU care will gain someone a few extra days or even a week more of sickness, who in peace of mind would want it? Even if it could mean another year of life, but is not available, it is not a tragedy, or even an inconvenience. In the absence of death, what difference does it make how long we tarry in our bodies until we await the general Resurrection? If we believe with Saint Paul that to live is Christ and to die is gain, and if we truly have confidence in God, what need have we to squabble over ICU beds? If God needs us to work further, as Saint Paul says, then He will see to it that we can. If we are not needed further in our bodies, better to lay them down and let them rest. We can continue our life in Christ as we await the Resurrection with or without our bodies; never being separated from those we love nor prevented from praying or praising God as before.

At the beginning, I proposed to speak from a common ascetical-mystical tradition that appeared to have maintained itself into modern Roman Catholicism. It may not in fact be true that this tradition is still intact. Father Paul Schotsman recognizes three commonly identified periods of Roman Catholic theology: (1) the period before John XXIII, (2) the period between John XXIII and John Paul II, and (3) the teachings of John Paul II (in this volume). It may well be that the theological trends following the serious upheavals in Roman Catholicism since the time of John XXIII have been so significant that Roman Catholicism no longer recognizes an enduring reality in the ancient, common ascetical, mystical tradition. If that be the case, all of my foregoing essay notwithstanding, it would therefore be impossible for the Orthodox to contribute anything to a Roman Catholic discussion concerning the use of intensive care. At best, they could analyze current commitments and draw out their implications.

The Roman Catholic Church may have developed in such a way as completely to eliminate from its life the apprehension of spiritual reality that once animated and informed all of Christian life and culture. If that is true, the Orthodox and the Roman Catholics speak from mutually unintelligible worlds. The reality of the ascetical, mystical tradition once was the presupposed ground beneath Roman Catholic theology and philosophy, as well as providing the basis for Roman Catholic moral theology. As has been pointed out by others, not only the great Cappadocian Fathers, but also Saint Jerome, Thomas Aquinas, Bonaventure, Ignatius of Loyola, and others were primarily ascetics and men of deep piety and prayer. They consciously supposed that their spiritual life was the source of their theological and philosophical understanding. Certainly this attitude persisted, however sporadically or marginally, until the time of John XXIII. The trends of Catholic theology and philosophy have in the past fifty years gone in radically other directions. It would seem that it may be futile for the Orthodox to speak of a common tradition with the Roman Catholics. Even though the present pope can speak of the East's maintaining the treasures of the faith, the bulk of his own theologians, philosophers, and scholars seem to find no real value in such "treasures." For them, and perhaps for the majority of Roman Catholics worldwide, their faith itself may have come to be something else than the pope and his vision may hold. Traditional spirituality, far from forming the basis of thought and understanding, is no longer relevant to modern discussions at all.

BIBLIOGRAPHY

Bartholomew, Patriarch of Constantinople. 1997. Address of His All Holiness Ecumenical Patriarch Bartholomew Phos Hilaron "Joyful Light." Georgetown University, Washington, D.C., October 21.

Breviarium Monasticum, Pars Altera. 1930. Bruges: Desclee De Brouwer.

Catechism of the Catholic Church. 1994. New Hope, Ky., and Rome: Libreria Editrice Vaticana, Urbi et Orbi Communications.

Chistodoulos, Priestmonk. 1998. *Elder Paisios of the Holy Mountain.* Athos: Holy Mountain.

Cyril of Jerusalem, Saint. 1977. *Lectures on the Christian Sacraments*, ed. by F. L. Cross. Crestwood, N.Y.: Saint Vladimir's Seminary Press.

Durasov, G. 1995. *Beloved Sufferer: The Life and Mystical Revelations of a Russian Eldress: Schemanun Macaria.* California: St. Herman of Alaska Brotherhood.

Guéranger, D. P., O.S.B. 1983. *The Liturgical Year.* Powers Lake, N.D.: Marian House.

Hapgood, I., trans. 1965. *Service Book of the Holy Orthodox Catholic Apostolic Church.* Brooklyn: Syrian Antiochian Orthodox Archdiocese of New York and All North America.

Harakas, S. S. 1990. *Health and Medicine in the Eastern Orthodox Tradition.* New York: Crossroad Publishing Company.

Ioannidis, K. 1997. *Elder Porphyrios: Testimonies and Experiences.* Athens: Holy Convent of the Transfiguration of the Saviour.

Lambertsen, I. E. 1991. *The Menaion in English.* Liberty, Tenn.: Saint John of Kronstadt Press.

Mary, Mother, and Archimandrite Kallistos Ware. 1977. *The Lenten Triodion.* London: Faber and Faber.

Maximus the Confessor. 1984. Quaest. Ad. Thal. In *The Philkalia,* ed. by Saints Nikodimos and Makarios, trans. by G. E. H. Palmer, P. Sherrard, and K. Ware. Boston: Faber and Faber.

Meyendorff, J. 1983. *Byzantine Theology: Historical Trends and Doctrinal Themes.* New York: Fordham University Press.

Miller, T. S. 1985. *The Birth of the Hospital in the Byzantine Empire.* Baltimore: Johns Hopkins University Press.

Paraklitiki. 1984. *Ekdoseis FOS.* Athenai.

Rohrbach, P.-T., O.C.D. 1961. *The Search for Saint Thérèse.* Garden City, N.Y.: Hanover House.

Schaff, P., ed. 1976. *Nicene and Post-Nicene Fathers of the Christian Church.* Grand Rapids, Mich.: William. B. Eerdmans.

Schmemann, A. 1974. *Of Water and the Spirit.* Crestwood, N.Y.: Saint Vladimir's Seminary Press.

———. 1982. Introduction to *Matins of Holy Saturday.* Syosset, N.Y.: Department of Religious Education, Orthodox Church in America.

Stark. R. 1996. *The Rise of Christianity : A Sociologist Reconsiders History.* Princeton, N.J.: Princeton University Press.

Theodosius, M. 1980. *Hear My Prayer, O Lord.* Syosset, N.Y.: Orthodox Church in America, Orthodox Prayer Movement.

Zander, V. 1968. *The Life of Saint Seraphim.* London: Fellowship of Saint Alban and Saint Sergius.

The Allocation of Medical Services: The Problem from a Protestant Perspective

Dietrich Rössler

The following remarks do not attempt to treat either Protestant ethics or the problems of allocating resources within the health care system in their entirety. Rather, my purpose is to draw attention to particular aspects of this broader issue that are of fundamental importance to Protestant ethics. One of the central insights of Protestant theology is the foundational need to develop health care policy that explicitly recognizes the fallen character of this world. Such a recognition allows us not to be tempted to seek to do the impossible. It focuses us on responsibly accomplishing what we can realize and, with respect to problems of allocation, leads us to seek an ethical program for those patients who will be directly affected.

THE BLESSINGS OF GOD ARE MANIFOLD AND UNEQUAL

Luther's teaching on the two kingdoms reveals the idea of the "perfect life" as an eschatological concept and concludes that the only means by which we can partake of it on this earth is "through faith." Thus, here on earth only a relative order is possible, the goals of which are essentially defined by the avoidance of discord. Within the framework of this worldly and temporal order, it is necessary for every Christian to accept his or her lot in life. As Luther points out, "No one should lament that he is poor or his estate too low." The blessings of God, he adds, are "manifold and therefore unequal" (1913; WA 49, 609, 15; WA 12, 334, 2).

Nevertheless, Lutheran theology and jurisprudence have always considered it a salient task to chart a design for the relative order of this world. A significant paradigm therein is necessarily the problem of the distribution of limited resources, especially the distribution of land. Likewise, there must exist a public order capable of protecting private property from arbitrary violations. Here, two models are of particular salience. The first is the contract model, as it originates primarily with Hobbes. Here, public peace is ensured by a monopoly of power in the hands of the state. However, the particular private holdings of individuals are left entirely to chance; all that is guaranteed is the protection of that which he or she possesses. In contrast, theoreticians of absolutism, following Grotius, differentiated the *dominium eminens* of the state from *dominium vulgare,* that is, the property of individuals. This was taken a step further in the *Preußische Allgemeines Landrecht,* the body of law instituted in Prussia in 1794, which guaranteed private property under the law. G. W. F. Hegel later provided a theoretical foundation for this guarantee in his philosophy of law (1970; §41 ff., §189 ff.) His theme was not the arbitrariness of distribution, but rather, the theoretical legitimization of existing conditions of ownership. As is well known, Marx finally demanded the abolition of private property altogether in order to achieve complete equality of circumstances, thereby rendering further thought on the equal distribution of such property irrelevant.

Since the nineteenth century, the main development in property theory has been in theories of legitimatization, which justify private property in its varying distribution and at the same time attempt to secure social welfare. These theories are indebted either more to the contract model or to that of positive law. They represent the mainstream in any public debate on issues of distribution. Therefore, it is not surprising that Protestant ethics in particular finds its position represented here. After all, it is one of the sources from which these theories arose. Nevertheless, egalitarian ideas have never played a role in Protestant theology, except insofar as they have received a religious interpretation: Equality is the equality of all men before God. However, using the theological concept of human dignity as a starting point, it is possible to call for a secular equality of all men within the framework of the relative order of this world: namely, equality before the law, from which political equality might then follow (Thielicke 1968, 333 ff.).

Insofar as the treatment of private property may be taken as an example of how the distribution of limited resources is regulated in a modern society on the whole, it may be assumed that we will not find any fundamentally different means of regulation when it comes to the allocation of limited resources within the field of health care. Protestant ethics has no cause, in any case, to expect or espouse an order in this area other than a merely relative order, which at best limits discord. In principle, the allocation of medical services can be only as just or unjust as the world to which this task is given.

THE SEARCH FOR A JUST MINIMUM

It is often claimed that health is not a commodity of the kind that can readily be compared with other goods, such as land or property. This is correct. Health is not necessarily one good that stands over against others. Rather, it is a "transcendental" or conditional good, like peace, freedom, monetary stability, or life, in that for such goods it generally holds true that while they are not everything, without them all else is nothing (Kersting 1997, 187). That health is a good that is a necessary condition of other goods could hardly be contradicted. In this discussion, however, the commodity that is scarce is not health itself. It cannot be, because health is not something that is available for distribution. It is rather health care—or more specifically, the treatment of disease and the restoration of health, as well as medical care for the chronically ill. The commodity in short supply is thus a service; it is the many services rendered by members of the health professions for the benefit of members of society.

In industrial and complex societies, services are also goods that must be distributed. Industrial societies have traditionally distinguished between those goods produced by skilled craftsmen and those manufactured by industry. Above all, however, cultural goods required regulation for access and participation. Such regulation was especially pronounced, for example, with regard to access to adequate education. In modern societies, a complete lack of access to education is not tolerated. Conversely, specialized education, though not precisely scarce, is of a very limited availability. In its most widespread form, the established regulation of access provides a general or basic education for all, whereas higher education is distributed to a small, especially qualified circle.

Analogous regulations pertain to access to medical services. The introduction of social insurance in Germany more than a century ago was intended to secure basic medical care for the entire German population. Since that time, a system of socialized medicine has developed which is supplemented by a great number of different kinds of private insurance. This system has led to the development of multitiered levels of medical care. Within the framework of socialized medicine, the level of medical care to which the patient has a right is substantially lower than that covered by private insurance. Thus we must speak of first- and second-class medical coverage, even if, in a narrow sense, the differences in medical treatment are rarely crucial. For the time being, the basic model still survives: Medical care, as a service of limited availability, is distributed according to rules that curtail differences in availability without completely eliminating them. Yet this system of socialized medicine has reached the limits of its capacity to care for patients. In the future, it will hardly be possible to continue to provide all medical services that may provide some benefit for each and every individual.

It is well known that this two-tier system of medical care contains a large number of gradations, each of which describes a level of allotment and quality of service; it is more properly referred to as a multitier system of health care. At the very top is that circle of patients who receive every needed attention under the best possible conditions, whereas at the bottom are those patients who receive only what is absolutely necessary, that is, "the minimum." The principles of a relative order do not necessarily stand in opposition to this different distribution of care. Considering the character of this world, a world in which the absolute justice of God does not yet rule unchallenged, it is of no great importance within the framework of a theological ethic how such differences are justified: individual achievement, need, or chance. Such differences are on the whole a sign and a consequence of the "Fall" of humanity.

In Germany, the relative order of this "fallen world" guarantees that no individual be denied basic minimum health care. The difficulty is that of defining the nature and extent of such a minimum standard. It is the responsibility of those who bear the burden of public trust, or, to use a term from the time of the Reformation, of the *magistracy* to determine acceptable minimal standards. In particular, a definition of the minimum fulfills its function when it can be accepted as the basis for social tranquillity.[1]

UNEQUAL DISTRIBUTION OF HEALTH CARE AS MORALLY ACCEPTABLE

It is widely held that social tranquility must be regulated by a system that is perceived as just. From such a point of view, the distribution of goods, including medical services, is seen as just if it follows from standards which are acceptable to all participants when considered from an objective standpoint (Kersting 1997, 187). Were we further to characterize such an "objective standpoint" as God's standpoint, then this might indeed constitute a statement of theological ethics. It would, though, still require an appropriate understanding of *justitia evangelica*, which the Protestant tradition teaches is not directly obtainable here on earth or in this life.

Theological ethics, in contrast, begins with the insight that conflicting interests will represent key issues in any discussion of *justitia civilis*, the relative order of this world. Even ethics, which merely seeks a relative or temporary and improvable order, may in the end seek consensus, but it begins with the clash of conflicting interests. Thus, within the framework of theological ethics, it makes sense first to differentiate among the various perspectives and special interests out of which conflicts arise. Therefore, with regard to the allocation of health care, we must consider the interests and needs of patients as well as of health care professionals, and of others in society.

Those who are ill, with few exceptions, already experience their illness as a form of injustice; they experience fate as unjust above all because it has selected them arbitrarily, without rhyme or reason for such suffering. "Why?" and "Why me?" are the most common questions asked by patients facing a serious illness. These are questions which include religious aspects, including theodicy, but which primarily thematize the patient's lived world and the priorities of that world. Patients typically expect to receive whatever care is possible based on the latest advances in medical science. As a rule, they will only perceive their allotment of health care as just if the entire range of medical possibility is put at their disposal. From this perspective, patients will view every curtailment of health care, every restriction or allocation, as unjust. This is especially the case when the patient knows that others may have received such care. From this perspective, a system of allocation would only be just if it guaranteed everyone equal care, the best of care, and unlimited access to all medical services.[2]

Obviously, patients will learn that in their case, as in many others, full and unrestricted access to medical treatment was not made available. Perhaps some patients will be able to accept such limitations; however, what would occasion one to call such circumstances just? From the standpoint of an objective observer, in order to allow the execution of a just policy on the whole, there may be reasons to deny particular patients certain services. But the patient, from his or her perspective, will hardly feel moved to accept this as just.[3] He experiences the medical world as unjust; moreover, the medical world mirrors the world he has always known. What might help him, what he is waiting for, is the effort of everyone involved to at least lessen some instances of injustice with regard to health care, thereby ameliorating the injustice represented by the whole of his life.

The perspective and special interests of medical professionals are by no means simply identical with those of their patients. Prima facie, however, they may appear to be in harmony. A physician may consider the distribution of his services just if he can give every patient he accepts all the treatment that he deems necessary. Indeed, the ancient Hippocratic principles of medical ethics appear to require just such an attitude. However, even if we leave aside the question of physical medical resources, it is not possible for a physician to follow these principles without restriction. Limitations are already inherent due to the personal nature of his services. A physician must not only budget his time, but also his energies; that is, he must allocate both in different proportions. This basic difficulty of personal allocation is especially pronounced when only limited external resources are available for the physician's use. To whatever extent he must budget, allot, and restrict these resources, he unavoidably runs into conflict with the interests of individual patients and with many of the goals of medical ethics.

Every form of rationing by the physician, even if it is only in the area of personal compassion, involves such a conflict. This is the case even if such rationing seems to be justifiable under the heading of priority setting (Kleinert 1998, 1244). In this way, injustice presents itself in the lived world of both doctor and patient. Both have already come to terms with this situation, but certainly not because they consider it just when one individual is treated better than another; rather, they have merely accepted the fact of injustice. In such a case, however, the physician can more easily retain the illusion that he at least comes close to providing just conditions if he follows objective standards. Even the theoretical legitimation of unequal and unjust treatment does not really alter the situation. Thus, the question remains whether there is a way to render such conditions acceptable.

A third area is represented by the perspectives and interests of society, which must regulate its health care system within the framework of its total order. Every society accepts inequalities of greater or lesser magnitude in all areas of life. "For as long as our society considers that inequalities of wealth and income are morally acceptable—acceptable in the sense that the system that produces these inequalities is in itself not morally suspect—it is anomalous to carve out a sector like health care and say that there equality must reign" (Fried 1982, 399). The health care system is organized by means of political decisions. The aggravation of the conflicts involved is proportional to the extent to which rationing must be made a general condition. Protestant ethics has no special reason to declare preferences in these matters. Since the time of Luther, it has demanded of the "magistracy," or of its equivalent in democratic societies, no more than that no one be denied basic minimum access. However, even in the case of regulatory measures which pursue these goals, conflict is unavoidable: conflicts with minorities, conflicts arising from unsatisfactory compromises, conflicts due to unavoidable discrimination, or perhaps, due to the preferential treatment of groups or individuals.

For Protestant ethics, such a situation full of conflict and clashing interests is just an ordinary instance of the type of constellation of problems commonly encountered in the area of social ethics. Its singularity lies in the topic alone: the allocation of medical services. Within the framework of Protestant theology, we are faced with a question of applied ethics: "Applications of ethics are descriptions of concrete cases with normative intentions" (Rendtorff 1991, 9). Thus, Protestant ethics begins in each case with the description of a specific situation and therefore with the observation of empirical reality and individual experience. For this reason, it was appropriate to go into the details of the patient's condition and environment. The normative intention of such description, within the framework of a merely relative moral order, can only be realized by determining what stands in the way of good and what, in the case of concrete injustice, can be corrected or reduced. It is not good in itself that will come within our grasp, or that can be used normatively, but only the relatively better, and thus in a concrete case we often seek to come to terms with the lesser evil.

For this reason, summary formulas as descriptions of specific situations have always been regarded critically in the Protestant tradition. Theoretical definitions of solutions to problems tend to give the impression of being able to formulate ideal circumstances, in which the problematic situation no longer exists. To such ideas, positivist criticism has already replied that "absolute justice is an irrational ideal" and that supposedly rational definitions of justice are completely empty formulas, which are useful neither for justifying nor criticizing actual existing systems of justice.

In its skeptical attitude toward ethical programs for the betterment of this world, theological ethics also attaches great importance to the criticism of illusory misunderstandings of reality. Protestant ethics must remind us that much as it is necessary and possible to improve the lives and circumstances of individuals, good itself cannot be obtained or produced by good works, no matter what their nature. All ethical reflection must begin with a recognition of the human condition as having a double aspect: Humans are finite and subject to chance, and this experience is to be interpreted through the fallen world.

In a theological context, moral processes can only be described in this manner, that is, in a relative manner. The question of how *justitia civilis* stands in relation to *justitia evangelica* will only receive an answer in the context of *justitia evangelica* itself. For Luther, the moral task was that of mediating between faith and ethos, both in the case of the individual and in the ordering of social-ethical problems (Elert 1932a, 48). Therefore, theological ethics is bound just as much to the empirical world as to the rational duty of at least avoiding that which is worse. If a good will rules the world as a whole, then given that this world is a "fallen world," it is just such a reduction of injustice that will allow this good will to show itself and will prepare the way for it.

Here, then, are the grounds for finding one's own situation acceptable. It is not the overcoming and dissolution of conflicts that renders the situation capable of consent, but rather the experience and insight that the prevailing order does not deny one access to the basic minimum and the recognition of the importance of the implementation of the normative principle of reduction of injustice. Thus, the impulse to accept one's own situation and its drawbacks does not arise from the insight into theoretical rules, but rather from the empirical process itself.

REASONABLE RESIGNATION

Protestant ethics cannot make a practical distinction between misfortune and injustice in view of individual experience. True, it is not the case that every misfortune is an injustice, but every injustice is rightly referred to as a misfortune. Illness is a misfortune; inadequate care is at times an injustice. For the sick, the true misfortune lies in the combination of the two. Protestant ethics, therefore, would guide us toward seeing as a whole the fate that burdens and makes unreasonable demands on individual experience. It is the individual's task to interpret this experience in ethical terms. For this purpose, two types of piety, which may be differentiated but not separated, have proven their worth in modern Protestantism.

First, as Kant pointed out, a consequence of moral reason is that all suffering and evil encountered by humanity should be seen as grounds for scrutinizing one's own convictions and for strengthening the moral will. Evil becomes a moral task. A person should always, but especially in the case of misfortune, do those things which will make one worthy of happiness. True happiness, which is seen as the suspension of all evil, lies in the far distance. But each step on the way there is a test of the moral conviction that accepts evil for the sake of good, precisely as a trail (1956 [1798], 180 ff.).

Second, Schleiermacher draws attention to the fact that reflection on experience and especially on the experience of evil reminds humans of the limits of their freedom. These reflections are fundamental aspects of human self-enlightenment. Misery and injustice lead us to realize that humanity is not completely identified either with them or with mere pleasure. The true self-enlightenment of humanity thus begins at the point where persons become aware of their limited freedom and their complete dependence. In this consciousness of the self's pure and simple dependence lies the final truth about humanity. Every experience that, when reflected upon, serves to bring about this insight must, therefore, be counted profitable for humanity and for life (Schleiermacher 1970, 112 ff.).

These two types of piety preserve the distinction between *vita activa* and *vita contemplativa*. Piety in the style of Kant makes evil into a moral task and refers to the duty always and everywhere to seek and do that which is one's duty. To this day, this tradition has continued to generate characteristic religious programs, which have become meaningful in other contexts, for example, as the theology of liberation, theology in socialism, or political theology. Protestant models for a *Gesinnungsethik*, ethics of conviction, or movements such as Moral Re-Armament also belong to this category. It is characteristic of all these that they are more representative of the moral type of piety than the reflective.

This reflective type of piety, which we have sketched in terms of Schleiermacher, has become a central ingredient in Protestant life as it is widely practiced. Here the emphasis is on the recourse to the questions that persons must ask in order to understand themselves, so that they need not shape their life blindly, but rather in accordance with the understanding they have won. The theology of cultural Protestantism belongs to this tradition, although it is not without connection to the moral aspect of piety. Of all the modern programs of ethics indebted to this school, the most important is that of Trutz Rendtorff. It defines ethics as "the theory of the conduct of human life" (Rendtorff 1986, 3).

For the sick individual, the contribution of Protestant ethics can consist in better enabling him or her to perceive the moral and reflective aspects of the situation. To the degree that he succeeds, he will, within the order of this fallen world, seek to accept fate as his own. It would be thoroughly in keeping with the nature of this world and that of human fate, if he or she would summarize the result in the simple and unadorned formula: reasonable resignation.

LIMITING ACCESS TO CRITICAL CARE

Intensive care is a form of therapy that cannot be offered everywhere and at all times to each patient in the same measure. Such very expensive therapy must be distributed and rationed. The general rule usually applied is that patients are admitted to the intensive care unit (ICU) in the order in which they arrive at the hospital. This rule is generally considered acceptable to all patients. Patients do not as a rule object to it, and physicians avail themselves of it, because it obviously guarantees that no patient is intentionally denied better therapeutic options.

In fact, this rule reflects conditions of the social lottery. It is in accordance with the accidents by which every individual biography is determined, for example, that for one patient the distance to the hospital is short and the ICU can be reached quickly, whereas for another patient the mere fact of the longer trip causes later arrival and thereby unavoidably worsens therapeutic prospects. This inequality of distribution is generally recognized and accepted, precisely because it is directly connected to inequalities in the circumstances of life. Conversely, it makes manifest a minimum of care on which everyone can rely; for, in the first instance, intensive care is equally available to everyone. This statement, however, is only valid in theory, not in practice. Nevertheless, this restriction of theory by shortcomings in practice is universally accepted. As long as intensive care is at least theoretically available to every patient, the minimum that each individual has a right to expect is still considered established, even if this care is not, for practical reasons, accessible in every instance. As long as the order of this world is understood as a relative order, there is no expectation that one must compensate for personal misfortune or individual disadvantages which are in some way due to "fate" or "acts of God."

In the narrower sense, however, the distribution of intensive care begins in the hospital. It is of ethical significance that here all distribution strategies focus on the patient's prognosis. It is always the prognosis that decides the issue in the triage of patients, even if one uses the APACHE system or most other types of likely cost-benefit calculators. It is the prognosis that must shoulder the burden of legitimating such strategies for limiting access to critical care.

The prognosis takes on deep ethical significance in at least three ways. First, we must remember that from an ethical perspective intensive care itself cannot be a valid treatment goal. Intensive care is only a means, the goal must be something different. Intensive care is a therapy that should be used in order to make itself superfluous. There may be circumstances that prevent this goal from being reached in particular cases, but there can be no moral grounds for deeming intensive care in itself desirable as an end. In this context, the prognosis is loaded with ethical significance from the outset; for it is on the basis of the prognosis that the decision is made whether to admit the patient to the ICU.

Second, the distribution of limited intensive care resources follows the maxim that preference is given to those with a better prognosis. This maxim is the basis of all distribution strategies. If the principle holds that intensive care should be provided primarily or exclusively to those patients where a successful result can be expected (Society of Critical Care Medicine Ethics Committee 1994, 1201), then the question arises as to whether patients with worse prospects are not being discriminated against. This applies especially to those patients whose prognosis is unclear. Patients with a very poor prognosis can understand foregoing treatment in the context of a fate which has been indelibly influenced by their illness, and in this they will be in agreement with their physicians and their next of kin. By contrast, patients with a promising diagnosis will expect to be admitted to intensive care and, indeed, will expect this as a right which may not be denied. In the case of a patient, however, who cannot on the basis of his or her prognosis be readily assigned to one group or the other, the question arises as to how injustice can be avoided or at least reduced. In the end, this patient must inevitably be assigned to one of the two groups. Depending on how the prognostic criteria for determining assignment to either of the two groups are defined, both options must be kept open as long as neither set of criteria has been satisfied, for in each case either alternative might represent the worse outcome. Thus, in the case of patients whose prognosis is such that both options must remain open, supplementary criteria should be given greater weight and in the end decide the issue. Here we are concerned with criteria in which the individuality of the patient is expressed (i.e., in which his or her own wishes are expressed), provided that these can be determined, together with the patient's value history and anticipated quality of life. Such factors must be closely evaluated within the framework of the patient's own life history. This supplementation of the prognosis by taking into account the biography of the patient may be understood as a contribution to the reduction of injustice, insofar as the personal pattern of the patient's life takes on a significance in dealing with his or her illness and the objective parameters of scientific prognosis are no longer the sole determiners of fate. In this context, we must of course include the possibility that the option of refusing therapy could constitute an ethically justifiable judgment on the part of the patient.

Third, the option of discontinuing intensive care, once begun, is as a rule also determined by the prognosis and changes in the prognosis. But here it is self-evident that such a discontinuation cannot be carried out solely on the basis of objective criteria, especially when such criteria formulate rigorous demands to justify the continuation of intensive care due to scarcity of resources. Discontinuation of therapy must be rendered explicable, not only by objective criteria, but also with a specific view to each individual case. It is necessary that the patient's family be convinced that the discontinuation of intensive care does not ensue as an unjustifiable and unreasonable demand dictated by arbitrary and extrinsic criteria, but rather, because it is perceived to have become the better option in specific consideration of the patient's medical history and personal circumstances. Such an explanation is the physician's responsibility during the medical consultation. If, however, all parties concerned are to reach an attitude of reasonable resignation, the physician must be equal to the task.

NOTES

1. Luther expresses himself regarding social welfare minimums and necessary benefits for individuals in his interpretation of the Magnificat (1913; WA 7, 584). In his catechism (*Großer Katechismus*), he recommends that princes use a loaf of bread rather than a lion in their coats of arms to remind them of their responsibilities (1913; WA 30 I, 204, 30). The Lutheran tradition has adopted the idea of the "common good" in its teachings on governance. See, e.g., Elert 1932b, 410 ff.

2. The disappointment of the sick person is not based on the mistake of demanding *justitia explectrix* (*arithmetica*) where it is only possible to proceed according to *justitia attributrix* (*geometrica*). The disappointment stems from the fact that expectations remain unfulfilled, whose fulfillment is or was known elsewhere. It stems, in short, from envy. The patient does not experience such circumstances as appropriately in line with what is to be acceptable from an objective standpoint for "all participants."

3. For example, small children can hardly be convinced that it is "just" to do without something to which they are convinced they are entitled just because their parents claim that it is, even if their parents are correct.

BIBLIOGRAPHY

Elert, W. 1932a. Schöpfungsordnung. *Morphologie des Luthertums* 2: 37–49.

———. 1932b. Wohlfahrtsstaat und Sozialismus. *Morphologie des Luthertums* 2: 409–29.

Fried, C. 1982. Equality and rights in medical care. In *Contemporary Issues in Bioethics*, 2d ed., ed. by T. Beauchamp and L. Walters. Belmont, Mass.: Wadsworth Publishing Co.

Hegel, G. W. F. 1970. *Grundlinien der Philosophie des Rechts, Auf der Grundlage der Werke von 1832-1845*, neu edierte Ausgabe. Frankfurt: Suhrkamp.

Kant, I. 1956 [1798]. *Die Religion innerhalb der Grenzen der bloßen Vernunft*. Hamburg: Felix Meiner.

Kersting, W. 1997. *Recht, Gerechtigkeit und Demokratische Tugend*: 170–212.

Kleinert, S. 1998. Rationing health care—how should it be done? *Lancet* 352: 1244.

Luther, M. 1913; 1891. *D. Martin Luthers Werke. Kritische Gesamtausgabe*. Weimar: Hermann Böhlaus Nachfolger.

Rendtorff, T. 1986. *Ethik I*. Stuttgart-Berlin-Köln: Kohlhammer.

———. 1991. *Ethik II*. Stuttgart-Berlin-Köln: Kohlhammer.

Schleiermacher, F. 1970. Die Gerechtigkeit Gottes. In *Kleine Schriften I*: 108–19.

Society of Critical Care Medical Ethics Committee. 1994. Consensus statement on the triage of critically ill patients. *Journal of the American Medical Association* 271 (15): 1200–1203.

Thielicke, H. 1968. Das Problem der Gleichheit. *Theologische Ethik* 3: 333–36.

PART VII

Critical Commentary

Between Secular Reason and the Spirit of Christianity: Catholic Approaches to Limiting Access to Scarce Medical Resources

Corinna Delkeskamp–Hayes

Intensive machinery ticking, nurses watching, pricking, poking, physicians deliberating, deciding, patients getting better or worse, families adjusting or protesting, lawyers considering, proceeding, hospital administrators calculating, patients on other floors ailing, waiting for their scheduled operation, patients refusing to get better or die, emergencies intruding, getting saved or dying, remaining unstable with expenses ticking, nurses getting overworked, standards of care decreasing, physicians referring or holding back, patients hoping or resigning, families fighting, considering costs, considering their obligations, insurance calculating, meting out reimbursements, negotiating, people generally accepting human finitude, people generally not accepting their own finitude, patients wishing to die, asking to be let die, physicians considering futility and their codes, nurses getting exhausted and hardening, the public considering costs and hardening, politicians committing themselves in mutually incompatible ways, ethics committees recommending, policymakers allocating, hopes being upheld against hope, values being defended, taxes being raised, rights being invoked, expenses skyrocketing, politicians feeling confident in public, emergencies being helicoptered around with patients dying in the process, the public being outraged, but just momentarily, while intensive machinery keeps ticking their units of help and hope and uncertainty and distributive justice into the silence of a ward that gets invaded by ever more emergencies . . .

How should scarce intensive care be allocated? The Roman Catholic authors in this volume draw on their tradition in order to lay out an understanding of proper health care allocations in a secular state. To accomplish this task, they must bridge the gulf between Roman Catholic moral theology and secular political theory. They must move from Christian insight to moral obligations defensible in general secular terms. In their own view, of course, there is no gulf and hence no bridge needed for crossing. Their particular Roman Catholic concept of moral theology places Christian morality in a continuum with secular justice, because the general lineaments of Christian morality are claimed to be open to natural reason, which guarantees access without belief and orientation without the assistance of the Holy Spirit. To secure this claim, they must show that the Christian moral message—when stated in secularly comprehensible terms so as to render it realizable through secular political structures—neither loses its Christian credentials nor disrupts the integrity of secular political morality.

The question I shall ask can be put even more radically. Is Christian culture Christian? Can the health care allocation policies of a secular state with a Christian history provide a possible context for the discharge of Christian moral duties? Can even an avowedly Christian culture in Western Europe and North America, left over from its former more explicitly religious commitments, but now officially secular, do without forcing Catholic moral theologians to betray, reduce, or pervert what is specifically Christian about their moral recommendations, once these are adjusted to the needs of political implementation? Will, on the other side, secular thinkers not find the Roman Catholic claim—that secular reasons are inadequate unless they conform to Christian commitments—unconvincing? One might think here of natural law arguments regarding contraception, which are suggested as rationally compelling by Roman Catholics but appear opaque and puzzling to outsiders. Will these latter not have to worry that Roman Catholics might impose their particular moral convictions on society as a whole, all the while maintaining in perfectly good conscience that they are simply realizing what social justice requires and what any goodhearted secular citizen should welcome?

In the course of this essay, I shall examine the difficulties of harmonizing Christian moral theology and secular politics. My bearing point will be Pope John Paul II's understanding of Christian morality, as summarized in this volume by Taboada: "(1) a subordination of the person and his acts to God; (2) the existence of a relation between the moral goodness of human acts and eternal life; (3) the imitation of Christ, who opens to the person the perspective of perfect love; and (4) the gift of the Holy Spirit, as source and strength of the moral life of Christians" (65). I shall try to expose the gulf that disrupts the supposed continuum between the search for salvation and the pursuit of justice in health care allocation, or between the interests of Christianity and those of the secular state. At the heart of these difficulties lie foundational issues regarding the relationship of grace and nature, which can only be touched in passing. Here I shall have to make do with considering the presuppositions the Roman Catholic authors would need to embrace in order to secure the plausibility of a Christian political competence for framing the health care policy of a secular state, rather than to restrict their efforts to the Christian community.

First, I shall address the plausibility of devising the moral obligations of modern secular polities along the lines of the moral obligations Christianity imposes on individuals. If one could establish an analogy between individuals' obligation to neighbor love and the polity's obligation to secure social solidarity, then at least the project of framing specifically Christian moral policy recommendations would make sense. The difficulty lies in the circumstance that recommendations devised according to this *analogical model*, had they ever been seriously based on the radical reinterpretation that Christ imposed on the Old Testament law of God, would disrupt the very purpose of a secular state.

Second, I shall examine the Roman Catholic claim for the rationality of the more basic-morality-oriented portion of Christians' moral duties, which are considered fit for political enforcement. Here I shall take account of the authors' methodological commitment to a separation of the Christian message into compartments of reason and revelation, as well as to their assumption that the obligations imposed by natural law, as that law can be verified by human reason as such, apply universally to all humans. The difficulty with this *applicative model* of political competence lies in the fact that the presupposed claim of universal rationality cannot be substantiated. Under this model, Christian moral theology would establish a system of force, whose justification will be unconvincing to many of those constrained to obey it.

Third, I shall proceed with a faith-bracketed version of the natural law theory, which allows for the specifically Roman Catholic understanding of morality and rationality to be advanced, in competition with other such understandings, in the struggle for political majority support. Here the endeavor toward the political implementation of the basic-morality portion of Christians' obligations will be understood as forming an integral part of their individual moral obligations themselves. Certain moral duties can be adequately realized by individuals, so it is assumed upon this *implication model* of Christians' political competence, only if they secure political enforcement on everyone. It will turn out, however, that precisely the quest for political implementation repudiates the regard for salvation that is integral to Christian morality, and that complying with that morality in terms of such implementation reduces what should have been a spiritual journey into a merely secular undertaking.

In the end, one will be left with a foundational contrast between the Christian pursuit of salvation on the one side, and secular moral concerns on the other—either with individual autonomy and human rights, as these permit people to do what Roman Catholics know to be wrong; or with the secularly political realization of the "common good" of solidarity and beneficence, as this in effect discourages people from meeting their obligation to love God with all their hearts and their neighbor as themselves. The authors' commitment to a Roman Catholic understanding of natural reason and moral obedience that is thought accessible and attainable without the assistance of the Holy Spirit has rendered them unable to take seriously the gulf that separates secular policy from the spiritual implications of Christian morality.

CHRISTIANITY AND SECULAR POLITICS: THE ANALOGOUS MODEL

Why should Christians be consulted about how to allocate medical resources? These resources, after all, do not concern individual patients' own moral, familial, and economic assets, which figure in customary Christian moral teachings on the limited value of this earthly life (Seifert, this volume) and the need to accept death (Taboada, this volume). Nor does the allocation issue address merely thoughtless misapplications of technology that violate medicine's ethos (Taboada, this volume), or the personalism support that this ethos might derive from contemporary Catholic moral reflection (Seifert; Taboada; both, this volume). Rather, the problem concerns the chronic insufficiency of societal resources, not just with regard to "luxurious" and "unlimited" care (Seifert; Schotsmans; both, this volume), but to necessary and beneficent health care: "medical options promising real and vital benefit will be denied to some people" (Boyle, this volume, 88). So how is Christian moral advice supposed to help?

The insufficiency not only hampers developing countries (Taboada, this volume) but also the technologically advanced "industrial world," and it hurts our political self-understanding. Modern democracies are morally justified by their securing respect for human dignity and protecting human rights. "Health care is . . . one of the basic human needs, or goods that are required for men and women to live in human dignity" (Wildes, this volume, 202).[1] The moral integrity of our polities is thought jeopardized when such care is not only as a matter of fact not granted (which could be remedied through better allocation schemes), but when that insufficiency is a matter of principle. The policy problem thus implies a moral challenge. Christianity has culturally shaped the past 2,000 years of Western history. It is generally thought to have provided the conceptual "raw material," the normative implications of which gave birth to the very notion of human dignity,[2] which came morally to found modern democracies. Even in secularized societies, Christianity is, therefore, not merely a historical influence. It provides a permanently acknowledged moral value-storage, where principles and norms are being tended, nurtured, and protected from pollution through narrow self-interest and the corrupting influence of secular utility calculations.[3] Accordingly, just as Christians are morally obliged lovingly to care for their individual human neighbors, so modern rights-based polities are morally obliged to respect and care for their individual citizens.[4] An analogy between the Christian love imperative and the democratic ideal-inspired imperative to respect human rights and dignity is thus supposed. It offers one reason why "a Christian ethical approach, which also may be called a kind of social personalism, can be developed that gives a foundation for a social health care system" (Schotsmans, 126; see also Wildes; both, this volume) or why Christians might in fact be consulted concerning the moral problems involved in societal resource allocation.

The Roman Catholic authors invoke three principles, which can be taken (according to John Paul II's understanding of Christian morality) to represent for them the "will of God":

1. *The unconditional prohibition on taking human life*: Christian individuals just as political institutions must acknowledge the "sanctity of human life" (Taboada, this volume)[5] as a Divine gift, of which humans are not free to dispose.[6] For the policy issue at hand, this should preclude permitting medical judgments about the quality of a life that might be saved to be influenced by the scarcity of intensive care resources. Such influencing could justify taking patients out of life-support systems and thus contribute to the termination of their lives (Taboada, this volume). Remedying the shortage of supply by such cuts on the demand side should be proscribed.

2. *The unconditional obligation to beneficence*: Humans' unique preciousness[7] not only prohibits acts against their life, but demands a positive concern for preserving and guarding their capacity to function according to their divine de-

sign.[8] Christian individuals just as political institutions are obliged to support the fullness of that functioning.[9] For the policy issue at hand, this should preclude any limitation of public health care to mere "basic and emergency care." As humans' design-hallowed flourishing also requires other social services (sanitary living conditions, food, shelter, and education), no limitation on redistributive taxation for the securing of such services should be defended.

3. *The love commandment*: Just as Christians individually are obliged to measure their neighbor love by their self-love (Boyle, this volume),[10] so societal solidarity should render any multiple-tier medical system morally unacceptable. This principle suggests a commonality of all the worldly goods of God's creation, as these were (anyway) granted by Him to "all humans" (Wildes, this volume). Insofar as human life (at least in its conscious form) is necessary for humans to fulfill their Divine design (and therefore must be protected out of second-principle respect), this third principle should discourage any limiting of the personal sacrifice every human is obliged to offer for the purpose of, for example, preserving any other human's life.[11]

By comparison with these high-strung principles, the authors' bottom-line policy recommendations, such as "[s]ome basic health care and emergency health care should be guaranteed" (Seifert, 112; see also Schotsmans; both, this volume)[12] are surprisingly stingy. As for intensive health care, most of the authors never question the existing consensus (Kaveny, this volume)[13] about the percentage of societal resources that should be spent on such care. Nor do they question the extent to which such resources have as a matter of fact been developed. There is a striking incongruity between the authors' introductory spirited idealism and their world-wise realism. It is hard to conceive how their meager policy conclusions could have been derived from their Christian premises. Considering the many good reasons advanced for the incomparable preciousness of human life as well as the requirement of a neighbor-love that is measured by self-love, the authors' bowing to the "economic necessities" (Seifert, this volume, 114) imposed by other societal priorities, people's "discretion over their lives" (Boyle, this volume, 90), or some objective "value hierarchies" (Seifert, this volume, 113)[14]—all of which limit the provision of medical resources—is disturbing.[15] Quite obviously, the political respect for human dignity, which was to impose an unconditional obligation for social solidarity, has been bracketed in a sense in which the private Christian love commandment is not meant to be bracketed. The supposed analogy between Christian and political morality has not been maintained.

As a consequence, the transcendent backing that analogy had been supposed to secure for dignity-respect is compromised. The safeguards that the Christian heritage was expected to provide against the utilitarian pursuits of group or majority interest have vanished.[16] The authors' policy conclusions (at least when one gets to the small print) do not differ from those that could have been reached on secular grounds.[17] But then it becomes once again difficult to understand why Christian moral theologians should be consulted on policy matters.

Perhaps the incongruity between Christian premises and secular policy conclusions can be repudiated. Perhaps the analogical model of Christians' political competence can be salvaged, if we attend to two further issues discussed by the authors, which I have so far neglected because they seemed beside the policy point: the need to accept human finitude and the moral significance of private property. The Christian neighbor-love premise was to justify considerably greater claims toward developing societal resources for closing the gap between intensive care demand and supply than the authors allowed. But perhaps their Christian regard for the afterlife and for the moral limits on taxation had been meant to considerably reduce the Christian justifiability of such claims. This would also reduce the supposed incongruity. Let us examine the authors' arguments in each case.

Human Finitude

Christians ought to be primarily concerned with their "eternal salvation" (Seifert, this volume). "[E]arthly life is neither an absolute nor the highest good" (Seifert, this volume, 111).[18] Health "has been strongly overvalued" (Schotsmans, this volume, 131). Pre-occupation with what can be technically achieved even amounts to an illegitimate idolization of earthly life and well-being (Seifert; Schotsmans; both, this volume).[19] Christians also should refrain from demanding too much for themselves. They should consider the needs of others and be willing to step back (Boyle, this volume). As such reasoning could be extended to any high-technology treatment of even non-life-endangering illnesses, further reductions in intensive care demand among committed Christians might be expected. Christians' legitimate drawing on societal resources thus is subjected to an internal self-limitation proviso.

The authors' prolonged discussions concerning when Christians may refuse medical help can thus be related to the policy issue after all. Their Christian principles, of course, should have justified going even farther: Although the authors consider limiting demand only in cases of borderline medical proportionality, committed Christians, having discharged their worldly obligations, might even understand themselves as obligated to renounce medically promising intensive treatment. Surely Christ's invitation that His followers should emulate His example of truly self-sacrificial love (John 15:12–14) would cover such understandings.

Unfortunately, no such demand-reduction would work well on the policy level. Imagine a regulation that encourages cost-conscious hospital managers, intensive care unit (ICU) gatekeepers or even physicians to hover over a Christian patient's bedside, to remind him of the salvific merit of sacrificial self-denial, or to urge his speeding up the reconciling-with-God process and to enhance his eagerness to join Him somewhat earlier than medically necessary. Clearly, such policies would not be morally acceptable for a Christian to recommend. The decision, when to renounce, out of a spiritual longing for union with God, any medically feasible and proportionate life-saving efforts, or when to renounce them out of concern for others, belongs to the eminently personal realm of spiritual development, which renders the hidden or overt constraint that comes with policy involvement inappropriate.

But if this is so, why did the authors discuss the human finitude issue in the first place? None of them explicitly draws the policy conclusions just sketched. Yet the case of Schotsmans is revealing. He starts out with the bold thesis that the best of care for all and with free choice of physician is economically affordable. The reader is tempted to suspect that Belgium harbors an underground battalion of unmercenary wonder-workers. But as

Schotsmans' reasoning unfolds, his definition of "best care" turns out to have already been custom tailored to that merely "basic" care, which a fairly self-denying Christian (well advanced in an "ethics of responsibility" motivated unconcern about his temporal well-being) ought to permit himself to demand. By labeling the care he in the end recommends as affordable "best care," he endorses a socialized health care system that permits "the prevention of some patients from having access to critical care" (126) and thus implicitly enforces a fairly ascetic Christian modesty concerning what Belgians should consider "best."[20] In a similar spirit, Taboada conflates (provider-centered) criteria concerning "an appropriate use" of ICUs with a (receiver-centered) affirmation of the "moral duty to accept death" (69). She thus fails to safeguard against ICU gatekeepers casting judgment about whether patients have fulfilled that moral duty. In both cases, insofar as Christians' ultimately obligatory after-lifeliness has been invoked for implicit enforcement of decreasing health care demand, these Christians have in effect been exposed to policymakers' utilitarian calculations. The very respect for their human dignity, which the Christian value heritage had been supposed to support, has been violated.[21]

Quite obviously, there are Christian moral obligations that an individual may impose on himself (and perhaps on those voluntarily associated with him), but not on others. But then the analogy between individual and societal Christian morality in the undifferentiated sense suggested by the authors' Christian premises is not tenable.

Personal Property

Respecting humans' dignity is incompatible with robbing them. There must be some limit to what a state can legitimately tax away (Wildes; Boyle; both, this volume). In that sense, the "economic limitations" invariably invoked at the end of the essays could be defended as guarding that very societal respect for human dignity that Christianity was to endorse. Conversely, property rights are said to be "limited by the needs of others" (Wildes, this volume, 205). But then it becomes again unclear, how much of the "freedom" or "discretion" over one's property the authors invoke should limit the charity-induced redistribution, and at what point that redistribution constitutes robbery in the sense of utilitarian disrespect.

Moreover, no specifically Christian theory of private property satisfies John Paul II's criteria of obedience to God's will and concern for salvation, unless it accounts for Christ's advice in Mattew 19:24: The rich young man, who is concerned about his salvation, is told charitably to give away all his worldly goods. Once again, it seems that no "economic-feasibility"-induced limit to charitable redistribution can be defended on private Christian principles.[22]

Nor is the Roman Catholic theory of the state helpful in this regard. The state is argued to be necessary and morally justified, insofar as it serves a "common good" (Wildes, this volume), which it finances through taxation. Yet, if that "good" is defined in Christian terms (Wildes, this volume) it ought to be salvation oriented. It should then be at least theoretically compatible with all Christians following Christ's enjoinder charitably to give away their worldly goods (and even charitably to sacrifice their lives to one another (John 15:12–14)). As secular polities are defined in terms of respecting human dignity by protecting human life and property, such a definition of their purpose would repudiate the rationale for their existence. Alternately, that "good" must be defined in secular terms. In which case, the safeguards against merely utilitarian construals of the common good (and thus the rationale for politically involving Christian morality in the first place) would have disappeared. Perhaps the "common good" of a secular state with room for such involvement should be composed of both ingredients. But then the principles governing their composition would have to be determined. One would have to explain which portions of Christian moral principles are relevant for given policy issues and which are not. Certainly, if one were to pursue such an apportioning middle course, the analogical supposition—that the individual person is entrusted to himself and to his neighbor-individual quite generally in (rather) the same Christian moral way as it is entrusted to solidaric polities—would (again) have to be given up.

As a result, the analogical model, in engaging the whole spread of Christian moral obligations, could secure the Christian credentials of Christians' political competence only at the expense of that model's political feasibility, and could secure its feasibility only at the expense of those credentials. It thus makes sense to drop such a whole-spread approach and consider the apportioning alternative just envisaged. The following two parts will pursue that option.

TWO-TIER ROMAN CATHOLICISM: THE APPLICATIVE MODEL

If only some Christian moral obligations are to qualify for policy implementation, these must be distinguished from the rest. The authors' methodological commitment to a distinctively Roman Catholic theory of natural reason and natural law provides the criterion. Natural law obligations are accessible to natural reason "prior to the life of religious faith" (Seifert, 106; see also Honnefelder, Boyle, and Wildes; all, this volume) and can be generally imposed on others. The more unreasonably demanding challenges of Christian revelation can be confronted or imposed only individually. Moreover, because what agrees with natural reason is supposed to be valid universally, it can also be politically enforced "by the state" (Seifert, this volume, 109). The second, applicative model for understanding Christians' political competence, therefore, is restricted to obligations of this latter kind.

This model promises to defeat the incongruity between the authors' sweepingly neighbor-loving premises and sensibly tight-pursed conclusions, which had hampered the analogical approach. One must merely allot the rigorous ideals that direct individual Christians' striving for holiness to revelation, and to the truths of reason that realistically concern all humans, whether Christian or not. The authors' patent unconcern with their mismatch now appears as a natural consequence of their methodology. Considering human life infinitely precious, endorsing an unlimited solidarity of neighbor-love, and being called to give away one's earthly possessions just as one looks forward eagerly to one's temporal death—all belong to the revealed and other-worldly-oriented higher-perfection criteria, whereas providing medical resources in general and intensive treatment in particular (as far as that is medically indicated, desired, and economically possible) seems reasonable enough to figure on the this-worldly-oriented basic-requirements level.

The fact, moreover, that both kinds of moral truths are invoked in the essays is accounted for by their triple interdependence. First, for truths of reason to be admitted onto the lower tier of Christian knowledge, they must have passed, as it were, the special entrance requirement of compatibility with the upstairs truths of revelation. They represent the certified selection of "right reason" (as distinguished from the many misguided products of error and prejudice) (Seifert, this volume, 97). Second, the truths of revelation provide a "deeper grounding." They play a "motivating" and "stimulating" role and give "meaning" to those selected truths of right reason (Honnefelder, this volume, 146).[23] Third, without such a reasonable downstairs prospective, converts "could not even consent" (Seifert, this volume, 106) to the revealed upstairs.

The most outspoken proponent of Roman Catholic two-tier Christianity is Seifert. According to him, the ban on killing any human life whatsoever is just as rationally universal a norm as is the obligation (if possible) to help humans in need. To justify the political enforcement of these norms (even on the non-Christian segment of a population), one has to prove that human life, from the moment of conception through all stages of prebirth immaturity, senility (including persistently vegetative existence) until death (holistically conceived),[24] possesses a dignity (Seifert, this volume), which grounds inalienable and globally accepted (Honnefelder, this volume) rights to bodily integrity as well as to basic benevolent care and protection.[25] Yet, precisely those rights cannot be rationally established as universally compelling. Two closely connected approaches to that establishment can be distinguished: natural religion and natural law.

Natural Religion

Roman Catholics invoke the rational knowability of not only the existence of a creator-God as such, but also of His benevolence, as endowing His work with normative implications.[26] Only this premise permits us to conclude that humans are not masters of human life, and that their universal brotherhood along with their social design constitute obligations toward solidaric sharing. This bare-bones presentation, of course, reveals at once that the benevolent-creator hypothesis proves too much: As humans' specially revealed "image and likeness" privilege (Genesis 1:26; just as their distinctly personal call to subduing and having dominion, Genesis 1:28) must be disregarded on the downstairs level of natural rationality, animal life, plant life, and even the pristine arrangement of rocks and rivers, would partake of the "sanctity" grounded in their benevolent design. Even disease and impending death would partake of such benevolent createdness and thus deserve respect in view of their running their natural courses. Moreover, as the difference between before-the-fall and after-the-fall creation belongs to revelation as well, on the level of "reason" anthropological facts concerning humans' natural collective egoism could hardly be kept from grounding their own (biologically adaptive) moral imperatives.

Even apart from such reductions, the very claim that the assumption of a benevolent creator-God constitutes "knowledge" (Seifert, this volume), or is rationally compelling, does not, as a matter of fact, invite universal agreement among those who consider themselves to be rational.[27] There is no argumentative strategy by which Roman Catholics could force all (big-bangers, say) into any such acknowledgment, and quite generally decide between conflicting interpretations of rational compellingness.[28]

Natural Law

Roman Catholics believe that universally compelling moral norms are grafted onto people's minds. Every human knows that killing is bad and helping those in need is good. To deny this is quibbling. For the purpose of justifying the authors' policy recommendations, of course, this does not prove enough. Even if all would agree that killing an innocent person (except in war) is wrong, people differ with respect to fetuses and the permanently unconscious. They differ also, as Taboada's example of Plato shows, with respect to the useless and burdensome.[29] A similar difficulty hampers the obligation to help those in need. Even if all would consider helping a neighbor in need (if the need is great and the trouble small) to be morally obligatory (Boyle), differences come with neighbors more removed from personal experience or responsibility, and when intensity of need squares poorly with chances and degrees of expected relief attending the sacrifices involved in helping. Surely many people feel no moral urge grafted upon their natural minds to pay taxes, regardless of their charitable design.

Roman Catholic defenders of natural law theory would likely denounce such opponents as morally defective, and their reasoning as misguided. Yet their competence for distinguishing right from wrong uses of reason forms part of their Roman Catholic self-understanding as Christians. Accepting this competence presupposes that one believes in the revelation generating that self-understanding.[30] As there is no secularly compelling reason to engage in that belief (in fact, there are secularly compelling reasons to abstain from belief in revelations altogether), no rational agreement can be expected.[31]

Obviously the assumption that the revealed truths of Christianity provide merely a deeper grounding, a firmer motivation, and a horizon of meaning for the truths of moral reason, and thus a kind of gratuitous addendum to something that can otherwise stand on its own rational feet, was too optimistic. It seems that in order to acknowledge the authors' claims to universal rationality, one must already be a partisan to their very particularly revealed understanding of rationality. But then any policymaker accepting their Catholic advice would find himself implementing, through political force, a moral goal that will not be accepted by many of those on whom the force is used. Such accepting, regardless of the moral intentions behind it, would disrespect the moral freedom of those whose moral freedom polities ought to respect.

Does this imply that no political competence remains for Christians? There is still one way open for conceiving that competence, once the rational universality claim has been dropped. The final part will investigate that option.

TWOFOLD CHRISTIAN MORALITY:
THE IMPLICATION MODEL

Just because Roman Catholics' claim of rational compellingness for their particular value priorities (including solidaric sharing vis-à-vis egoistic enjoyment of property and of holding all human life sacred vis-à-vis reserving protection for persons) is illicit, it does not follow that appealing to all rational minds, and inviting them into what Roman Catholics know through revelation to be the right reason behind those priorities, should be illicit as well. They could simply confess and advertise their specifically reason-transforming faith.[32] This would not by itself defeat political action in the sense in which this is generally accepted today.[33] If it could be shown that influencing secular polities so as to render them ever more responsive to Roman Catholic moral norms is implied in what those norms require, then the offering of policy advice would itself be an expression of Roman Catholics' spiritual commitment. It would involve a politically unobjectionable claiming of one's right to the free exercise of religion. Roman Catholics would understand themselves as one of those value communities within modern democracies that compete or seek cooperation with one another in influencing public opinion about what human dignity implies and how policies should respond. It is this implication model for understanding Christians' moral competence that will now be examined.

Such an understanding can, in fact, be traced as a further argumentative layer within the essays under examination. Boyle derives the moral justification of the secular state not only from its providing service for "people . . . pursuing . . . the goods of life," as was considered by the analogical model, but also from its service for people "fulfilling their prepolitical obligations . . . to provide . . . assistance to the ill" (89). According to the subsidiarity theory, individuals' moral obligations toward charitably relieving those in need can be fulfilled more efficiently by means of the state (Boyle; see also Kaveny; both, this volume).[34] This morally required efficiency, so we may add, is not held to be warranted by the merely increased numbers of individuals contributing, as would be the case with voluntary cooperative endeavors.[35] For Roman Catholicism, committed to a moral reconstruction of the state that disregards fallen human nature (see note 25), only the optimal efficiency that arises from universal cooperation and is secured by political force will morally do.[36]

With the secular unobjectionableness of such a more modest, party-interest promulgating involvement in politics conceded, it remains only to check its Christian morality-credentials. In what sense does advocating health care policies for the relieving of basic medical need within the limits of what is politically and economically feasible relate to salvation, obedience to God's will, the imitation of Christ, and the necessity of spiritual assistance? As the authors have not considered this question,[37] we shall have to check the sources of the tradition they invoke.

Regarding salvation, Matthew 25:31–46 is helpful: Charitably relieving others' basic needs[38] is declared to be both the necessary (verses 45–46) and the sufficient condition (verses 34–36) for attaining eternal salvation at the Final Judgment. Such relieving, thus, even appears to be Christians' only relevant moral duty. As it responds to Christ's enjoinment, the obedience-to-God's-will condition is satisfied as well. One may conclude that what (optimally) increases the efficiency of such relief, namely the creation of public social services, should also increase the salvation-and-obedience credentials.

Of course, salvation is rather a substantial reward. And, of course, Christian morality differs from secular morality in that the latter takes moral effort to generate desert (and increased moral efficiency to increase the desert), whereas the former renders desert (and its subsequent reward) a matter of grace. It is this feature that renders the assistance of the Holy Spirit condition of Christian morality crucial. Only if moral achievement involves such assistance does the required Christian abstaining from desert-claims make sense. Policy advocating, conversely, is directed toward implementing what is humanly achievable. Hence it seems that no political involvement can satisfy the crucial criterion of Christian morality.

However, even if particular policies must be restricted to what is humanly achievable at any given moment (such as "providing a decent level of intensive medical care as far as possible"), the advocating itself could be thought to pursue a more ambitious, "moral ideal" (Seifert, this volume), like achieving an ever more encompassing relief of peoples' (medical) needs. It would envisage developing more effective technology as well as increasing the solidaric generosity of voting publics. We could recognize such a properly utopian concern in the authors' ideally humanitarian premises, while their modest policy conclusions would point to the presently feasible next steps toward its attainment. Such a view is captured in Schotsmans' commitment to realizing "the Kingdom of God in the world." The final achievement of adequate societal respect for human dignity would always remain beyond human capacities. The Holy Spirit's assistance in support of the relevant progress would be (*Weltgeist*-style) indispensable. The temptation to desert-claiming could thus be evaded: Whether one had labored enough toward politically meeting one's moral obligation in furthering such a progress, after all, would remain for God to judge.

The *imitation of Christ* condition, finally, looks easy to satisfy: We are to love the least of Christ's brethren just as He loved them. Loving means relieving someone's needs. Hence, advocating policies for ever better relieving needs imitates Christ. Yet on closer inspection, Christ did not exactly express His love through the relieving of basic needs. To be sure, He healed and fed many. He was not concerned with securing efficiency, though. Perhaps He wished to leave that to His followers. More important, the biblical texts indicate a rather different goal of His love. When sending the Apostles (Matthew 10:7), Christ orders them not only to heal the sick (etc.), but also to preach that "the kingdom of heaven is at hand."[39] He decrees that those who will not receive them will not be saved. We must conclude that not relieving others' needs is not (as was supposed before) the only route to nonsalvation. It seems that Christ wished to express His love when healing the sick (etc.) specifically in conjunction with conveying the fact that the kingdom of heaven is at hand. This also fits with Paul's treatment of charity: What counts in the end is not just that needs have been relieved but also that God gets glorified (2 Corinthians 9:13). Glorifying God, then, seems integral to realizing that the kingdom of heaven is at hand. The concern about efficiency in need-relieving, which motivated the involvement of political constraint, does not pertain to the glorification part. Rendering such efficiency-securing a Christian moral cause amounts to chopping a whole into two, and withholding one half. Although the state can be invoked to get the hungry fed and the sick basically cared for, the state cannot be invoked to imitate Christ.

Anyway, the Christian morality-credential of Schotsmans' vision of "God's Kingdom in the world" is challenged by Christ's declaration "My kingdom is not of this world" (John 18:36), especially considering that He specified (in answering John's disciples) the essentials of His mission as the poor having "the Gospel preached to them" (Matthew 11:5). Moreover, Paul emphasizes that bestowing all (not even merely some of) one's goods "to feed the poor" profits nothing, unless one loved them too (1 Corinthians 13:3). Although clearly linking charity with imitating Christ, this suggests that political redistributive constraint even damages the goal of distinctively Christian charity. Its value, so we must conclude, does not exclusively reside in what the receivers get, but equally in how the givers become. This fits with a peculiarity of Matthew 25:35–40, 45: Christ does not even speak of "others'" needs, but of Himself: "I was hungry, and you gave me food" (verse 35; see also Matthew 11:40). What renders charitable giving salvific, then, is that the giver recognizes in the face of the receiver Christ Himself, who is a brother to the ones in need first. The provider, in lovingly imitating Christ, is asked to include in his personal love for Christ the receiver personally as well, as the one who is personally loved by the one whom he loves. Drawing one's neighbors into one's own love-relationship with Christ, then, understandably contributes to that "kingdom," which is "near" whenever such personal charity is extended. Or that kingdom is realized when God is glorified not merely as a result of a need having been relieved, but in the very process of personal love-including. If this is what Christian charity is about, then the enhanced receiver-efficiency gained by political constraint (very much in contrast to that of voluntary Christian cooperation), in imposing impersonal sharing, hinders the provider-efficiency of growth in love.

In addition, the final judgment context of Matthew 25:31 refers back to the preceding parable of the talents (verses 14–30). As John Chrysostom observed,[40] the "talents" are what God out of love for us presented us with, whether property or capacities or even just bodily skills. Their required multiplication arises from their being used for charitable presentings on our side. In making such presents in the process of relieving others' needs, we thus cannot even flatter ourselves with supposing that we are sacrificing something of our own. We are merely using a foreign deposit the way in which we are ordered.[41] This precludes not only our counting such acts as moral achievements. It also enjoins us to disassociate ourselves from what we identify with: our property, our capacities, and even our bodily skills. Charity, when extended in the spirit of this parable, not only frees us from our worldly-goods egoistic possessiveness. It also presents a spiritual exercise, again not only in unselfishness (which still acknowledges an identifiable self and merely disregards it), but in genuine selflessness. This implied self-negation, in disrupting humans' mortality-induced self-enclosure, goes "against the grain" of fallen humans' very nature. It thus becomes understandable in a much more profound sense, why the assistance of the Holy Spirit is indispensable for every step we take on the way of turning from self to God.[42] It also becomes understandable why imitating Christ's love is placed in the horizon of ultimately learning how to lay down our lives for one another, as Christ commands.

But if the point of Christian morality is that spiritual journey, then even the merely conceptual (and faith-bracketed) division of moral obligations into a generally manageable downstairs concern for getting saved and an ascetically heroic upstairs concern for becoming holy is morally counterproductive. If the purpose of Christian moral life is to grow in the love of God, even Boyle's distinction between "basic" or "intrinsic" and "witness to Gospel" values, which corresponds to that division, is profoundly misleading. Christians' moral project cannot be to single out certain goods that "one always has a reason" to pursue, unless this is morally wrong (80). Their project is to understand that we have no reason to pursue any good whatsoever, unless this is spiritually right.[43] But then, *a fortiori*, the very notion of any "natural" common good, from the furthering of which the secular state could derive its (positively) moral justification, is incompatible with Christianity's specific morality. There is nothing wrong with Christians morally approving of the state's merely negative function for opposing (specified forms of) social discord, and thus for securing (some aspects of worldly) peace. But the political, and thereby merely superficial, obedience to Christ's positive salvation-related precepts transforms a spiritual therapy for worldly possessions-possessed humans into a finite management problem. This reduction betrays the link that Christ's demands establish between the nitty-gritty of bodily needs and the truly "basic need" for salvation. The distinction between what a Christian may demand of himself and what may be imposed on others, and thus between what is publicly enforceable and what is privately voluntary, turns out to be untenable. This distinction had been assumed at the end of part I in order to render Christians' involvement with secular policy conceivable. We shall have no choice, so it appears, but to give up the idea of such involvement.

Pope John Paul II's criteria for Christian morality are compatible with Christians realizing their moral responsibility in this world. They encourage Christians' cooperating for the realization of God's kingdom. They are incompatible, however, with engaging secular polities for this purpose. Secular polities can successfully function only if their use of constraint is morally acknowledged, to be sure. Ultimately, however, it is constraint through which they function. Even if Christians throughout history have helped render such constraint moral, their own morality is spiritual. Although constraint may secure compliance with moral dos and don'ts, it fails to secure spiritual growth. Looking back at the Roman Catholic authors of this volume, it appears that insofar as many of them mostly evade the policy issue, they follow their healthy Christian intuitions. Insofar as most of them assume policy advocating to be a Christian moral concern, either they are not Christians in the sense of John Paul II, or the present pope is not Roman Catholic after all.

NOTES

1. See also Schotsmans on "the human person, created in the image of God and endowed with unassailable dignity" (127).
2. See Wildes, this volume. Only Heisig vigorously opposes this general consensus among the other Roman Catholic authors, and there is a reserve even in Taboada.
3. See Seifert's opposition to consequentialism and Taboada's discussion of "proportionalism."
4. Schotsmans quotes von Nell Breuning on "the duty of the community to give all individuals the opportunities to develop as persons" (129). Boyle justifies "the socialization of health care" in view of (among other things) its service for "people in pursuing responsibly the goods of life and health" (89).
5. Taboada concludes that "nobody is allowed intentionally to kill or otherwise injure . . . a . . . person" (63).
6. Seifert quotes *Evangelium Vitae*: "Human life is sacred and inviolable at every moment of its existence" (99).
7. Seifert speaks of humans' "unique dignity" and the value of incomparable depth that belongs to each person, because God Himself became man (96).
8. Seifert contends that the person who saves a human life is to be compared to someone who has saved the entire world. Kaveny adduces the "essential dignity" of "a being created in the image and likeness of God" and translates "respect" into "beneficence" (79).
9. Schotsmans even includes the "growing possibilities" that attend the "historicity of the person" in the requirements for the "promotion of the human" for the "proper develop-

ment of life" (128). In a similarly generous spirit, Wildes quotes John XXIII on the societal common good as "the conditions . . . whereby men are enabled to achieve their own integral perfection more fully and easily" (207).

10. The fact that health care makes "infinite" demands (Boyle) and thus creates an inescapable "scarcity" should not be permitted to obscure the fact that Christian neighbor-love requires in principle open-ended sacrifices precisely in terms of one's "discretion over one's life" (which is, after all, usually not exhausted by moral projects). Boyle shifts his moral attention to the issue of fairness with respect to any existing "reality" of health care, and thus neglects Wildes' warning that the issue of social justice (which might motivate demands for increasing that "reality") is easily confused with that of distributive justice (which settles for any such "reality").

11. These three principles are of course not even specifically Christian. They reflect what has been revealed about God's will in the Old Testament already, and thus cover a common ground with Jewish moral thought. But because Christ claimed not to have abolished "the law" but rather to have fulfilled it (Matthew 5:17), these principles belong to the Christian moral tradition as well. Moreover, as Christ even attenuated what "the law" requires (such as extending the ban on killing to mere anger, Matthew 5:21–22; and having "love of neighbor" include enemies, Matthew 5:43–44; and assume the form of complete self-sacrifice, John 15:12–14), the policy conclusions will certainly not be weakened once we include regard for what is specifically Christian.

12. Although Seifert (normally) includes life-saving efforts, for Kaveny "basic health care . . . does not mean . . . any form of medical treatment that could . . . ameliorate . . . life-threatening problems" (179). Wildes contrasts his "dignity of the human person" with "what is needed for a minimally decent human life" (205). A helpful middle term is offered in the end as "basic human dignity" and illustrates his sudden decline of neighbor-loving commitment. But even this does not answer the question whether and under what circumstances life-saving intensive care, even though devoted to the truly "basic" good of preserving human life, may count as a "basic" need, if it is considered costly. For Seifert, "even life-saving measures" can be withheld because of "forbidding expenses" (114). Although this sounds reasonable enough in terms of affordable policy framing, merely invoking the threat of "economic collapse" should not relieve Christians from investigating how much "imitation of Christ," self-sacrificial love, could still be afforded just this side of "collapse."

13. Thus, when Taboada refers to "given communities" when preferring smaller effective ICUs to bigger mediocre ones, she seems to assume such set percentages. Quite in contrast to her emphatic affirmation of human dignity, she concludes that "the decision of having an ICU cannot be simply justified on the basis of eligible patients and suitable personnel and facilities" (70). She never questions the political will to not satisfy "a population's present need" and merely affirms that "individual members of the hospital are not morally responsible," when the needed resources are not allocated (70). Similar reasoning is found in Boyle: "then our duty does not apply" (92). Boyle once steps forward toward taking a clear moral stand: "If . . . facilities . . . are compelled regularly to ration . . . then the allocation . . . seems indefensible," but from the very next paragraph onward he softens the moral sting of this remark by considering only the unfairness of using expensive resources on patients who might benefit less in comparison to others; that is, by again attending to distributive rather than social justice in Wildes' terms (92).

14. He opposes the demand for an unlimited distribution of public means and invokes the importance of culture, art, and education. Although Christian principles certainly are unfit for grounding even moderate demands on public resources, it is not clear whether

it is patients' own commitment to culture, art, and education (or, in the case of Wildes, to freedom and creativity) that generates the economic necessities (or Wildes' balancing efforts) invoked here, or perhaps the commitment (and efforts) of tax-paying majorities. In the latter case, it seems difficult to maintain any specifically Christian sacrificial-neighbor-love credentials for the resulting limitation of intensive care.

15. Admittedly, in what concerns the first principle concerning the taking of human life, the authors have altogether taken a powerful stand against much that is practiced within secular society (Seifert, this volume). Yet Taboada quotes a *Charter for Health Care Workers*, which permits "to interrupt the application of [life support] when the results disappoint the hopes placed in them, because there is no longer due proportion between the investment of instruments and personnel and the foreseeable results" (61). She endorses actions that are causally linked with the patient's subsequent death, as though the Sixth Commandment would not quite pertain. Others (Honnefelder, this volume) invoke the distinction between primary (intended) and secondary (unintended) consequences. Obviously, in the process of conquering a dying patient's tormenting pain, no responsible physician would withhold necessary pain suppressors just because they might hasten the approaching death. But that general understanding should not render Christian moralists insensitive to the fact of that causal connection. The distinction emphasizes its tragic nature, but is not sufficient to repudiate the connection. An unjustified moral complacency that is built up concerning such "clear" cases will all too easily be transferred into situations that are less clearly determined. Decisions about "futility," even in the strictest medical sense, depend on what counts as "accepted practice," which in turn reflects existing societal choices about "investment of instruments and personnel" (Taboada, 61; see above), or adequate resource allocation (Kaveny, this volume). That latter ingredient of contingent (and decidedly non-Christian) societal decisions gets merely hidden by definitional adjustments (such as between primary and secondary causes), and thereby rendered inaccessible to moral scrutiny. (It should be noted that Honnefelder, in quoting Pius XII, clearly classifies the "renunciation of intervention" as "choice of unavoidable evil" and considers the scarcity of medical resources as a test case for the "moral standards" of a society (152). But then he restricts his discussion to the comparatively cheap care for patients in a persistent vegetative state. It is unclear how his Christian commitments would fare in the case of intensive care.)

16. Seifert justifies limiting health services in view of the "proportionally greater harm on society" that would be inflicted by helping suffering individuals (114). Similarly, Schotsmans endorses a "careful balancing between macro- and microethical considerations" with the goal of cost containment (133).

17. To be sure, Taboada's and Schotsmans' explicit option for the poor, and Kaveny's option for "the weakest and most needy" (see also Honnefelder, this volume), are clearly motivated by Christian moral principles (Matthew 25:40, 45), which causes them to set distinctively different priorities in health care, such as for improving general sanitary conditions (Wildes, if only very hypothetically) and for concentrating on the obligation to care for those who can no longer be cured (Schotsmans; Honnefelder; both, this volume). But with regard to the central issue of scarcity in medical resources, this implies a sacrifice of intensive care investments, and thus a failure to take seriously the avowed loving concern for those whose life might be saved.

And Kaveny's emphasis on physician-patient fidelity in her analysis of a just distribution of units of intensive care, as well as Taboada's emphasis on dying as a human accomplishment and Boyle's vocational reconstruction of what can be presumed to underlay proxy consent for incapacitated patients clearly betray the spiritual experience of a life in Christ. Yet because neither that fidelity goes beyond what even secular medical ethics should proscribe, nor that emphasis amounts to more than alerting physicians to their secular professional obligation of attending to patients' wishes, nor finally that concept of vocation implies more than what people may happen to consider their life-plan, the conclusions of these authors are not distinctively Christian.

18. See also Taboada: "there is a moral duty to accept death" (64).
19. Accordingly, intensive care physicians are enjoined to resist the temptation of aggressive treatment (Taboada, this volume).
20. See, e.g., Schotsmans' argument that "the necessary restrictions on the investments in medical treatments" are justified as not really serving "adequate goals" of health care systems, which have already internalized the moral constraints of his Christian personalism (133).
21. Schotsmans' "critique of the dominant role being given . . . to the principle of self-determination and autonomy" (131) illustrates his insensitivity to the distinction between areas in which individuals must be protected against societal pressure or instrumentalization and areas where it would be morally desirable that individuals would use their autonomy in more responsible ways: "Excesses of patient autonomy must be made impossible by favoring more important values as authentic responsibility and solidarity" (136). The same insensitivity to the difference between what society may impose on individuals and what individuals may decide for themselves characterizes Seifert's entire discussion of limiting health care. (See, e.g., his discussion of organ transplantation.)
22. Of course, if, as Wildes quotes Leo XIII, "every man has by nature the right to possess property as his own," then the relevance of Christ's advice to the rich young man would have to somehow be explained away and limits on redistributive charitably taxation could again be defended on Christian grounds. Yet Leo's reference to Thomas Aquinas (1953, II IIae, question 66, 2) does not prove that property is necessary in a sense that would warrant such discounting. The supposed necessity of a *potestas procurandi et dispensandi* is based on merely pragmatic reasons (that people care more about what is their own, that confusions in caring responsibility should be avoided, that peace is better preserved and quarrels avoided), the first and third of which (egoism, and quarrelsomeness) relate not to humans as originally designed by God but to their fallen nature, and the second of which could be circumvented by assigning caring responsibilities (as in Christian monasteries). Moreover, Thomas himself specifies that with respect to use, external things cannot be had as *proprias*, but have to be shared according to a "need" that is in Thomas's texts nowhere earmarked as "merely basic" in a sense that would justify withholding resources for the saving of a human life (regardless how expensive the effort). Quite in general, Thomas is concerned with the necessity of property not as such, but as an unavoidability that keeps the commonality of the goods of creation from rendering the concept incoherent. Moreover, this unavoidability pragmatically relates to humans' fallen nature in precisely the sense in which the human establishment of property rights as an element of the legal order does. Quite in contrast, after all, to Wildes' supposition of the state as "part of the natural order of creation" (205), Thomas, whose question 96 (1962, I IIae) Wildes quotes, affirms the opposite in question 95: Considering whether the establishment of human laws is useful, Thomas argues that these are necessary in order to keep people by constraint and fear from committing evil: "necessarium fuit ut per vim et metum conhiberentur a malo. . . ." This seems hard to reconcile with Wildes' "the state is not established simply because of humanity's fallen nature."

23. John Paul II's criteria for a specifically Christian morality are then no longer relevant for the downstairs reason compartment. The fact that almost none of the Roman Catholic authors is concerned with such criteria thus becomes understandable. (The exception is Taboada, and her reasoning is restricted mostly to the medical ethics plane anyway, not to that of policy implementation.)

24. Seifert opposes even organ explanation from brain-dead donors.

25. If modern democracies are morally justified in their use of political power by reference to a human dignity, without the acknowledgement of which the very quest for moral justification would not make sense, then any political restriction of autonomy rights (including discretion over property), the respecting of which is implied in that reference, must be justified as indispensable for that respect. This requires exposing the universal compellingness of those human rights, the corresponding societal obligations of which justify restricting that to-be-respected autonomy. For a more thorough development of this argument, see Delkeskamp-Hayes (in press).

26. It is these implications that underlie the possibility of an ontological foundation for ethics, as invoked by Seifert, Kaveny, Schotsmans, and Wildes.

27. Even within Christianity, this claim cannot be substantiated. As master source for this theory, Honnefelder quotes Romans 1:19–22: "What can be known about God is plain to them, because God has shown it to them. . . . Ever since the creation of the world His eternal power and Divine nature, invisible though they are, have been understood and seen through the things he has made." Yet the immediate context shows that the people about whom it is said that God showed what is knowable about Himself are people against whom His wrath is directed, because they suppressed the truth in unrighteousness (verse 18). The truth they suppressed becomes clear from the following verses: They failed to glorify and thank Him, even though they knew Him (in the sense of being "*gnontes*," i.e., of having been able to be drawn toward, or to appreciate Him). Instead, they became futile in their reasoning and their senseless heart was darkened by exchanging the immortal God for idols. So the "truth" at stake here is not a theoretical one and concerns not whether natural (qua secular) reason can climb up the chain of causes and ascertain from the order of natural things their benevolent design. The issue at stake is the practical one of acknowledgement and obedience. [This is supported by Saint John Chrysostom (1995b, 352), who quotes Jeremiah 2:13 as a parallel, and adds as an explanation of humans' failure in both cases: "They trusted everything to their reasoning." That is: when they destroyed the Divine light in their hearts, their reasoning became vain.] For a thorough refutation of a merely secularly rational rendering of Paul's natural religion, see Engelhardt (2000, 164 f.).

28. Even among the Roman Catholics of this volume, Heisig defends the validity of alternative rationalities.

29. Honnefelder valiantly defends the close connection between soul or person and body, thus claiming that what is illicit to do to a person (killing) is also illicit to do to a human body (with permanent loss of person-capacities or soul-expression). Yet secular minds will insist that ultimately, and how handy so ever bodies are for distinguishing persons or securing their identity, bodies provide only a necessary condition for to-be-respected personhood and thus are not entitled, once their sufficient-condition counterpart is missing, to that respect.

30. Even among those who agree concerning revelation, within Catholic moral theology itself, Seifert must admit profound differences of opinion.

31. The thesis that humans possess a natural knowledge of good and evil is usually derived

from Romans 2:14–15: "When Gentiles, who do not possess the law, do instinctively what the law requires, these, though not having the law, are a law to themselves. They show that what the law requires is written on their hearts, to which their own conscience also bears witness. . . ." Thomas Aquinas (1962, question 91, 2) adds: "Etsi non habent legem scriptam, habent tamen legem naturalem qua quilibet intelligit et sibi conscius est quid sit bonum et malum." He further establishes the universal validity and Divinely binding power of that natural law by saying that it means "participatio legis aeternae in rationali creatura." Yet Thomas also refers to Psalm 4:6, where the question "who will show us the good" is answered by "the light of your countenance has been manifested in us." Thomas paraphrases this with "quasi lumen rationis naturalis," thus linking the moral law in our natural consciences with the light of natural reason. Such a transition, of course, is possible only because he previously has translated God's loving providence for His creation into a distinctively more impersonal, more (as it were) value-neutrally rational "lex aeterna." But in the next Psalm verse the result of the "light of God's countenance on us" from which Thomas's rendering started out, is not at all described as knowledge (in the epistemological sense of this English term), but as "gladness which is put in our heart." Thus the question for "ta agatha" is answered not with respect to "the morally right" in some intellectual insight shape. Rather, it is answered in terms of that "euphrosyne."

A similar shift of meaning happens, when the same verse from Romans 2:15 is discussed by Thomas in (1953) question 93, 2, where the issue is whether the eternal law is known to all. Thomas refers to Augustine's treatise on the free will as a backing for his statement: "quod aeternae legis notio nobis impressa est." But Augustine (1995a) in this book does not discuss that verse with respect to the epistemological question concerning the knowability of good and evil for humans at all. (He is concerned only with establishing the fact of humans' free will, and he proves this fact by referring to God's habit of spinning off moral imperatives, which would make no sense if there were no such will.)

The verse in question is treated epistemologically by Augustine in *Of the Spirit and the Letter* (1995b, 101 f.). Here Augustine's central intention is to argue that the (epistemological) knowledge of good and evil requires an additional act of grace. Either, he claims, the people who "by nature" know good and evil are the ones to whom the Gospel was given (and along with it God's grace). Or else, if that original knowledge that humans possessed before the Fall was not quite eradicated by that Fall, it must have been already renewed by grace. In either case, Thomas, on whom the Catholic authors of this volume rely as their natural authority, in turn relies on Augustine as his natural authority in a way that in no way supports the theory of a natural knowledge of good and evil, independently of any religious commitment (or Divine grace) and rationally accessible even to secular minds (independently of grace, and thus) in a universally compelling manner.

Even more so, that surprising *euphrosyne* from Psalm 4:7 becomes understandable (in a way that further weakens the natural law theory as it is used by the authors), if we consider how the knowledge of good and evil is treated in Gregory of Nyssa's (1995) account of *The Making of Man*. To a natural law theorist, it should, after all, be a puzzling detail that the forbidden tree was "of (understanding—the *Septuaginta* adds an *eidenai*—and of) knowledge of good and evil": Why, if it belongs to humans' special excellence (and likeness-to-God prerogatives) to have a moral sense, should what provides moral knowledge have been forbidden them? Gregory's answer (409 ff.) distinguishes "knowledge" from "discernment." By investigating the biblical uses of the former (*gignoskein*), he translates it (in a quite nonepistemological manner) as "being favorably disposed towards." He reserves the epistemological "knowing" to discernment (*katakrinein*). Under that interpretation, the tree in question is forbidden because it offers fruits of a mingled quality (good and evil not set side by side, but intertwined with one another). The fruits seem beautiful and good, but they are in truth evil. Thus, it makes sense that God's verdict was designed to keep Adam from coming to know in the sense of being favorably disposed or drawn toward such dangerous food. At the same time, this makes better sense of the *euphrosyne* from the psalm-verse 7: The light of God's countenance reveals to us "the good" as that which we should be drawn toward, or which we should enjoy. Accordingly, the light of reason should not be rendered as a purely epistemological affair but involves a kindling of one's love for God. (Again a more complete treatment of the question of natural law is found in Engelhardt 2000, 170 ff., 245 ff., 293 ff.)

32. In spite of himself, Seifert implicitly does acknowledge that Roman Catholics' use of the terms "reason" and "philosophy" are somewhat idiosyncratic: What secular understanding of rationality, after all, could settle for Jesus Christ, perfect in deity and perfect in humanity in two natures, without being mixed, transmuted, divided or separated.

33. Even though modern democracies are morally justified in their use of political power only with respect to their protecting human dignity in a quite narrow, but universally compelling sense, as a matter of fact they fulfill this function everywhere in a much more comprehensive (and philosophically unjustifiable) sense. What is rationally compelling (and demands corresponding restrictions in the use of political power) is not what is generally believed. What is generally believed is that human dignity ought to be politically protected in a much fuller sense, even though the particulars of this fuller sense are disputed among various groups of believers.

    This difference between rational compellingness and factual acknowledgment concerns especially (though of course not exclusively) property rights, as these are implied in the right to autonomy. In proportion to the extent to which moral dignity is thought to encompass "dignified living conditions" or "equality of opportunity" and so on, more or less extensive redistributive taxation schemes are generally held to be acceptable. (For a more thorough exposition of this reasoning, see Delkeskamp-Hayes, in press.)

    In that sense, then, Catholic moral advocacy of more extensive redistribution can be protected against the charge of advocating disrespect of autonomy by an appeal to common consensus: If common practice anyway "justifies" the use of political power much beyond what is rationally compelling, the (secular) proof that Catholics' political norms are not rationally compelling (either) loses political weight. If it is anyway the opinion of voting majorities, to whom the interpretation of human dignity, as the basis for justification, is entrusted, why not let Christians advertise their party opinion as well! Moreover, in the context of what is thus generally accepted, even the demarcation between legitimate interpretations of human dignity and utilitarian compromising that dignity, which was impossible on strictly rational grounds, can be granted. Legitimate interpretations satisfy what is acknowledged by international declarations on human rights. Thus, Christians' involvement in influencing that interpretation can also be at least pragmatically freed from the charge of such compromising.

34. In a similar vein, Schotsmans speaks of the "common good" that is realized by the state, as that "task to which every responsible member should contribute" (127), or Wildes:

"Government should act when the actions of individuals are not sufficient to meet the basic needs of all men and women" (203).

35. This alternative option to efficiency enhancing has been admirably developed by Hughes.

36. The fact of such constraint does not by itself have to repudiate the moral character of the cooperation, and advocating constraint therefore does not amount to depriving others of their chance of acting morally: Not only is constraint (e.g., in a Kantian context) quite generally compatible with moral desert. Within a limited redistribution scheme individuals also retain, as Boyle has rightly observed, sufficient resources for the discharge of private and strictly voluntary charity. And anyway, as the subsidiarity justification of the state rests on a teleological ethics (basic needs get satisfied), one might consider the means employed for the moral goal to be of secondary importance.

This politically amplified understanding of Christian morality, so one should note, is widely recognized today. Private acts of charity are even considered deficient, as merely patching up symptoms, unless they be included in political programs for attacking what is taken to be the deeper causes of human's suffering. Private charity is even suspected of mere moral self-satisfaction at the expense of receivers, who are being rendered "objects" of others' beneficent urges. By contrast, the political advocacy of "rights" to social support and solidarity, in avoiding such implicit humiliation, is believed to betray a more considerately humanitarian love-of-neighbor. The state, then, is seen to endow private charity with enhanced efficiency not only on the quantitative level (more people receiving more help), but also on the qualitative level (the help is less counterproductive for receivers' self-esteem).

37. Taboada is an exception here, but she applies these criteria only to the medical ethics aspect, not to the political issue.

38. The sick, admittedly, come in only for visiting. Yet in the New Testament, *episkopein* signifies "helpful looking at someone," like with a doctor's visit. And then the underdeveloped state of medicine in Christ's time may have caused Him to be conservative about ordinary Christians' charity duties (as opposed to the healing powers granted to the apostles (see Matthew 10:8)). In either case, progress of medicine having increased its efficacy, we may (and this seems to be understood by the authors as well) conclude that providing medical treatment also qualifies as act of Christian charity. It is, then, especially the resource-demanding intensive care variety of medical treatment that renders the indispensability of the state's closing the efficiency-deficiency of private charity obvious.

39. If He was thinking of Schotsmans' kingdom, which took some 2,000 years to arrive, this must have involved an instance of divine thousand-years-into-a-day time-compressing.

40. John Chrysostom even points to the nonfertility of the "children" that are set to the left in verse 33 as referring back to the obligation toward "multiplying" in the talent-parable (1995a, 475).

41. Considering charity as using God's talents according to His will also takes away the temptation of self-righteous superiority feeling, and thus of humiliating the object of such charity (see note 40). Rather, the giver himself is called to feel ashamed about the fact that he still keeps possessing something that he should have given away long ago.

42. For example, the unwillingness of the rich young man to even consider wishing to get into the process of ever so slowly and painfully beginning to "empty himself of his possessions." John Chrysostom (1995a, on the Gospel of Saint Matthew) accordingly illustrates a failure not just in achieving special moral excellence. It concerns a failure in

readiness to practice an art of self-sacrifice that permeates, in the Christian spirit, even the seemingly most basic moral requirements.

43. Boyle himself is aware of this, when he says: "The pursuit of any human good is likely to be harmful and wrong if not integrated into . . . allegiance to the kingdom of God." He restricts this insight to "the revealed plan of God," however, and proceeds to consider nonintegrated "natural human concerns" exclusively. He does not seem to see the conflict between trying to respond to what is revealed and at the same time living "naturally" (79).

BIBLIOGRAPHY

Aquinas, T. 1953. *Summa Theologica II IIae*, ed. by A. F. Utz. Heidelberg: Gemeinschaftsverlag F. H.Kerle, Anton Pustet.

———. 1962. *Summa Theologiae I Iiae*. Matriti: Biblioteca de Autores Cristianos.

Augustine of Hippo. 1995a. On Grace and Free Will. In *Nicene and Post-Nicene Fathers*, 2d ed., vol. 5, ed. by P. Schaff. Peabody, Mass.: Hendrickson Publishers.

———. 1995b. On the Spirit and the Letter. In *Nicene and Post-Nicene Fathers*, 2d ed., vol. 5, ed. by P. Schaff. Peabody, Mass.: Hendrickson Publishers.

Chrysostom, J. 1995a. Homilies on the Gospel of Saint Matthew. In *Nicene and Post-Nicene Fathers*, 2d ed., vol. 10, ed. by P. Schaff. Peabody, Mass.: Hendrickson Publishers.

———. 1995b. Homilies on the Epistle of Paul to the Romans. In *Nicene and Post-Nicene Fathers*, 2d ed., vol. 11, ed. by P. Schaff. Peabody, Mass.: Hendrickson Publishers.

Delkeskamp-Hayes, C. 2001a. Global Biomedicine, Human Dignity, and the Transformation of European Democracy: A Selectively Kantian Approach to Moral Justification. In *Individuals, Community and Society: Bioethics in the Third Millenium*, ed. by J. Tao. Dordrecht: Kluwer Academic Publishers.

———. In press. *The Moral Justification of Political Power*. Dordrecht: Kluwer Academic Publishers.

Engelhardt, H. T. 2000. *The Foundations of Christian Bioethics*. Lisse: Swets and Zeitlinger Publishers.

Gregory of Nyssa. 1995. The Making of Man. In *Nicene and Post-Nicene Fathers*, 2d ed., vol. 5, ed. by P. Schaff. Peabody, Mass.: Hendrickson Publishers.

Catholicizing Health

James W. Heisig, S.V.D.

I wish to argue here for an adjustment of the Catholic perspective on technologically intensive medical care. The immediate context for these remarks is the effort under way to produce a set of moral guidelines, based on Catholic principles, to govern the apportionment of limited critical care facilities to a surplus of patients. I would like to take a step back from the complexities of that question to consider what it means for Catholicism to put the weight of its tradition and institutional presence behind such guidelines. In particular, I mean to suggest that the primary audience for Catholic moral guidance in matters of health has been eclipsed by excessive attention to the problems generated by the medical profession. I have no illusions about the irrelevance of these remarks to the question as framed. No doubt, for many of those who devote themselves to the management of intensive care units (ICUs), the skepticism in these pages will ring hollow and out of touch with the realities of health care. I ask only that they listen between the lines for the faint echoes of a rising chorus of voices looking for another kind of guidance altogether, and consider whether this clamor is really as secondary a concern for Catholic moral reflection as their professional interests lead them to believe.

QUESTIONING THE MEDICAL MYTHOS

The ICU is more than an ensemble of equipment and technicians designed to perform a specific range of tasks for a specific class of patients. It is a metaphor for a wider set of beliefs about the place of science and technology in health. Independently of whom the wires and tubes happen to be attached to at any given moment, the whole kit is permanently attached to a wider network of ideas. Whatever the rate of efficiency of the tools and techniques of the unit, the very fact that it is functioning at all implies a commitment of resources from outside the ICU itself that could have been committed otherwise. And those decisions in turn rest on a set of assumptions and decisions about what things are more valuable than what other things.

For those committed to providing high-technology intensive care, the ICU is an index of the state of medical science as a whole. Whatever goes on within its walls testifies to the level of progress that has been achieved and justifies further expenditure for what has not yet been achieved. This symbolism is real enough, and its meaning is hardly lost on anyone devoted to the betterment of intensive care. But this symbolic meaning is itself wrapped in a wider creed, less clearly articulated, perhaps, but no less firmly adhered to. It is this creed that defines the boundaries for moral concern. In a word, the ICU is assembled, used, and maintained on the basis of the belief *extra ecclesiam nulla salus*: "No health outside of the system." Though not a blind belief, neither is it without its blind spots.

To anyone with firsthand experience, whether on the giving or receiving end of critical care, it is clear that detachment from the experts and gear assembled in the ICU means all but certain death for the terminally ill, whom such units are designed to save. This is why the fact of having more patients than available space in such units becomes a moral issue. Whom do we save and whom do we let go? And on what grounds? As long as these units remain at the cutting edge of the healing sciences, there will always be a disproportion of equipment to patients. But the more the question of morality focuses on the appropriate or inappropriate use of available facilities, the stronger grows the conviction that in the best of all possible worlds everyone would have equal access to such treatment. The contradiction is easier to accept than the possibility that the ICU could be grounded on a creed unworthy of belief. In order, therefore, for patients and caretakers to believe that the only real health is health that has been certified by the established medical profession, they must first accept the idea that the presence of scientific validation adds to the value of things, even as its absence devalues things. The ICU is a metaphor of this wider myth.

"Let no one be deceived," writes Origen in the middle of the third century. "Outside this house no one is saved." In matters theological, the words have become by *consensus fidelium* an embarrassment to Catholic tradition, but in matters related to institutionalized medicine they have all but the strength of an infallible dogma. Healing outside of the system is real only by analogy; the history of medicine and diversity of traditional medical practices are valued as a kind of pre-evangelium. The problem with this creed, as with its soteriological parallels, is not that it aims to be as comprehensive as possible. Neither science nor religion would be served by reining in the will to teach its truth to all nations. The problem is rather that it does not know how to view its own faith except as certitude and how to view other faiths except as heresy. Neither science nor religion is served by this sort of dogmatism.

If the ICU is indeed a metaphor whose significance depends on a broader set of beliefs in the background, a different background implies a shift of meaning in the foreground as well. As ludicrous as it may seem to those who see intensive care medicine as the best that civilization has to offer humans facing certain death, the fact is, only a minority of the world subscribes to the creed on which it is based. This is not just a reflection of the demographics of technology, which relieve most of the world's population of any choice in the matter. There is growing evidence that even those within arm's reach of the latest equipment and methods of medical practice are going through a crisis of faith. In 1997, for the first time the expenditures for alternative therapies in the United States exceeded that paid for primary care services, and the number of actual visits to providers of alternative medicine surpassed that of visits to regular physicians. According to research published in the *Journal of the American Medical Association*, "Extrapolations to the U.S. population suggest a 47.3% increase in total visits to alternative medicine practitioners, from 427 million in 1990 to 629 million in 1997" (Eisenberg et al. 1998). The therapies showing the most marked increase include herbal medicine, massage, megavitamins, self-help groups, folk remedies, energy healing, and homeopathy. More and more insurance companies are agreeing to cover these expenses, and knowledge of alternative medicines is growing among the younger generation of doctors,[1] which can only further weaken the monopoly of allopathic medicine. Clearly, the myth of scientific medicine that forms the backdrop to intensive care medicine may not have quite the hold over the popular imagination that the medical establishment has taken for granted.

Trust in the healing powers of one's physicians has long been known to be a key ingredient in curing illness. Although trust in prayer and religious faith (which may still be, as Rustom Roy suggests, "the single most powerful pill in the world's pharmacopoeia"[1999]), tends to recede in the modern clinic, it is quickly replaced by trust in scientific expertise. Still, despite the sophisticated methods at the disposal of doctors today and the vast amounts of data amassed to put those methods on a solid basis of objective and verifiable fact, faith in the healing powers of today's medical profession is far from absolute. And there is no reason to suspect that better equipment, better medications, better surgical techniques, and more and more research will ever make it so. As is the case with all practical science, there will always be cracks in the method through which superstition and nonscientific ideas can leak into an otherwise solid trust in the medical profession; as with all human institutions, there will always be political and economic motives for distracting its functionaries from the highest aims and full potential of their profession. But rarely does such mistrust of the establishment touch the core belief in the primacy of medical science as the guardian of health in an advanced and civilized society. Nor does the concern with norms for the proper use of equipment and the proper allocation of resources. More often, they are absorbed into the concern with preserving the integrity of the profession and weeding out anything that might compromise the fundamental trust of the patient in the system.

The turn to alternative medicine in technologically advanced countries and the continued reliance on traditional medicine in technologically backward cultures must not be understood simply as the mistaken response of the disillusioned or ignorant. More than a mere loss of faith, it testifies, at least in part, to faith of a different sort altogether. This faith thinks in terms of wholes greater than the sum of body parts; it is not ashamed to talk of forces unknown to and uncontrollable by reason; it values felt affinities with the plants and animals of the natural world more highly than it values their taxonomy or genetic manipulation. The very achievements that faith in science holds up as metaphors of true health, it sees as metaphors of spiritual infection. Because the discourse of this faith is closer to the archaic languages of religion and philosophy than it is to the contemporary idiom of science, it is easily classified as the remnant of a prescientific mindset that is destined to be reformed as the evidence against it accumulates in the academies and eventually filters down to the masses. What seems to be happening is rather that the evidence in its favor is beginning to seep into the medical establishment itself.

The spectrum of beliefs marked off by allopathic medicine at one pole and wholistic medicine at the other seems to be more densely populated in the middle than at the extremes. Despite the growing interest in alternative medicines, it is caricature to think in terms of mass migrations from rationalism to spiritual awareness or from science to magic. For most people who live within reach of technologically advanced medicine, it is more a question of drifting a measured distance away from doctors and hospitals and standard medication in order to see what else might be out there. For such persons, the symbolism of the ICU is as ambivalent as is their faith in science. All of this, I insist, cannot be a matter of indifference to Catholic moral reflection on health.

THE CATHOLIC MORAL COMPASS

The questions of medical ethics that occupy Catholics moralists are real problems that require careful attention. I am suggesting that there are *more* questions which, if ignored, bias the Catholic perspective in a morally unacceptable way. I will further suggest that the failure to widen the field to include these other questions can only further weaken the already seriously debilitated authority of the Catholic tradition. Nothing would be served by narrowing the focus of Catholicism's moral concerns to exclude the issues raised by technologically intensive scientific medicine, especially not in response to complaints that the medical profession can manage certain areas of health quite well on its own without the moralizing interference of nonspecialists. The problem is rather to determine where the needle points north on the Catholic moral compass.

Introducing the critique of present-day medicine and the viability of alternative medicines into the Catholic moral outlook is not meant to set up a choice between contradictories, but only to ensure that the choice is not biased by tacit assumptions that run counter to Catholic tradition. The principal such assumption is the idea that the general advance of science and technology as such marks an irreversible stage of human civilization fated to cleanse the human spirit of its age-old addiction to superstition and magic. The role of Catholic moral reflection, accordingly, is to direct the use of the tools of science and technology (as well as their institutional superstructures) to the benefit of humanity and to resist abuses that offend the fundamental dignity of the human person. The spread of tools and institutions from a core of industrial nations to the masses of people in underdeveloped countries across the globe is therefore seen as a necessary and irrevocable fact of history. To belong to the present is to accept this fact; to belong to it as a Christian is to seek out its spiritual significance for the emerging global culture. The efforts of indigenous spiritualities and cultures to subsist apart from what is thought to be the very essence of human being— or at least to reserve the right to participate in the process at their own pace and in accord with their own values—are taken to be an affront to common sense and a deliberate disorientation from reality.

In a recent address, Cardinal Josef Ratzinger voiced these views in an explicit attack against the influx of alternative spiritualities into what he calls "universal Christian culture," an uncritical flood of primitive ideas that risk infecting the achievements of global, technological culture with "magic" and "cruelty":

> It is not only the case that the convergence of mankind towards a single community with a common life and destiny is unstoppable because such an inclination is grounded in man's essence, but also because the diffusion of technological civilization is *irrevocable*. . . . But since technology, like natural science, appears to be neutral, the thought suggests itself: Why not accept the achievements of the modern age while, however, at the same time keeping the indigenous religions? This seemingly so enlightened notion, however, does not work. For in reality modern civilization . . . alters the interpretation of the world at its base. It changes standards and

behavior. The religious cosmos is *necessarily* moved by it. . . . The division of Western heritage into the useful, which one accepts, and the foreign, which one rejects, does not lead to the salvation of ancient cultures. (Ratzinger 1994, 683–84)

As for the sacred texts of Asia's high religions (the address was delivered in Hong Kong), he welcomes them as serious resources in the battle against materialistic elements in Western technology, but not as a foundation for serious cultural alternatives. So not only Christianity but the achievements of Western Christian culture are to remain permanently on loan to the 200 million Christians of Asia, their own ancient cultures having outlived their usefulness for directing the relentless progress of globalization.

Fortunately for Catholicism, though perhaps unfortunately for its current leadership, the words of the Cardinal Prefect of the Congregation for the Doctrine of the Faith are not in accord with the growing consensus of theologians around the world about the role of Western culture in non-Western Christianity. I cite them here because they articulate the perspective within which Catholic moral reflection on scientific medicine tends to move when it comes to questions such as the allocation of ICU facilities for the terminally ill.

Once we broaden our view to take into account the way most of the world heals its sick and the broad range of spiritual meanings attending sickness and death, health and healing, it is by no means self-evident that moral questions surrounding the ICU require universal guidelines valid in principle for all health systems, let alone that the Western Catholic Church, in collaboration with the Western medical establishment, is in a position to provide them. The idea of solving local problems with global norms is every bit as culturally specific as the culture of high-technology medicine that generated these problems in the first place. The leap to universal relevance conceals a failure to ask if one culture of health, and a relatively recent one at that, should be allowed, even in a limited number of cases, to redefine for all of humanity what it means to resist sickness and die a good death. The side effects of scientific-technological medication reach far beyond the body parts it aims to repair, beyond the entire medical and pharmaceutical professions that administer the reparation. It is a kind of artificial culture produced in a controlled environment, immunized against threats to its homeostasis, and released on the open market for universal consumption. For Catholic moral reflection to serve the spread of this culture, even where it seems to be working according to design, without at the same time keeping these wider side effects in view is nothing short of a betrayal of its heritage.

It is not enough for Catholic morality to pose as a representative of worldwide culture. It must also proclaim as one collective voice the rich variety of vernacular cultures being swept along by historical tides not of their own choosing. The distinctively Catholic presence in creating guidelines for problems like high-level critical care should be to insist that they are not allowed to justify underlying biases inimical to the health of the masses of living persons who fall outside the purview of science's latest achievements. At some point, this will mean shifting the weight of its tradition and its resources toward protecting and encouraging alternative models of the healthy person and the medical vocation. Unlike medical science and the medical ethicists who serve its interests, Roman Catholicism cannot, without risking its soul, excuse itself from such questions on the grounds that there is no financial base to support alternatives, that the more "primitive" cultures of the world will have to succumb to the more "advanced" in matters of science and technology, or that the leaders of the world's "poorer" countries are poised to devour as much of the technology of the "richer" countries as they can. It cannot see things so simply and be faithful to the plurality of conditions in which its faith is lived around the world. Better the church were criticized for being out of touch with who is winning the clash of civilizations than that it stand accused once again of having failed to speak for those whose voices were being drowned out by the current arrangements of power and wealth.

It may be objected that the moral authority of the Catholic Church will be weakened in proportion as it aligns itself with critics of the pillar institutions of the modern world and encourages alternatives. It seems more accurate to say that its authority is already being weakened because it does *not* do so. The time has come, it seems, to ask to what extent the teaching authority of Roman Catholic moralists can any longer expect to reach a substantial majority of its own believers, let alone the public at large, with its moral message. It is also time formally to decanonize the doctrine that there is no salvation for the church outside the cultures of the world's ruling economies. No doubt there are certain moral issues today that by their nature override cultural differences, such as the reality of nuclear weaponry and industrial destruction of the environment. But when it comes to problems related to sickness and health, the Catholic Church cannot discard viable alternatives to the dominant models of medicine and at the same time retain its teaching authority toward those who pursue those alternatives. Readjusting the Catholic perspective on technologically intensive medical care requires an idea of Catholicity different from global uniformity and a view of death and suffering broader than the unconditional commitment to their alleviation. On both counts, the Catholic tradition is more likely to find stimulus in secular and primal spiritualities than in science and industry.

THE ILLOGIC OF UNIVERSAL GUIDELINES

The attempt to formulate norms to govern the operation of ICUs in the world's hospitals brings into clear relief the problem of grounding Catholic morality on universal principles that transcend cultures and institutions. Both logically and existentially, there are reasons for misgivings.

Regarding the logic of universal guidelines, a basic flaw has already been touched on: abstraction from the superstructure of the beliefs and institutions that generate the moral questions at hand, and the side effects of that abstraction on cultures and individuals that do not share those beliefs and institutions. Clearly the universal applicability of ethical conclusions is seriously compromised if the very formulation of the question can be shown to exclude relevant moral data from the picture. In the case of traditional Catholic moral argumentation, this reduction of the moral field is supported by the appeal to "natural law" that in principle excludes the possibility of historical relativity from matters of ultimate concern. But when it comes to the application of universal moral principles to the use of technologically intensive medical equipment, the leap over time and place and culture to an objective order of truth and morality is more than an act of philosophical faith, principled or otherwise. It is a means of controlling the production of those values that support the "globalization" of particular ideas of sickness and health care. This is not a separate moral question, to be decided on other grounds. It is as essential a part of the ICU as the equipment, the technicians, and the cost-benefit analysis of the procedures.

In his philosophical essays, Alfred North Whitehead was fond of chiding Western rationalism for what he formally called the "fallacy of misplaced concreteness" (1925, 52–56). By this he meant the tendency to attribute concrete reality to what are in fact mental abstractions. Plato fell into it when he forgot the abstractness of pure form and ascribed being to ideas; Aristotle, when he forgot the abstractness of simple individuality and argued for a primary substance; seventeenth-century science, when it assumed as concrete data the two abstractions of observing mind and observed matter. By and large, Western philosophy has accepted Whitehead's criticism as a commonplace (it had been so in the Buddhist philosophies of the East before the first philosophical idea had dawned in Plato's head), but fallacies with so long and noble a pedigree have a way of holding on. The idea of an objective moral order belonging to a natural law knowable in principle, though under no theoretical obligation to commit the fallacy, frequently does.

Universal moral principles are abstractions from culture, and as such always require reference to the relative values and aims of a culture to become concrete. Their universality is always mediated, never direct. To think otherwise is to read back into nature what has been drawn out of culture. We may call this sleight of logic "the fallacy of misplaced universality." By this I mean the tendency to attribute universal validity to what are in fact culturally specific values. In so doing, the interests of particular statements of universal morality are turned into laws of nature, and what would seem an anachronism to the philosophy of science is swallowed whole in ethics.

The history of colonialism provides ample evidence of how universal principles, particularly when reinforced by religious doctrine and technically superior equipment, can be evoked to disorganize one local culture and replace it with another. But even in the more enlightened, postcolonial age of the early twenty-first century, the fallacy survives in subtler though hardly less potent forms. On the face of it, there seems little to object to in establishing general norms to ensure distributive justice in critical medical care. On the one hand, we have the basic dignity of the human life; on the other, particular individuals of every shape and stripe, but all equal in their humanity. Hammer and anvil, these are, it would seem, tools enough with which to forge moral values of service to the whole of the human community. The only problem is, concrete human beings do not exist as particular examples of a general equation, and human life is nowhere to be found among the haphazard of items that make up the world. The particular and the universal are everywhere mediated by the specificity of human society, which cannot be abstracted from without forfeiting the concreteness of that which is being moralized about.

Without the specific, the relation of the individual to the community is merely a question of deciding the size of the relevant community to which one must answer. Surely the range of the community whose interests need to be taken into consideration when making decisions about appropriate medication is not irrelevant; it is crucial. But this does not exhaust the meaning of the specific. In such a scheme, communities, whether immediate family, the nation, the local township, or the whole community of nations, are aggregates of persons. The value of the culture that shapes both communities and individuals is ranked both below the value of the universal human and below the value of the individual person. As a result, not only is the cultural environment that shapes particular forms of rationalism and philosophic expression left out of the picture; so, too, is the value of protecting cultural plurality in the dissemination of Catholic moral values.

In questions related to medical care, to speak of the dignity of the human person regardless of culture, it seems to me, is to fall into a basic methodological error. To posit individual subjects and then lift the foundational ideas of human dignity and the sacredness of life up to the surface in order to cloak those individuals in "Catholic" moral value is to make a foundational idea perform a task it cannot perform—or at least cannot perform without falling into rationalism in the glum sense of the term. Not that religious values have nothing to do with universal human dignity, any more than medical science has nothing to do with universal human anatomy. But by identifying values as Catholic because of their universal applicability is to turn things inside out. If anything qualifies as Catholic, it cannot be simply in virtue of a universal judgment about a particular reality. It requires inclusion of the philosophically neglected category of the specific that necessarily mediates the relation between the universal and the particular.[2]

MORAL AND CULTURAL PLURALISM AND THE MEANING OF HEALTH

This much can be extrapolated, it seems to me, from the logical fallacy of misplacing the universal. But recognition of the fallacy at work within the realm of faith and morals, and the determination to correct it, are neither prompted nor secured by contemplating the rules of logic. These are efforts of hindsight exerted in the attempt to appropriate more immediate, existential intuitions. If there are reasons to be suspicious of the true universality of moral guidelines governing equitable access to sophisticated medical technology, there are also reasons to question the idea that the foundations of these guidelines have been deduced from faith or reason. Insofar as they are of any consequence at all to moral choice, they need to be seen as interpretative paraphrases of faith and reason based on the awareness that violence is being done.

Appeals to principles such as the dignity of the human, the value of life, and the right to a good death are not, therefore, the foundations of conscience but an expression of conscience. The purpose of this expression is to alter certain habits of thought and action while maintaining continuity with others. The significance of these general principles, whether they be formulated in nonsectarian philosophies or in the scriptural and theological idiom of a particular religious tradition, lies in critically widening our perspective on immediate, living moral questions to prevent them from being expropriated by conventional social institutions. Their primary claim to authority over practical conscience is a function not of their provenance in faith or reason, nor of any innate transcendent truth in the formulation, but of the level of perception of the particular violence they address (Maldonado 1997, 9–28).

The perception of violence that present-day Catholic thinking brings to problems of medical care is no longer restricted to the treatment of the individual. It includes the social consequences of the institutions that provide the treatment. Whereas the imagination of those dependent on access to the latest medical technology seems by and large to have resigned itself to the institutional contours that define the pursuit and practice of modern medicine, and provide a framework for dealing with particular issues, there is something in the Catholic vision that feels cramped and uncomfortable in these same circumstances. Attempts to work within the existing institutionalization of medicine in order to try to rein in its excesses and protect it from injustice and oppression, for all the enthusiasm with which they are made, yet leave a residue of dissatisfaction. I am not talking about the accusations of inadequacy, incompetence, and ineffectiveness that those at the cutting edge of science often use to bleed the enthusiastic temper of its less-informed critics. I mean something more in the nature of an uneasy sense of those structural disorders that have been excluded from the picture. True, the suspicion of structural disorder is a distinctively contemporary preoccupation that religious ethics has inherited from secular social criticism; but its place in Catholic self-understanding has been secured by a generation of theological reflection. That said, it is still engaged in a tug-of-war with elements in the tradition that persist in isolating the health and salvation of the individual from the reality of social violence.

The allegiance to technological civilization begs the question of cultural pluralism by assuming that a basic, uniform, global cultural form pedals in tandem with the tools of modern Western society and its view of the cosmos. On such an assumption, the business of organized religion is to ensure that the whole package, the tools and the cultural forms in which they are embedded, does not infringe on basic human rights but enhances the quality of life. This very identification of technological civilization with its Western form introduces a colonial dimension to any Catholic morality that supports it without serious question. The accomplishments of modern medicine do not as such justify the cultural and institutional form in which those tools have been embedded. Nor do they gainsay the possibility that the aims of medicine might as well be served if wedded to radically other forms of civilization with histories different from that of Europe and the United States.

Mere dismantling of the offending structures and a simple transfer of the tools of modern medicine into the hands of societies that did not participate in their invention and development is naïve. Even were the transfer to succeed, it would likely do so only by reimporting the structures in a subtler form. At the same time, the hope of awakening moral conscience for the totality of the structure in all those on whom the structure leans for its existence is unrealistic. Quantitatively speaking, most of our sin, like most of our virtue, takes the form of cliché. Most of the common courtesies of everyday life that make human intercourse pleasant, as well as most of the prejudices that keep us at a distance from one another, are the result of unwitting force of habit. As important as consciousness of sin and willfully cultivated virtue are, they are no match for the power of structural evil. But to see our institutions as no more than necessary evils, doomed one day to fall prey to their own darker nature, is a caricature of culture itself. They must be seen as experiments with belief in our ideals, the ultimate goodness of our humanity, experiments that can only be radically corrected by the encounter with other, alternative experiments. Without wishing to deny the reality of the issues that surround critical care at the edge of medical science today, it does not seem fair to exclude alternative models or to assume that they will all embrace the same questions with the same sense of "emergency" that surrounds the dominant health culture.

Again, it is not a question of asking the church to divest itself outright of Western civilization. Rather, insofar as the church is determined to participate in the production of moral guidelines to lead the technological civilization of the West, let it just as far participate in supporting alternative forms for wielding the technology. The imbalance of resources devoted to the former amounts to a denial of the latter. In such circumstances, every step taken to Catholicize health ends up catholicizing a culture of health that for vast numbers of the human family is still parochial and foreign.

Now for all the trust we have in the pillar institutions of contemporary society, our understanding of the way they transform our perception of the world is still meager in comparison with our understanding of how to manage them at home and export them abroad. Clearly, we are caught in a bind. On the one hand, we look with alarm at what transformations in schools, hospitals, agriculture, financial markets, mass transport, and even organized religion have done to traditional values in the societies where progress has been most marked. On the other, our dependency on these institutions prevents us from standing in the way of their continued expansion.

To make matters worse, the damage a particular society can sustain through the unchecked development of its central institutions is compounded and accelerated, not checked and balanced, when the cultural diversity of societies around the world is made subservient to the mechanisms of a globally interconnected world. Like the media for the exchange of information, which parade an unlimited variety on the surface even as they canonize an underlying structural uniformity, the internationalizing of those institutions to which we entrust the major dimensions of our lives advances steadily away from supporting the cultures they were intended to uphold and enhance. The plurality of cultures cannot survive unconnected from one another, and yet their connections seem to pressure them into a uniformity that trivializes the meaning of pluralism.

As with a greater concentration of power, a greater accumulation of information and perfection of technique are no guarantee that an institution will not promote the frustration of its original purpose. In this regard, the poverty of insight into alternative ideas of health—not just alternative forms of medicine or alternative forms of organized care, but alternative ideas of what it means to be healthy and of what are the limits of resisting suffering and death—seems to be in inverse proportion to the wealth of knowledge about the latest advances in medical science. From the ordained experts of the health industry, to the functionaries who administer it, to the recipients who have come to depend on it, the measure of physical well-being is simply assumed to be as transcultural and universal as the periodic table of the elements. Within the course of our own lifetimes, traditional ideas of health around the world have been redefined as a sickness, the cure to which lies in the hands of those with knowledge and equipment so far superior that it seems folly to resist. Evidence that the quality of human life has been enhanced as a result, even where the dominant model of health has taken strongest root, is flimsy.

Data gathered during the past two decades on iatrogenic illness, namely, diseases contracted through the very services that set out to cure disease, seem to have had a certain sobering effect on the health industries. But the idea that "health" itself may be an iatrogenic malady specific to certain societies and inflicted on others is all but unthinkable. Modern medical care is too much part of the "package" of modern life to be isolated as a particular colonial construct that economically backward cultures are free to take or leave. Intensive care, the exchange of organs, and other high-order surgery are no longer viewed as luxury items but as the legitimate right of all people everywhere. Despite the complexities involved in providing such care and the economic superstructure needed to sustain the equipment and personnel, it has come to be seen as a basic resource of all human culture.

Together with food, clothing, shelter, literacy, and work, it has become one more item on the moralist's agenda for distributive justice.

There is no denying the moral dilemma for those who stand at arm's length from the very best equipment medical science has to offer and having to decide where to apply it and where to withhold application. Nor is there any doubt that such decisions require carefully reflected norms and guidelines. It is quite another thing, however, to allow such examples to beg the question of whether the dilemma and its ethical resolution, together with the whole medical culture to which they are specific, should simply be accepted as the inevitable fate of all people everywhere. Policing the morals of a civilization where the poor cannot get the same care as the wealthy, and where the financing of health has made higher health care impossible without dedicating a sizable part of one's income to insurance against the harsh realities of hospital costs, is work enough without bothering about the more basic question of whether the goal of providing everyone everywhere with the same high level of care is a worthwhile goal at all.

In short, the thoughts of a certain portion of the human community about health and longevity have become the form of all thoughts about health. The rich plurality of beliefs, rituals, and even superstitions surrounding sickness and death has lost its power to the imperial myth of modern health care. Like all empires, it is a specificity masquerading as a universal. And like all myth, it has seeped into common sense so that it is virtually transparent to opinion polls and ordinary decision making. In matters of the gravest consequence, the distinction between what is indigenous and what imported has become irrelevant. One of the richest sources of human diversity, the practices and attitudes surrounding death and illness, has been sacrificed to a worldwide campaign for uniformity regarding what it means to be well and what it means to die.[3]

The very fact of insisting on the inclusion of "alternative" models to health care in the field of discussions about medical ethics entails some degree of cultural anarchy, in the sense of breaking with the *archaí* or ruling principles. Awareness of the threat of structural violence in the medical professions demands that this be done. Of all the great religious traditions of the world today, perhaps none is as well prepared, as missiologically alert, and as self-reflective as the Catholic Church to commit the weight of its tradition to meet this demand.

CONCLUSION

Not only those who continue to identify themselves with one or another form of organized religion, but also the greater part of those who run the organizations trying to keep them there, are relying more and more on the moral sensitivities of those outside of religion for guidance. The fact is that the major moral enthusiasms of the age, for the preservation of the natural world, for the eradication of slave labor, for freedom of thought and expression, for the protection of minorities against the democratic majority—were neither inspired by organized religion in the first place nor have they depended on organized religion for their vitality. Quite the opposite: It is only by tapping into this enthusiasm that organized religion can maintain any moral authority at all toward the contemporary world. I do not see the retreat of the Catholic from the construction of a global, universal world order as submission to the rising dark tide of secular paganism, but rather as a call to purge Catholic tradition of its colonial vestiges and to turn the considerable resources of the church toward preserving cultural pluralism and alternative models of social order. In the context of moral reflection on health and medication, the Catholic viewpoint would see conventional institutions, however strong or however weak they happen to be in a particular setting, as more like local churches than like local branches of an ecclesiastical multinational. The difference is not trivial. In the former, the question is always how to wrestle what is best from vernacular culture and at the same time pry open its conscience toward the world beyond it; in the latter, the question is rather how to maintain uniformity in essential modes of thought and behavior while allowing for variation in the accidentals.

Before committing itself to the formulation of universal guidelines for access to critical care, the Catholic moralist must at least take into account two interrelated facts. First, the health care systems of most of the world are likely to embrace a code of universal principles governing the application of critical care only if they perceive it as one of the conditions for receiving the latest medical technology or for being allowed access to it as the need arises. Once they have the technology firmly in their own grasp, the authority of the principles is exhausted. Second, the truly Catholic perspective on health always opens up a horizon wider than the medical complexes of Europe and the United States; these latter never represent more than a minority opinion. We cannot, as Catholics, simply make principles based on one set of cultural norms and then ask that others adjust them to their own conditions. This is what I mean by claiming that the ethical imagination is constrained to a perspective that deprives the Catholic tradition of its fullest contribution.

At all levels—of universal principles, of institutional structure, and of individual spirituality—the Catholic moral imagination needs a kind of cultural refund from the advances of the medical industry. It is an industry that brings to the medication of the individual patient the authority of the knowledge, the facilities, and the organization it has at its command. As such, it is a kind of new church universal, whose values justify themselves in statistical effectiveness of healing illness. But it is not, and can never be, a *Catholic* church. To allow the industry to pose the questions in its own terms, and not radically to overturn them in the light of religious tradition, is not only un-Catholic, it is irreligious. This is how I understand the summons to join you in discussing the problem of allocating critical care in the light of Catholic belief.

NOTES

1. According to Wetzel, Eisenberg, and Kaptchuk, the majority of medical schools in the United States now offer courses on alternative medicine (1998, 784–87).
2. One of the most sophisticated philosophical arguments on this neglect of the specific— posed in the language and sources of Western philosophy—is to be found in the works of the Japanese philosopher Tanabe Hajime. His idea is that the specificity carried by culture mediates between universal humanity and the individual person, providing not only values and the parameters of reason, but also the fund of ethnocentric thinking and irrationality that feeds isolationism and colonialism alike. I have outlined this in several essays, including "Tanabe's logic of the specific and the spirit of nationalism" (1995b, 255–88) and "Tanabe's logic of the specific and the critique of the global village" (1995a, 198–224).
3. See John (1996).

BIBLIOGRAPHY

Eisenberg, D. M., R. Davis, S. Ettner, S. Appel, S. Wilkey, M. Van Rompay, and R. Kessler. 1998. Trends in alternative medicine use in the United States, 1990–1997. *Journal of the American Medical Association* 280: 15690–775.

Heisig, J. W. 1995a. Tanabe's logic of the specific and the critique of the global village. *Eastern Buddhist* 28 (2): 198–224.

————. 1995b. Tanabe's logic of the specific and the spirit of nationalism. In *Rude Awakenings: Zen, the Kyoto School, and the Question of Nationalism*, ed. by J. W. Heisig and J. C. Maraldo. Honolulu: University of Hawaii Press.

John, P. C. 1996. The millennial migraine: Health care and the poor in the 21st century. Nagoya University, Graduate School of International Development.

Maldonado, C. E. 1997. *Human Rights, Solidarity, and Subsidiarity: Essays toward a Social Ontology.* Washington, D.C.: Council for Research in Values and Philosophy.

Ratzinger, J. Cardinal. 1994. Christian faith and the challenge of cultures. *Origins* 24: 683–84.

Roy, R. 1999. Whole person healing. Keynote address to the Third Yōkō Civilization International Congress. Takayama, Japan, August 18.

Wetzel, M. S., D. Eisenberg, and T. Kaptchuk. 1998. Courses involving complementary and alternative medicine at U.S. medical schools. *Journal of the American Medical Association* 280: 784–87.

Whitehead, A. N. 1925. *Science and the Modern World.* New York: Macmillan.

Roman Catholic Theology and the Allocation of Resources to Critical Care: The Boundaries of Faith and Reason

Mary Ann Gardell Cutter

This essay addresses methodological questions concerning what or who provides access to knowledge about how Roman Catholic institutions and individuals ought to allocate resources to critical care.[1] In focusing on methodological issues, it does not forward specific guidance regarding how to allocate critical care resources. Rather, it maps the range of responses offered by Roman Catholic authors in this volume. The essay argues that differences among Roman Catholic views regarding the allocation of resources to critical care turn on how authors understand the boundaries of and relation between faith and reason in the acquisition of knowledge.

ACCESSING TRUTH: THE CONTRIBUTIONS OF FAITH AND REASON

Nearly all Christian thinkers, including Roman Catholics, agree that humans have a supernatural knowledge revealed by God and accessed by faith, though they do not at all agree about the contribution of natural knowledge or reason. The problem of faith[2] and reason[3] in its Christian version amounts to the following question: Inasmuch as God has revealed Himself in a supernatural self-disclosure, what role, if any, does natural reason play in the quest for theological knowledge? Two ancient church fathers, Tertullian of Antioch (ca. 160–230) and Clement of Alexandria (ca. 150–215), illustrate that from the beginning of Christian theology there existed two distinctly different answers to this question.[4]

Tertullian took as his point of departure Saint Paul's declaration that

> Jews demand signs and Greeks seek wisdom, but we preach Christ crucified, a stumbling block to Jews and folly to Gentiles, but to those who are called, both Jews and Greeks, Christ the power of God and the wisdom of God. For the foolishness of

310

> God is wiser than men, and the weakness of God is stronger than men. (I Corinthians 1:22–25)

Armed with this, as well as with Paul's warning "See to it that no one makes a prey of you by philosophy . . ." (Colossians 2:8), Tertullian set out to vindicate the divine foolishness of Christianity while denouncing philosophy as the demon-inspired mother of heresies. No better evidence is found for Tertullian's contempt for philosophy and vain philosophy than his rhetorical challenge, "What indeed has Jerusalem to do with Athens, the Church with the Academy?" (*Prescription Against Heretics*, 7; Baird and Kaufmann 1994, 40), and his famous outburst concerning the death and resurrection of Christ, "I believe because it is absurd; it is certain because it is impossible" (*On the Flesh of Christ*, 5; Baird and Kaufmann 1994, 41). For Tertullian, it is sufficient that God has spoken. The Scriptures must be our guide and standard in all matters pertaining to faith and doctrine, and we must be on constant guard against those who seek to ensnare us with sophisticated reasoning and to corrupt the pure and simple Christian teachings. For Tertullian, then, faith provides access to metaphysical truths.

Clement of Alexandria, conversely, was an early representative of those who saw in pagan philosophy a direct access to Christian faith. According to Clement, Christ is the *Logos*,[5] the instructor of *all* humanity. We should, therefore expect that even the pagans have apprehended something of God's truth. More specifically, Clement taught that philosophy was perhaps even a divine gift directly bestowed upon the Greeks, a position Saint Paul endorsed concerning the Law given to the Jews (Galatians 3:24). Philosophy lifted and turned the Hellenic mind toward Christ and helped to set the stage, historically and culturally, for the advent of the Gospel. God's will is that the believer should, as much as possible, know, and philosophical activity equips him in his progress from faith to understanding or genuine *gnosis*.[6] Thus, Clement calls philosophy a "contributory cause of the truth" (*Stromateis*, I, 20; Baird and Kaufmann 1994, 39), one of the ways in which God has made the word responsive to the Gospel and a useful tool through which Christian understanding is cultivated and established.

Clement supports his position with numerous passages from Scriptures, often allegorized, drawing especially upon the wisdom literature of the Old Testament. For example,

> "Now," says Solomon, "defend wisdom, and it will exalt thee, and it will shield thee with a crown of pleasure" (Prov. 4:8–9). For when thou hast strengthened wisdom with a cope by philosophy, and with right expenditure, thou wilt preserve it unassailable by sophists. The way of truth is therefore one. (Clement, I, 5; Baird and Kaufmann 1994, 38)

Concerning Saint Paul's warning against philosophy (Colossians 2:8), Clement explains that the full statement reveals Paul's true intent: "See to it that no one makes a prey of you by philosophy and empty deceit, according to human tradition, according to the elemental spirits of the universe and not according to Christ" (Clement I, 2 ff.; Baird and Kaufmann 1994, 39). That is, according to Clement, Paul is not denouncing philosophy as such, but rather the return to philosophy by one who has already passed through its elemental, rudimentary, and preparatory counsels. Once having served its preparatory function in the life of the believer, human philosophy can be left behind for the higher knowledge that is given by God. For Clement, then, reason provides access to metaphysical truths.

Tertullian and Clement represent divergent positions on the contributions faith and reason make in accessing theological knowledge. In the middle, so to speak, are Christian thinkers who assign a central role for *both* faith and reason in the provision of truth. Put another way, neither faith nor reason are sufficient to access metaphysical truths. Saint Augustine (354–430) and Saint Thomas Aquinas (1225–74) represent thinkers within the Christian tradition who, although acknowledging the final authority of revelation, theologize with a distinctly intellectual character. Their theologies are classic examples of *fides quaerens intellectum,* "faith in search of understanding."[7]

Aquinas inherited from Greek philosophy an interest in humans as rational beings. According to this tradition, and especially Plato (ca. 428–348 BC) (1992) and Aristotle (ca. 384–322 BC), there is implanted in all humans a natural appetite for knowledge, and it is by virtue of their reason that humans are elevated above all other creatures. Everything has its proper good or end, and the proper end of humans is rational activity. Contemplation and the pursuit of knowledge actualizes, enhances, and perfects essential human nature and happiness. It is clear that Thomas adopts this understanding of humanity when he says, "Among all human pursuits, the pursuit of wisdom is more perfect, more noble, more useful, and more full of joy" (1994a, *Summa Contra Gentiles,* I, 2). More specifically, he derived his doctrine from the Aristotelian conception of reality that came to exert much influence over the entire Thomistic system. God, the highest reality, is purely form or actuality; in Him there is no matter or unrealized potency. This means, in a word, that God is pure intelligence. Now, insofar as man is possessed of intelligence, he partakes in the life of the gods. It behooves us to soar as high as our intellect can take us, thereby realizing and exercising as much as possible the divine element within us.

With respect to Christian truth, Aquinas insists on the necessity of special revelation. Even knowledge about God that lies within reach of natural, unaided reason would, due to the difficulty of the subject and the weaknesses of human nature, be grasped by only a few, and after a long time, and with the admixture of many errors. Indeed, "if the only way open to us for the knowledge of God were solely that of reason, the human race would remain in the blackest shadows of ignorance" (1994a, *Summa Contra Gentiles,* I, 4). If revelation is required for an adequate knowledge of truths that reason can know, how much more is it required for a knowledge of those truths that would otherwise lie forever beyond the reason of all human understanding? Still, though many divine truths utterly exceed our ability to understand (such as the truth of the Trinity), some knowledge of God is yet attainable, however imperfectly, through the natural light of reason (e.g., knowledge of His existence and many of His attributes). In this way, Aquinas offers a twofold notion of truth, requiring both faith and reason for its acquisition.

Now the Christian individual ought, as much as possible, to pursue philosophical knowledge concerning the Divine since, being human, he or she possesses a natural desire and proper inclination to understand what he or she already accepts on faith. Reason is necessary for the clarification and explanation of revealed doctrines, the refutation of opposing and erroneous teachings, and for the apologetic purpose of reasoning with those who do not accept the authority of Scriptures. With respect to the last motivation, Aquinas reminds us that Saint Paul himself (as is recorded in Acts 17:28) documented one of his sermons from a Stoic philosopher, showing that he was willing to meet the pagan thinkers on their own ground (1994a, *Summa Contra Gentiles*, I, 2 ff.; 1994b, *Summa Theologica*, I, Q1, A8).

Aquinas's influence on contemporary Roman Catholic thought is significant. The *Catechism of the Catholic Church* (U.S. Catholic Conference 1994) is considered the encyclopedia of reference for contemporary Roman Catholic believers. With regard to the contribution of faith and reason, the *Catechism* states that "What moves us to believe is not the fact that revealed truths appear as true and intelligible in the light of our natural reason: we believe 'because of the authority of God himself who reveals them, who can neither deceive nor be deceived' (*Dei Filius* 3: DS 3008)" (U.S. Catholic Conference 1994, 42). In other words, faith (as the human reception of revelation) grants knowledge. Yet faith is always in accordance with reason: so "'that the submission of our faith might nevertheless be in accordance with reason, God willed that external proofs of his Revelation should be joined to the internal helps of the Holy Spirit' (*Dei Filius* 3: DS 3009)" (U.S. Catholic Conference 1994, 42). Although faith is in accordance with reason, it is nonetheless "above reason," a position that does not lead to a contradiction, as the following passage indicates: "'Though faith is above reason, there can never be any real discrepancy between faith and reason. Since the same God who reveals mysteries and infuses faith has bestowed the light of reason on the human mind, God cannot deny himself, nor can truth ever contradict truth'" (*Dei Filius* 4: DS 3017). (U.S. Catholic Conference 1994, 43). Applied to the human search for knowledge (e.g., science), the *Catechism* states: properly and morally executed "'methodological research in all branches of knowledge . . . can never conflict with the faith, because the things of the world and the things of faith derive from the same God' (GS 36 SS 1)" (U.S. Catholic Conference 1994, 43). The *Catechism* supports a methodology that relies on both faith and reason to achieve knowledge. Faith and reason are not opposing concepts but rather complementary ones. Such is the legacy of Aquinas and a dominant approach in contemporary Roman Catholic theology, as the majority of authors in this volume illustrate.

SHARED BUT COMPLEX METHODOLOGIES

One of the goals of this volume is to explore the extent to which Roman Catholic theology provides guidelines concerning the allocation of resources to critical care. This entails determining what constitutes a Roman Catholic method or approach, and how the approach can be applied to the problem at hand. The foregoing historical discussion provides a background to compare and contrast Roman Catholic authors in this volume (i.e., Boyle, Heisig, Honnefelder, Kaveny, Schotsmans, Seifert, Taboada, and Wildes). In terms of comparison, one notes that authors (despite suggestions to the contrary; see Heisig) share a commitment to the roles faith and reason play in responding to the problem involving the moral boundaries of allocating scarce resources to critical care from a Roman Catholic perspective. All are committed to Roman Catholic teachings. All develop their positions in discursive style, by means of concepts, language, and argument. That is, all employ reason to persuade themselves and others of the boundaries of the interpretation of Roman Catholic theology on the question of resource allocation to critical care.

Nevertheless, there are significant points of difference between and among authors regarding how Roman Catholicism provides knowledge concerning the moral boundaries of allocating resources to critical care. Differences turn on a number of issues, including (1) what constitutes a distinctively Roman Catholic methodology and (2) how one is to apply the method to the resolution of the problem of resource allocation to critical care. Both issues lead us to reflect on the boundaries of and relation between faith and reason in the acquisition of knowledge.

On Method

Consider what according to our authors constitutes a Roman Catholic methodology that can be used to address the critical care allocation problem. Given that essays are not focused primarily on this topic, authors cannot be expected to develop their views at length. Nevertheless, many do set forth their approach, at times quite explicitly. Upon inspection, one sees that authors line up along a continuum, ranging from those who limit the role reason plays to those who grant reason a significant role in the acquisition of knowledge. From Tertullian to Clement, so to speak, we begin with Heisig, who argues "for an adjustment of the Catholic perspective on technologically intensive medical care" (297). This is a call to employ Catholicism in critique and in light of a "Catholic moral imagination." As he puts it, "if anything qualifies as Catholic, it cannot be simply in virtue of a universal judgment about a particular reality. It requires inclusion of the philosophically neglected category of the specific that necessarily mediates the relation between the universal and the particular" (304). In this way, he calls Catholic thinkers to "question the idea that the foundations of these [medical allocational] guidelines have been deduced from faith or reason." He offers the following alternative response: "Insofar as they [foundations] are of any consequence at all to moral choice, they need to be seen as interpretative paraphrases of faith and reason based on the awareness that violence is being done" (304).

Heisig's call to recapture "Catholic moral imagination" complements Taboada's call to imitate Christ. For Taboada, the Catholic understanding of therapeutic proportionality, when applied to the problem of resource allocation, "must also take into account whether or not the act itself represents a subordination of the person to God's will . . . and an imitation of Christ's example." She continues: "It is only with regard to the existence of higher, transcendental values, which the person is invited to respect, and taking also into account the assistance of the Holy Spirit, that it is possible to judge an action as morally obligatory (proportionate). . . ." (63).

The call by Heisig and Taboada to consider what is grounded in specific expressions of Catholic belief is echoed as well by Schotsmans. He employs a so-called personalist approach, one that is "inspired by the Louvain personalist model, which may be considered identical to the theology of the *Pastoral Constitution on the Church in the Modern World* of the Second Vatican Council" (126). More specifically, "[i]t explains the fundamental and constant aspects or dimensions of persons. . . ." These aspects include "a subject, not an object; a subject in corporeality . . . ; a part of the material word . . . ; essentially directed toward each other . . . ; created in the image of God . . . ; a historical being . . . and also a social being. . . . " (128). The call here is to treat patient as person.

With Schotsmans, Kaveny and Wildes draw from the Roman Catholic tradition a commitment to human dignity and social unity. For Kaveny, the two essential features of the Roman Catholic tradition are: (1) "each human person, embodied and ensouled as a psychosomatic unity, possesses an essential dignity as a being created in the image and likeness of God" and (2) "human persons are essentially social, called not to live in splendid isolation, but to contribute their God-given gifts and talents to the community, even as they draw strength from the gifts and talents of others" (179). Likewise, for Wildes, "basic human dignity is at the heart of the Roman Catholic moral tradition and social teaching. The common good is the set of necessary conditions for the realization of this dignity" (209). Although Taboada and Schotsmans stress the Roman Catholic obligation to respect the person, Kaveny and Wildes focus on the social justice themes (e.g., proportionality, ordinary versus extraordinary, and common good) Roman Catholicism forwards and supports in the development of its tradition.

Boyle, Honnefelder, and Seifert illustrate how the Roman Catholic tradition of natural law assists in thinking through matters of deliberation. As Boyle explains: "My approach takes seriously the teaching of the church, and treats respectfully the methods, reasoning, and consensus of scholars working within the Catholic moral tradition." He continues: "My rationale for such an approach is that like many Catholic moralists, I believe that Catholic moral teaching reveals God's will, and plainly states easily accessible moral truths which, nevertheless, often are obscured or set aside" (78).

With Boyle, Honnefelder and Seifert stand in clear support of reason's role in theological investigation. As Honnefelder puts it, "revelation and the faith based on it do not contain any immediate norms for human action; instead they form the horizon within which reason has to search for those norms." He qualifies: "On the basis of Romans 1:20 (and following) and the philosophical ethics of antiquity, reason is seen as participating in God's law in such a way that reason *as reason* can grasp what is morally required. . . ." He continues: "that grasp of the natural law (*lex naturalis*) is restricted to first principles, i.e., metanorms which are both nonarbitrary and open to active interpretation and thus require concrete elaboration through human law (*lex humana*)" (145).

Similarly, for Seifert, faith is in accordance with reason: "The Catholic Church disagrees profoundly with such a despair of reason and philosophical knowledge as well as with such a radically fideistic position. . . ." Further, it "insists on the validity and universality of rational knowledge and on a rationally knowable, moral, and pre-positive legal 'natural law'. . . ." He qualifies: "this knowledge is clearly recognized, by many Catholic thinkers and magisterial church documents, to be imperfect and threatened in sinful man" (97). Yet, for Seifert, faith is not reducible to reason: "I rather think that all genuine epistemology, axiology, and so on, unites Christians with non-Christians. Christians just know many more things than can be understood through secular reason alone. Indeed, they can know the things known by reason much more deeply" (105).

In short, the Roman Catholic authors in this volume agree that Roman Catholicism provides a method to address issues regarding resource allocation in critical care. Yet they illustrate a range of methods historically employed in Roman Catholicism. These include: commitment to nonviolence, imitation of Christ, respect for the person, social personalism, social justice, and the natural law tradition.

Toward Concreteness: Pitfalls and Possibilities

A second issue that divides authors is the extent to which Roman Catholic theology in its present state grants guidance in questions concerning the allocation of resources in critical care. Upon inspection, we see that authors again line up along a continuum, ranging from the negative to the affirmative.

To begin with, Heisig claims that universal prescriptions regarding the allocation of resources to critical care are not forthcoming. "The attempt to formulate norms to govern the operation of ICUs in the world's hospitals brings into clear relief the problem of grounding Catholic morality on universal principles that transcend culture and institutions" (302). He finds logical and existential objections to forwarding a universal solution to the problem of allocating critical care resources. As he puts it, "every step taken to Catholicize health ends up catholicizing a culture of health that for vast numbers of the human family is still parochial and foreign" (306). In its replacement, Heisig calls for Catholic "specificity," which means that guidelines regarding the allocation of critical care resources will vary between and across cultures, in keeping with their objections to the perpetuation of violence.

Confident of the ability of Roman Catholicism to offer concrete guidance in matters of resource allocation are Kaveny, Wildes, and Seifert. Yet these thinkers agree that additional work is needed in applying Catholic principles to matters of resource allocation. As Kaveny says, "In this essay, I assume that the Roman Catholic tradition's perspective on justice and health care can indeed shed some light on the vexing moral issues involved in the just distribution of intensive care resources." She continues: "I will argue, however, that the tradition needs to be developed in specific ways if it is to have the necessary subtlety to tackle the problem. . . ." (178). Kaveny goes on to develop in detail how the Roman Catholic principle of distribution needs to be supplemented by additional reflections of how intensive care goods are specifically distributed and redistributed. Likewise, for Wildes, the derivation of prescriptions regarding the allocation of critical care resources is possible given further reflections. He calls us to consider "Roman Catholic reflections on taxation, the common good, and social justice" and how they "give guidance to a society in developing and allocating goods in health care" (202).

Seifert similarly calls for further work on thinking through how Roman Catholicism can give guidelines regarding the allocation of critical care resources. As he says, "much further work has to be done to present the general relevant factors for the distinction between good and bad forms of and reasons for limiting access to medical treatment" (115). Nevertheless, Seifert provides an extensive analysis of legitimate and illegitimate forms of resource allocation in health care, indicating his confidence that Roman Catholic theology in its present state can provide important guidance in such matters.

Boyle, Taboada, Honnefelder, and Schotsmans stand in contrast to Kaveny, Wildes, and Seifert in that they see that Catholic theology provides guidance in matters of resource allocation, and this guidance is a matter of careful interpretation of percepts already available. As Boyle puts it, the "combining elements of the traditional moral theology of withholding treatment with the implications of Catholic social teaching concerning social authority and scarcity provide a basis for a systematic analysis of the issues raised by the need to limit the treatment offered to patients." He cautions, however, that "this systematic analysis is not sufficient to generate detailed directives for all who must make decisions in this area; rather it is meant to highlight the considerations relevant for morally assessing the full range of moral issues which decision makers must address" (78).

Likewise, Taboada holds that Roman Catholicism provides the basis for developing specific allocational guidelines. As she says, "the virtue of prudence, understood as practical wisdom trying to discern God's will, plays a key role in disclosing the way in which the different elements involved in therapeutic proportionality have to be weighed in individual situations" (64). Honnefelder also sees practical deliberation performing a central role in applying Roman Catholic theology to concrete problems. As he says, "the concrete moral norms . . . cannot simply be deduced from the framework criteria but must be won in a process of practical deliberation" (145). Likewise, Schotsmans claims that guidelines regarding the allocation of resources in critical care can be derived from Roman Catholic theology. As he says, "in a personalist approach, the promotion of the patient in all his or her dimensions and relationships, adequately considered, is the central dynamic orientation. In the context of critical care, this can be translated in very precise guidelines" (133).

Taken together, these Roman Catholic authors provide a range of responses to the question of whether Catholic moral theology in its present state provides concrete guidance regarding allocating scarce medical resources to critical care. These responses range from reorienting the Catholic moral perspective to voice objection to occurrences of violence (e.g., Heisig) to introducing new considerations into Catholic moral deliberation (e.g., Kaveny, Wildes, and Seifert) to applying Catholic moral theology in its present state to matters of resource allocation (e.g., Boyle, Taboada, Honnefelder, and Schotsmans). Nevertheless, all agree that Catholic moral theology has something to say about the ways in which critical care resources are distributed.

A RESPONSE

The foregoing sets forth a geography of agreement and difference among Roman Catholic authors in this volume regarding the extent to which Roman Catholicism provides guidance regarding the allocation of critical care resources. How does one respond to noted differences?

One way to respond to differences is to lament them, to claim that there is something quite confusing about contemporary Roman Catholicism, in that it cannot decide upon an agreed upon methodology and application to a pressing contemporary dilemma. One could go back in history and blame ancestors for the divisive debates and separations of churches, and church and state, and political structures. One could blame present-day Catholic leaders for their inability to lead, to provide guidance, to discern truth, and to stand up against cultural and political forces. One could attack natural theology for its bankruptcy and join the popular postmodern movement.

This reaction is, I submit, problematic. It presumes that difference is bad and necessarily leads to irreconcilability and chaos. It presumes that anything goes and nothing matters. This position is nondefensible, for both conceptual and practical reasons. Conceptually, relativism is self-defeating, for it undermines taking seriously any position that is offered, including its own. Practically, relativism does not portray how humans actually live their lives. Humans care. They care because they must. They care because they are limited and limited beings must choose between and among options. Most choose what they care about.

Perhaps at this point we can respond to the noted differences among Roman Catholic authors as von Balthasar (1987) does: "a variety of perspectives by no means implies a 'pluralism' of new Testament theologies. 'Pluralism' here is a misleading term because it insinuates that the various theological approaches are irreconcilable with one another" (von Balthasar 1987, 66). They are not irreconcilable. Rather, "they complement each other in tension, as a statue viewed from different angles presents ever new aspects, obviously complementing one another and advancing the viewer's understanding" (von Balthasar 1987, 66).

This is not to suggest that there are no limits in interpretation. For von Balthasar, the inflation of knowledge becomes dangerous "when, ceasing to be concerned about the integrity of the figure (i.e., Jesus Christ), it reproduces itself like a laboratory culture and regards its own hypotheses . . . as equal or even superior to the knowledge of faith" (von Balthasar 1987, 66–67; also see von Balthasar 1980). In this way, von Balthasar calls us to orient our perspective toward Christ and his teachings, a call that is echoed in Taboada's essay.

At this point, then, one might think about the relation between faith and reason as one that is dynamic and "uncovers the inchoate and essentially incomplete character of philosophies and world views" (von Balthasar 1987, 53). In this way, differences are to be expected among Roman Catholic thinkers, and these differences reflect those of earthly existence, human limits on interpretation, expressions of truth, and mysteries of life. The challenge, then, is not to forget what it means to be human (Taboada; Schotsmans), our differences (Heisig), the incompleteness in our analyses (Seifert; Boyle; Honnefelder), and the importance of continued dialogue (Kaveny; Wildes).

CONCLUSION

In thinking about the allocation of resources to critical care from a Roman Catholic perspective, we are confronted with questions concerning what or who provides access to knowledge about how distributions ought to take place. In investigating how authors address the methodological questions, we are presented with differing options. In addressing how one is to respond to this diversity, we are reminded that difference is not bad, but rather a sign of a similar struggle to map a complex terrain of thought and action. We end where we began, with mystery, with mystery that breeds reverence and continued dialogue, as modeled by the authors in this volume.[8]

NOTES

1. For analysis of the resource allocation problem, see Suter (1994), Society of Critical Care Medicine Ethics Committee (1994), Halevy and Brody (1996), and Engelhardt and Khushf (1995).
2. The term "faith" has developed in Catholic theology to designate something rather narrower than it does in the New Testament—a matter that has led to discussions between Protestants and Catholics. When Protestants speak of salvation by faith alone, faith has for them the broad New Testament sense of acceptance of Jesus as Lord and Savior and full self-disclosure of God. This acceptance is a total personal response. When Catholics speak of the theological virtue of faith, they more usually refer to an analysis of what is involved in that total personal response in which the word "faith" stands for one aspect. That aspect is the intellectual or cognitive. By faith in this sense, one opens up one's perception, imagination, and understanding to the truth of God revealing Himself. One allows God's revelation to shape one's vision of reality. One receives this revelation with an

open mind as it is given in the person of Jesus Christ and through the mediation of the church (Hellwig 1981, 161–62).

3. The term "reason" denotes the mind's logical, rational, or discursive activity, which is to be distinguished from sense experience.

4. The goal here is to set up a geographical map of positions, not to advance any novel historical thesis.

5. *Logos* is a Greek word applied to Christ by the writer of the Fourth Gospel (John 1:1 ff.) and understood by Clement to mean "reason," one of its several possible meanings.

6. *Gnosis* is a Greek word meaning "knowledge" that Clement borrowed from the heretical Gnostics, who professed a kind of secret wisdom concerning things divine.

7. The roots of this expression are found in Saint Anselm, "faith seeks understanding" (Prosl. Prooem. PL 153, 225A) (Barth 1960).

8. I am indebted to the Monsignor George Schroeder, Pastor of Holy Name Catholic Church, Steamboat Springs, Colorado, for discussions on these and related matters.

BIBLIOGRAPHY

Aquinas, Thomas, Saint. 1994a. *Summa Contra Gentiles.* In *Medieval Philosophy,* ed. by F. S. Baird and W. Kaufmann. Englewood Cliffs, N.J.: Prentice Hall.

———. 1994b. *Summa Theologia.* In *Medieval Philosophy,* ed. by F. S. Baird and W. Kaufmann. Englewood Cliffs, N.J.: Prentice Hall.

Aristotle. 2000. *Nicomachean Ethics,* trans. by T. Irwin. Indianapolis: Hackett.

Baird, F. S., and W. Kaufmann, eds. 1994. *Medieval Philosophy,* Englewood Cliffs, N.J.: Prentice Hall.

Barth, K. 1960. *Anselm: Faith in Search of Understanding.* Cleveland: World.

Engelhardt, H. T., Jr., and G. Khushf. 1995. Futile care for the critically ill patient. *Current Opinion in Critical Care* 1: 329–33.

Halevy, A., and B. A, Brody. 1996. A multi-institution collaborative policy on medical futility. *Journal of the American Medical Association* 276 (7): 571–74.

Hellwig, M. K. 1981. *Understanding Catholicism.* Saddle River, N.J.: Paulist Press.

Plato. 1992. *The Republic,* trans. by G. M. A. Grube. Indianapolis: Hackett.

Society of Critical Care Medicine Ethics Committee. 1994. Consensus statement on the triage of critically ill patients. *Journal of the American Medical Association* 271 (15): 1200–03.

Suter, P. 1994. Predicting outcome in ICU patients. *Intensive Care Medicine* 20: 390–97.

U.S. Catholic Conference. 1994. *Catechism of the Catholic Church.* New York: William Sadlier.

von Balthasar, H. U. 1980. *Does Jesus Know Us? Do We Know Him?* San Francisco: Ignatius Press.

———. 1987. *Truth Is Symphonic: Aspects of Christian Pluralism.* San Francisco: Ignatius Press.

Contributors

Joseph Boyle, Ph.D., Professor, Department of Philosophy, Saint Michael's College, Toronto, Ontario, Canada.

Mark J. Cherry, Ph.D., Assistant Professor, Department of Philosophy, Saint Edward's University, Austin, Texas.

Mary Ann Gardell Cutter, Ph.D., Associate Professor, Department of Philosophy, University of Colorado at Colorado Springs, Colorado Springs, Colorado.

Teodoro Forcht Dagi, M.D., M.P.H., M.T.S., F.A.C.S., F.C.C.M., Professor, Department of Surgery, the Medical College of Georgia, Atlanta, Georgia.

Corinna Delkeskamp-Hayes, Ph.D., European Programs, International Studies in Philosophy and Medicine, Freigericht, Germany.

H. Tristram Engelhardt, Jr., Ph.D., M.D., Professor, Department of Philosophy, Rice University, Houston, Texas; Professor Emeritus, Baylor College of Medicine, Houston, Texas.

James Heisig, S.V.D., Ph.D., Nanzan Institute for Religion and Culture, Nagoya, Japan.

Ludger Honnefelder, Dr. Phil., Professor, Philosophisches Seminar, Universität Bonn, Bonn, Germany.

Very Reverend Edward Hughes, Saint George Institute, Antiochian Archdiocese, Methuen, Massachusetts.

M. Cathleen Kaveny, J.D., Ph.D., Professor, Department of Law, University of Notre Dame, Notre Dame, Indiana.

George Khushf, Ph.D., Associate Professor, Department of Philosophy, University of South Carolina, Columbia, South Carolina.

Michael A. Rie, M.D., Associate Professor, Department of Anesthesiology, University of Kentucky, College of Medicine, Lexington, Kentucky.

Dietrich Rössler, Dr. Theo., Dr. Med., Ethik-Kommission der Medizinischen Fakultät, Universität Tübingen, Tübingen, Germany.

Paul Schotsmans, Dr. Theo., Professor, Centrum voor Bio-Medische Ethiek en Recht, Universität Leuven, Leuven, Belgium.

Josef Seifert, Ph.D., Professor, Internationale Akademie für Philosophie, Schaan, Liechtenstein.

Paulina Taboada, M.D., M.A., Professor, Department of Internal Medicine, Center for Bioethics, Pontifical Catholic University of Chile, Santiago, Chile.

Kevin W. Wildes, S.J., Ph.D., Associate Professor, Department of Philosophy, Georgetown University, Washington, D.C.

Index

von Nell-Breuning, O., 129
von Planta, M., 54

W
Wagner, D., 93, 160–62
Waltzer, M., 180
war, 284
Ware, K., 242
waste management, 25
Weil, M., 54
welfare, 90, 125, 130, 264
Wetzel, M., 308
Whitehead, A. N., 303

Wiesel, E., 48
Wildes, K., 3, 9, 23–24, 35, 49, 54, 64, 70, 109, 174, 196, 201, 239, 278–79, 281–82, 289–92, 294, 313–18
Wise, S. I. M., 220
withholding health care, 77
Wood, K., 20, 44
World War II, 48

Z
Zander, V., 242
Zoloth, L., ix